T0332724

Lower-Limb Prosthetics and Orthotics

CLINICAL CONCEPTS

Lower-Limb Prosthetics and Orthotics

CLINICAL CONCEPTS

Joan E. Edelstein, MA, PT, FISPO, CPed

Special Lecturer, Columbia University

New York, New York

Alex Moroz, MD, FACP

Director of Residency Training and Medical Education, NYU School of Medicine

Director of Musculoskeletal Unit, Rusk Institute of Rehabilitation Medicine

New York, New York

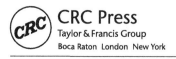

CRC Press

Taylor & Francis Group

Boca Raton London New York

CRC Press is an imprint of the
Taylor & Francis Group, an **informa** business

First published 2011 by SLACK Incorporated

Published 2024 by CRC Press
2385 NW Executive Center Drive, Suite 320, Boca Raton FL 33431

and by CRC Press
4 Park Square, Milton Park, Abingdon, Oxon, OX14 4RN

CRC Press is an imprint of Taylor & Francis Group, LLC

Library of Congress Cataloging-in-Publication Data

Edelstein, Joan E.
  Lower-limb prosthetics and orthotics : clinical concepts / Joan E. Edelstein, Alex Moroz.
    p. ; cm.
  Includes bibliographical references and index.
  ISBN 978-1-55642-896-8 (alk. paper)
  1. Artificial legs. I. Moroz, Alex. II. Title.
  [DNLM: 1. Artificial Limbs. 2. Lower Extremity. 3. Amputation--rehabilitation. 4. Gait. 5. Joint Prosthesis. 6. Orthotic Devices. WE 172 E21L 2011]
  RD756.4.E34 2011
  617.5'8--dc22

                    2010023047

ISBN: 9781556428968 (hbk)
ISBN: 9781003524922 (ebk)

DOI: 10.1201/9781003524922

DEDICATION

For David, Benjamin, and, always, Haskell.
JEE

For my safe harbor: Marina, Ryan, Justin.
AM

CONTENTS

ACKNOWLEDGMENTS

We offer profound thanks to our family and friends for their encouragement and forbearance during the creation of this book. John Bond, Brien Cummings, Debra Toulson, and Alanna Jones of SLACK Incorporated provided unfailingly helpful guidance for realizing our vision. Timothy Evans, CPO; Roger Chin, CPO; Jonathan Glasberg, DPT; and William Goldberg, CPO, generously contributed to the book's illustrations. Our teachers, patients, and colleagues shaped our professional insights, for which we are most grateful. Finally, we acknowledge the contributions of our students and residents whose ongoing challenges inspire us to harmonize the practical with the research aspects of clinical experience.

ABOUT THE AUTHORS

Joan E. Edelstein, MA, PT, FISPO, CPed is a world-renowned authority in prosthetics and orthotics. Beginning clinical practice in the Children's Division of the Institute of Physical Medicine and Rehabilitation, subsequently named the Rusk Institute of Rehabilitation Medicine at New York University, she then joined the faculty of the University of Wisconsin. Returning to New York, she became senior research scientist in New York University's Prosthetics and Orthotics Program, originally part of the College of Engineering, later under the joint aegis of the Department of Orthopedic Surgery in the School of Medicine and the Department of Prosthetics and Orthotics in the School of Education. The program awarded the world's first baccalaureate in prosthetics and orthotics. She conducted research on prostheses and orthoses for the upper and lower limbs, as well as trunk orthoses. Following the closing of the department, she became Associate Professor of Clinical Physical Therapy at the College of Physicians and Surgeons, Columbia University and served as the Director of the Program in Physical Therapy there. Highly regarded for her spirited instruction, she is a special lecturer at Columbia University and adjunct faculty member at New York University, Husson University, Touro College, and Eneslow Pedorthic Institute. Professor Edelstein presents postgraduate and continuing education courses throughout North America, Europe, Africa, Asia, and the Middle East. Her numerous publications include journal articles, book chapters, monographs, and books, particularly *Orthotics: A Comprehensive Clinical Approach* and *Prosthetics and Patient Management: A Comprehensive Clinical Approach*, both published by SLACK Incorporated. A certified pedorthist, Professor Edelstein is a Fellow of the International Society for Prosthetics and Orthotics.

Alex Moroz, MD, FACP, is an experienced educator in the field of disability and medical rehabilitation. Dr. Moroz graduated from Brooklyn College and New York University's School of Medicine, then trained in rehabilitation medicine at the world-renowned Rusk Institute of Rehabilitation Medicine, where he was invited to join its faculty in 2000, and is a full-time Assistant Professor of Rehabilitation Medicine at the School of Medicine, New York University. Prior to focusing on medical education, Dr. Moroz worked at Bellevue Hospital Prosthetic and Orthotic Clinics for several years. He has directed over 30 educational courses for physicians at New York University over the last decade, including 22 courses in prosthetics and orthotics where more than 1700 rehabilitation and orthopedic physicians have benefited from his educational leadership. He has also developed a Lower Extremity Prosthetics and Orthotics course for orthopedic surgery residents. An editor of the textbook *Medical Aspects of Disability*, he is also a contributing editor of *Rehab in Review*. Dr. Moroz has authored numerous peer-reviewed studies published in *Archives of Physical Medicine and Rehabilitation, American Journal of Physical Medicine and Rehabilitation, International Journal of Rehabilitation Research, Topics in Geriatric Rehabilitation,* and *Journal of the American Geriatric Society,* among other periodicals.

CONTRIBUTING AUTHORS

Richard A. Frieden, MD is Medical Director of the Mount Sinai Medical Center Amputation Specialty Program, the first Commission on the Accreditation of Rehabilitation Facilities-accredited program in New York State. He is also an Assistant Professor in the Department of Rehabilitation Medicine at the Mount Sinai School of Medicine. Dr. Frieden directs the Prosthetics and Orthotics Clinic at the Mount Sinai Hospital, where he has been on staff for over 23 years, after completing residency training at the Rusk Institute of Rehabilitation Medicine/New York University. Clinicians in many specialties praise his lectures and publications about the etiologies of amputation, prevention of amputation in people with circulatory compromise and diabetes, functional mobility after amputation, gait deviations, and aging with an amputation. Dr. Frieden has the privilege of caring for people with limb loss in both inpatient and outpatient settings, and continues to pursue excellence in care across the continuum.

Joan T. Gold, MD has been a pediatric physiatrist for over 3 decades. She graduated from New York University with an AB in Chemistry, received her MD from State University of New York Downstate, and trained in Pediatrics and Rehabilitation Medicine at Beth Israel Medical Center and the Rusk Institute of Rehabilitation Medicine, respectively. She is a Clinical Professor of Rehabilitation Medicine at New York University School of Medicine and the Clinical Director of Children's Rehabilitation Services at the Rusk Institute/New York University Langone Medical Center. Her areas of interest include providing care to the limb-deficient child and caring for physically challenged children with a variety of conditions including cerebral palsy, spina bifida, traumatic brain injury, and other diagnoses, all with an emphasis on family-centered care. In addition to her clinical responsibilities, Dr. Gold is a celebrated educator and prolific contributor to the professional literature.

PREFACE

Prostheses and orthoses are integral components in the rehabilitation of many patients, particularly those with musculoskeletal and neuromuscular disorders. Optimum management involves interaction between knowledgeable clinicians, the patient, and the individual's family. *Lower-Limb Prosthetics and Orthotics: Clinical Concepts* provides the basis for prescribing a wide gamut of contemporary appliances. Clinical experience, together with scientific evidence, informs our recommendations for selecting particular devices. We believe that each patient is best served when fitted with a prosthesis or orthosis that facilitates optimum function.

This book is intended as both a text for the student and a reference for the clinician. We assume that the reader understands the biomechanics of normal and pathological gait, as well as anatomical terminology. We begin with a summary of normal gait and then proceed to a detailed exploration of the care of patients with lower-limb amputation, following patients through the early, nonprosthetic, phase of rehabilitation through selection of prosthetic components. Comprehensive presentations of transtibial and transfemoral prostheses include analysis of the biomechanical aspects of prosthetic design, instructions in evaluating prosthetic fit and function, and gait disorders attributable to various departures from established practice. We describe amputations and disarticulations at the foot, as well as knee and hip disarticulations and special considerations for children and those with bilateral amputations. Instruction in gait and activities training is applicable both to the frail elderly patient and the vigorous athlete.

Our strong belief in the concept of lifelong management is reflected in this book. The section on prosthetics concludes with research documenting the functional outcome of people with various levels of amputation caused by many etiologies, wearing a wide range of prostheses.

Orthotic intervention is approached in a similar fashion, beginning with establishing principles of orthotic design, including their purposes, means of increasing the wearer's comfort, advantages and drawbacks of a wide gamut of contemporary materials, and other design considerations. This leads to detailed discussions of foot orthoses through trunk-hip-knee-ankle-foot orthoses, together with instructions for evaluating the fit of the orthosis and the patient's function when wearing it. Ensuring that the orthosis fits and functions properly is essential in order that the patient obtain the maximum benefit. We approach pathological gait analysis from the dual perspectives of physiological and orthotic effects on the patient's style of walking. Because orthotic prescription aims to improve the wearer's function, examination of the functional outcomes achieved by people wearing various types of orthoses can guide the clinician. The section concludes with a detailed discussion of orthotic management of people who have the most common musculoskeletal and neuromuscular disorders. The book concludes with an extended presentation of both prostheses and orthoses for children.

Although the popular media may splash a headline or sound bite extolling the latest development in the field, most patients are better served by more established devices for which scientific evidence exists. Consequently, we present the broad range of prostheses and orthoses, ranging from relatively simple devices to sophisticated computerized models. We hope to inspire broader thinking about clinical management and a deeper understanding of rehabilitation so that patients may achieve the highest level of function and well being.

Chapter 1

Normal Gait

A major purpose of lower-limb prostheses and orthoses is enabling patients to resume or improve their ambulation. Consequently, understanding the key features of normal gait[1-9] is fundamental to prescribing these devices. An increasing number of people who wear prostheses are engaging in sports, many of which incorporate running into the activity. Thus, differences between walking and running deserve exploration.

The gait pattern can be described in terms of the following:

> *Time-distance factors:* Divisions of the gait cycle that can be measured by a chronometer or other timing device and by a measuring tape or similar tool.

> *Kinematics:* The branch of physics concerned with the origin, direction, and extent of motion without regard to the cause of the motion. Watching passersby stroll in a park or observing a patient walk in the clinic are both examples of kinematic analysis. Video cameras are customarily used to record gait kinematics.

> *Kinetics:* The branch of physics concerned with the forces that cause motion. A moment of force, also known as *torque*, refers to force acting at a distance from the center of rotation. Unbalanced moments result in movement. To remain upright, one must balance the external forces by internal forces. The floor (ground) reaction, measured with force plates, is the principal external force. The most important internal force, muscle contraction, is measured with electromyography.

> External forces
>> ¤ Ground reaction force
>> ¤ Inertial forces caused by moving body segments

> Internal forces
>> ¤ Muscles
>> ¤ Tendons
>> ¤ Ligaments
>> ¤ Joint capsules

> Internal forces act on bones, which provide lever arms with joints as the axes.

> Power is the product of all internal moments multiplied by joint angular velocity.

> Generation: Joint moment and joint angular velocity in same direction:
>> ¤ Concentric

> Absorption: Joint moment and joint angular velocity in opposite direction:
>> ¤ Eccentric

TIME-DISTANCE (TEMPORAL-SPATIAL) FACTORS

Walking can be described in terms of the duration of its various aspects and the distance the walker travels.

Gait Cycle

Normal walking is a repetitive, rhythmical, symmetrical activity. The *gait cycle* includes all of the body's activity from the time one foot strikes the floor until the same foot strikes the floor again (Figure 1-1). Gait cycle is synonymous with stride, which can have its duration timed and its distance measured. Nomenclature referring to the subphases of normal gait varies[7]; the most popular terms are those originated in the post-World War II Artificial Limb Program of the National Academy of Science—National Research Council and those developed at Rancho Los Amigos, in Downey, California.[1,9] Consequently, alternate terms for the same episode are juxtaposed.

Edelstein JE, Muroz A.
Lower-Limb Prosthetics and Orthotics: Clinical Concepts (pp 1-10).
© 2011 Taylor & Francis Group.

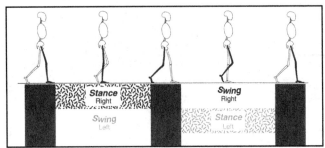

Figure 1-1. Gait cycle. (Reprinted with permission from Perry J, Burnfield JM. *Gait Analysis: Normal and Pathological Function*. 2nd ed. Thorofare, NJ: SLACK Incorporated; 2010.)

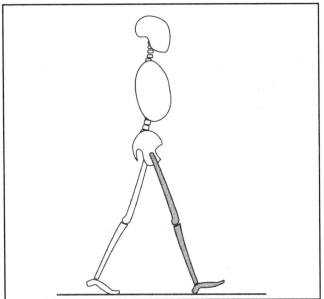

Figure 1-2. Initial contact. (Reprinted with permission from Perry J, Burnfield JM. *Gait Analysis: Normal and Pathological Function*. 2nd ed. Thorofare, NJ: SLACK Incorporated; 2010.)

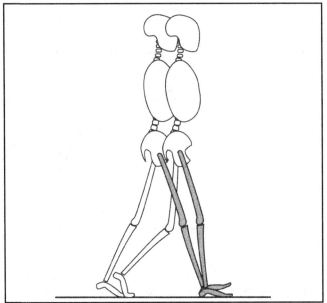

Figure 1-3. Flat foot/loading response. (Reprinted with permission from Perry J, Burnfield JM. *Gait Analysis: Normal and Pathological Function*. 2nd ed. Thorofare, NJ: SLACK Incorporated; 2010.)

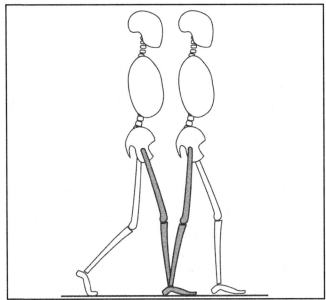

Figure 1-4. Midstance. (Reprinted with permission from Perry J, Burnfield JM. *Gait Analysis: Normal and Pathological Function*. 2nd ed. Thorofare, NJ: SLACK Incorporated; 2010.)

Stance Phase

Stance phase refers to the portion of the gait cycle during which some portion of the reference foot contacts the floor. At comfortable walking speed, stance phase is approximately 60% of the gait cycle.

Heel contact, also known as *heel strike* or *initial contact*, occurs when the heel contacts the floor (Figure 1-2). *Foot flat*, also known as *loading response*, takes place when the entire plantar surface contacts the floor (Figure 1-3). During *midstance* the foot is directly beneath the lower trunk (Figure 1-4). *Heel off*, also known as *the beginning of push-off, propulsion*, or *terminal stance*, occurs when the heel lifts off of the floor (Figure 1-5). *Toe off*, also known as *the end of push-off, propulsion*, or *pre-swing*, is the last part of stance phase when the forefoot lifts off the floor (Figure 1-6).

Swing Phase

Swing phase is that portion of the gait cycle during which no part of the reference foot is in contact with the floor. Normal walking is characterized by having a swing phase that is always briefer in duration than a stance phase.

During *early swing*, also known as *acceleration* or *initial swing*, the leg and foot move forward from behind the trunk (Figure 1-7). *Midswing* occurs when the foot is

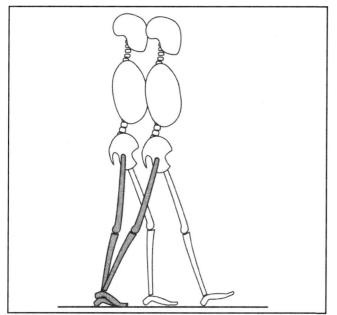

Figure 1-5. Heel-off. (Reprinted with permission from Perry J, Burnfield JM. *Gait Analysis: Normal and Pathological Function.* 2nd ed. Thorofare, NJ: SLACK Incorporated; 2010.)

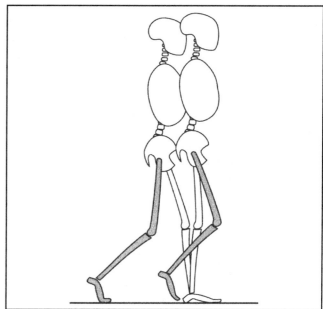

Figure 1-7. Initial swing. (Reprinted with permission from Perry J, Burnfield JM. *Gait Analysis: Normal and Pathological Function.* 2nd ed. Thorofare, NJ: SLACK Incorporated; 2010.)

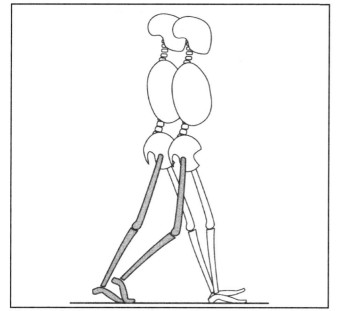

Figure 1-6. Toe-off. (Reprinted with permission from Perry J, Burnfield JM. *Gait Analysis: Normal and Pathological Function.* 2nd ed. Thorofare, NJ: SLACK Incorporated; 2010.)

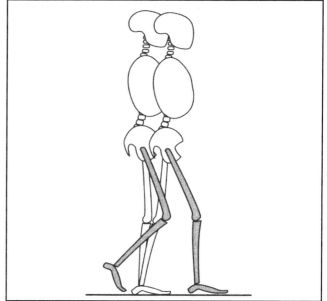

Figure 1-8. Midswing. (Reprinted with permission from Perry J, Burnfield JM. *Gait Analysis: Normal and Pathological Function.* 2nd ed. Thorofare, NJ: SLACK Incorporated; 2010.)

directly beneath the lower trunk (Figure 1-8). *Late swing,* also known as *deceleration* or *terminal swing* is the last part of swing phase and occurs when the leg and foot move ahead of the trunk (Figure 1-9).

Double Support

Normal gait always includes 2 periods of double support during the stance phase when portions of both feet, typically the rear foot on one side and the forefoot on the other side, are contacting the floor simultaneously. The first episode occurs at the start of stance phase on the reference foot, and the second is at late stance on the same foot. At usual walking velocity, double support occurs during approximately 20% of the gait cycle.[10] The slower one walks, the longer the duration of double support.[11]

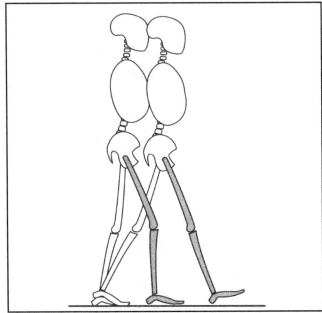

Figure 1-9. Late swing. (Reprinted with permission from Perry J, Burnfield JM. *Gait Analysis: Normal and Pathological Function*. 2nd ed. Thorofare, NJ: SLACK Incorporated; 2010.)

Stride

Stride refers to the entire gait cycle, both in duration and distance. At normal walking speed, the stride duration is approximately 650 ms and is about 1.3 m long.

Step

Each stride is composed of 2 *steps*. A step begins when the reference foot contacts the floor and ends when that foot leaves the floor. During normal walking, the left and right steps are equal in distance and duration (Figure 1-10).

Cadence

The number of steps per measurement of time is referred to as *cadence*. Customarily, cadence is determined by counting the number of steps taken per minute. During normal walking, cadence is approximately 115 steps per minute,[6] varying from approximately 87 to 123 steps per minute for able-bodied walkers.[2]

Velocity

The average walking speed for young and middle-aged adults is 5.4 kph (3.4 mph, 1.5 m/s).[5,10,12] The environment, whether urban or rural, as well as the walker's age, height, and weight, influence velocity. Most walking, however, occurs in brief bouts of less than 30 s.[13]

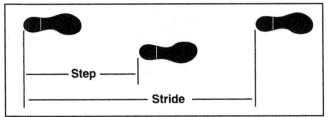

Figure 1-10. Step and stride. (Reprinted with permission from Perry J, Burnfield JM. *Gait Analysis: Normal and Pathological Function*. 2nd ed. Thorofare, NJ: SLACK Incorporated; 2010.)

KINEMATICS

The following discussion refers to an able-bodied young man walking barefoot on a level floor. Angular values represent an average of multiple gait laboratory studies.[1-9]

- ➤ Sagittal metatarsophalangeal joints

Heel contact:	Neutral
Foot flat:	Neutral
Midstance:	Neutral, moving to 20 degrees hyperextension
Heel off:	Hyperextended 30 degrees
Toe off:	Hyperextended 60 degrees
Swing:	Neutral

- ➤ Sagittal ankle[14] (Figure 1-11)

Heel contact:	Neutral
Foot flat:	Plantar flexed 15 degrees
Midstance:	Neutral, moving to dorsiflexion
Heel off:	Dorsiflexed 5 degrees
Toe off:	Plantar flexed 20 degrees
Swing:	Neutral

- ➤ Sagittal knee (Figure 1-12)

Heel contact:	Neutral
Foot flat:	Flexed 15 degrees
Midstance:	Flexed 5 degrees
Heel off:	Flexed 5 degrees
Toe off:	Flexed 30 degrees
Swing:	Flexed 60 degrees

- ➤ Sagittal hip (Figure 1-13)

Heel contact:	Flexed 30 degrees
Foot flat:	Flexed 25 degrees
Midstance:	Neutral
Heel off:	Hyperextended 15 degrees
Toe off:	Neutral
Swing:	Flexed 25 degrees

- ➤ Frontal/transverse foot

Heel contact:	Supinated, then pronated
Foot flat:	Pronated
Midstance:	Supinated
Heel off:	Supinated
Toe off:	Neutral
Swing:	Supinated

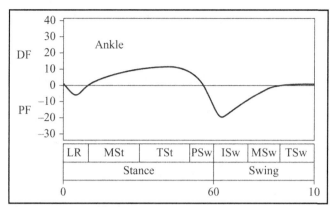

Figure 1-11. Ankle kinematics.

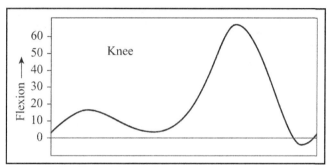

Figure 1-12. Knee kinematics.

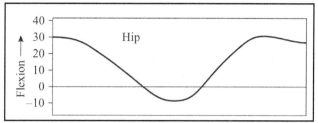

Figure 1-13. Hip kinematics.

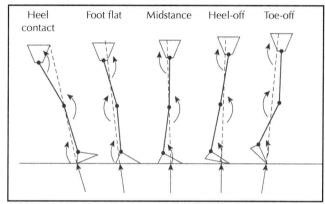

Figure 1-14. Floor reaction throughout stance phase.

➤ Transverse trunk: Trunk rotation lengthens the stride. The pelvis is maximally rotated forward to achieve a longer step length, producing less horizontal velocity.

Heel contact:	Forward rotation
Foot flat:	Forward rotation
Midstance:	Posterior rotation
Heel off:	Posterior rotation
Toe off:	Posterior rotation
Swing:	Forward rotation

Shoulder and elbow flexion and extension occur in the opposite direction to leg motion. Thus, left forward step is accompanied by right shoulder and elbow flexion.

➤ Walking base: The normal walking base is 2 to 4 inches (5 to 10 cm) between the heel centers.[5]

KINETICS

Walking occurs primarily as the result of internal forces, principally muscular contraction, and external forces, especially the floor (ground) reaction. In addition to kinetic factors, other internal influences affecting walking include pain, emotions, restricted range of joint motion, weakness, hypertonicity, vision, hearing, and cardiopulmonary status. Relevant external factors include footwear and other clothing; orthoses; prostheses; assistive devices; terrain contour, surface, and resilience; climate; other people and animals; lighting; and noise.

Floor (Ground) Reaction

"Every action has an equal and opposite reaction." Newton's Third Law of Motion is relevant to understanding walking. As the individual applies body weight to the floor, the floor applies force to the person. This force is the *floor reaction* (*ground reaction force*), which has a vertical component equal to the weight applied to the floor, a horizontal component indicative of the force of forward motion, and a fore and aft component caused by lateral movement of the walker. The result of these components is the floor reaction, which has a profound effect on joint motion and muscular action. For example, at the time of heel contact, the floor reaction passes posterior to the knee. The knee flexes slightly and the quadriceps muscle group contracts strongly to control knee stability (Figure 1-14).

In quiet walking, the floor reaction equals approximately 120% of body weight both in early and in late stance, reflecting the walker's acceleration. Floor reaction declines to about 75% of body weight during midstance.[4,15]

Rapid walking or running increases the floor reaction, confirming Newton's Second Law of Motion; namely, force equals mass times acceleration. Though the walker's mass, measured as body weight, does not change appreciably in a single session, fast walking, with its increased acceleration, magnifies the floor reaction force.

> Ankle and foot[7,9,14-16]

Heel contact:	Posterior floor reaction, eccentric contraction of dorsiflexors
Foot flat:	Minimal floor reaction, minimal dorsiflexion contraction
Midstance:	Anterior floor reaction, eccentric contraction of plantar flexors
Heel off:	Floor reaction anterior to metatarsophalangeal joints Plantar flexor contraction
Toe off:	Floor reaction anterior to metatarsophalangeal joints Toe flexor contraction, followed by dorsiflexor contraction
Swing:	Dorsiflexor contraction throughout swing phase

> Knee[7,9,14]

Heel contact:	Posterior floor reaction, quadriceps contraction
Foot flat:	Minimal floor reaction, minimal quadriceps contraction
Midstance:	Anterior floor reaction, gastrocnemius contraction
Heel off:	Posterior floor reaction, gastrocnemius and hip flexor contraction
Toe off:	Posterior floor reaction, hip flexor contraction
Swing:	Early swing: viscoelastic resistance to knee flexion provided by quadriceps Late swing: hamstrings decelerate knee

> Hip[7,9,14]

Heel contact:	Anterior floor reaction, hip extensor contraction
Foot flat:	Anterior floor reaction, minimal hip extensor contraction
Midstance:	Minimal floor reaction
Heel off:	Posterior floor reaction, hip flexor contraction
Toe off:	Posterior floor reaction, hip flexor contraction
Swing:	Late swing: hamstrings contraction

ENERGY CONSERVATION

Walking is a relatively efficient activity. The average adult consumes approximately $0.8 \text{ kcal} \times 10^{-3}$ per kilogram of body weight per meter walked.[17] Oxygen utilization increases when the person walks slower or faster than the comfortable walking speed. Efficiency results from a smooth transition of body weight through the gait cycle with relatively little wasted effort moving the body. Unlike a wheel, which does not move its center of gravity vertically or laterally, human beings walk on 2 legs jointed at the hips, knees, and ankles. Consequently, the center of gravity, located approximately at the second sacral vertebra, shifts upward and down and side-to-side during each stride. Normally, however, displacement of the center of gravity is minimal. Contrary to previous analysis,[18] the energy cost of walking increases when the vertical movement of the center of gravity decreases because of the greater mechanical work required to control the joints of the lower limb.[19]

Potential energy stored in ligaments and tendons is later released as kinetic energy. Biarticular muscles, including rectus femoris, hamstrings, and gastrocnemius, transfer energy from one body segment to another. Pelvic motion maximizes acceleration of the body's center of gravity in early stance. The pelvis acts as a pivot so that rotation of the lower limb is balanced by rotation of the shoulders and arms. As the shoulder rotates forward, the lower limb rotates posteriorly. Effective interchange between kinetic energy and gravitational potential energy facilitates effective use of the mechanical energy supplied by muscles.

Though the amount of oxygen required for an able-bodied or a disabled person to walk a given period of time is similar, marked differences exist when oxygen consumption is related to walking velocity. Someone with a disability compensates by walking slower and thus covering less distance in a given time period. Oxygen consumption per unit time and per unit distance is greater in a disabled person than in a normal person who is walking at the same speed.[17]

Vertical Displacement of the Center of Gravity

Vertical displacement of the center of gravity normally follows a sinusoidal curve, which peaks at 5 cm at midstance and midswing and is lowest at early and late stance phase.[11,20,21]

Factors limiting vertical displacement[18]:

> Foot roll-over shape
> Step length
> Pelvic rotation
> Plantar flexion

Pelvic obliquity and knee flexion during stance phase serve primarily to absorb shock, rather than modify the center of gravity excursion.

Lateral Displacement of the Center of Gravity

Lateral displacement also follows a sinusoidal curve, which reaches its extreme point at 5 cm at midstance on the left side and 5 cm at midstance on the right side.

Factors limiting vertical displacement:
> Hip adduction
> Lateral pelvic shift

OTHER AMBULATORY CONSIDERATIONS

Age

The 9-month-old usually cruises, shifting weight from one foot to the other, while supporting the body with the hands on furniture. Weight is usually borne on the forefeet. Goal-directed ambulation begins at approximately 10 months.[22] Clambering up stairs and low chairs demonstrates the child's ability to flex the hips independently and use the upper limbs for assistance. Transition from crawling and cruising to walking usually occurs at 11 months. Early walking is characterized by shoulder abduction, hip abduction, knee flexion, and initial contact with the entire plantar surface.[23] Cadence is rapid; however, short steps cause velocity to be slow. The new walker steps diagonally forward and sideward, which widens the walking base. Independent walking is flat-footed with considerable trunk waddling. Lateral trunk bending also serves to advance the leg. The beginning walker is somewhat top heavy. The center of gravity is closer to the xiphoid process than to the sacrum, necessitating holding the arms in "high guard" to aid stability; consequently, carrying a toy is difficult at this age. Collapse into a fall is common, but the child is proficient at resuming upright balance. The early walker takes short steps and keeps the trunk and limbs stiffly extended.

At 18 to 20 months of age, the toddler relinquishes high guarding and parental hand support, and with less shoulder abduction for balance becomes able to carry a toy while walking. Initial contact matures to heel loading. The base is narrower as hip abduction reduces. Cadence diminishes as steps increase length, resulting in a more rapid walking speed.[6,24-26]

Mature gait occurs at 7 years of age, although the child, being shorter than an adult, still has a greater cadence, shorter steps, and thus slower walking velocity.

Age-related changes are reflected in elder gait, particularly more cautious balance control and reduction in joint range. Steps are shorter, speed is slower, and propulsion is less forceful. Hip excursion, both flexion and hyperextension, diminishes. Knee flexion in stance phase increases but decreases during swing phase. Heel contact is present but flatter than with younger people. Toe-out is greater, as is the walking base. The range of plantar flexion is less than for younger adults. Energy consumption is greater.[27-33]

Women

Subtle differences distinguish the walking pattern of healthy women from that of men.[32] With adults of the same height, women demonstrate a greater cadence than men.[34,35] Women use more hip flexion and less knee extension before heel contact. In late stance, the knee flexes more acutely.[36] Muscle activity, particularly gluteus maximus, also differs slightly.[37] Hip internal rotation and adduction are greater in women.[36]

Footwear

The type of shoes worn by the walker has a profound effect on gait. High heels restrict the range of ankle dorsiflexion and active plantar flexion; consequently, propulsion is diminished, as is step length and walking velocity. These shoes also maintain the metatarsophalangeal joints in maximum hyperextension, further limiting propulsion. Knee flexion occurs much sooner than when walking in low-heeled shoes.[38-40]

Slippery, firm soles reduce traction during stance phase, impeding the individual's ability to control the horizontal component of the floor reaction. Uncontrolled forward movement is *skidding*, which can lead to a fall. Firm soles do not absorb the shock caused by the vertical component of the floor reaction. Consequently, greater-than-normal stress is transmitted to the joints of the lower limbs and trunk.

Stiff boots hinder ankle motion, particularly dorsiflexion. Steps tend to be shorter and negotiating steep ramps more difficult.

Ramps

> Forward ramp
  ¤ Ascending requires greater dorsiflexion.
  ¤ Descending demonstrates greater ankle dorsiflexion and plantar flexion and knee flexion range. Steps are shorter. More gastrocnemius and quadriceps contraction is needed.
> Side-banked ramp
  ¤ The uphill lower limb shows greater hip adduction and foot inversion, whereas the downhill lower limb has more hip abduction and foot eversion.

Stairs

Ascending requires greater dorsiflexion, knee flexion, and hip flexion range, as well as more prolonged quadriceps and hip extensor contraction as the climber pulls the body up from one step to the next.

Stair descent also places a high demand on the quadriceps and hip extensors to prevent inadvertent collapse as the individual lowers his or her body weight. The foot remains in plantar flexion during swing phase with gastrocnemius contraction throughout. Reliance on one or bilateral handrails reduces the muscular demand on both ascent and descent. Conversely, the higher the stair, the greater the effort needed to climb.[41-44]

REFERENCES

1. Perry J, Burnfield JM. *Gait Analysis: Normal and Pathological Function.* 2nd ed. Thorofare, NJ: SLACK Incorporated; 2010.

2. Craik RL, Oatis CA. *Gait Analysis: Theory and Application.* St. Louis, MO: Mosby; 1995.

3. Kerrigan DC, Edelstein JE. Gait. In: Gonzalez E, Myers S, Edelstein JE, et al, eds. *Downey and Darling's Physiological Basis of Rehabilitation Medicine.* 3rd ed. Boston, MA: Butterworth-Heinemann; 2001:397-416.

4. Kirtley C. *Clinical Gait Analysis: Theory and Practice.* Oxford, UK: Churchill Livingstone; 2006.

5. Ayyappa E, Mohamed O. Clinical assessment of pathological gait. In: Lusardi MM, Nielsen CC, eds. *Orthotics and Prosthetics in Rehabilitation.* 2nd ed. St. Louis, MO: Saunders; 2007:41-68.

6. Whittle MW. *Gait Analysis: An Introduction.* 4th ed. Oxford, UK: Butterworth Heinemann; 2007.

7. Norkin CC. Examination of gait. In: O'Sullivan SB, Schmitz TJ, eds. *Physical Rehabilitation.* 5th ed. Philadelphia, PA: F.A. Davis; 2007:317-372.

8. Wellmon R. Gait assessment and training. In: Cameron MH, Monroe LG, eds. *Physical Rehabilitation: Evidence-Based Examination, Evaluation, and Intervention.* St. Louis, MO: Saunders; 2007:844-876.

9. Perry J. Normal and pathological gait. In: Hsu JD, Michael JW, Fisk JR, eds. *AAOS Atlas of Orthoses and Assistive Devices.* 4th ed. Philadelphia, PA: Mosby; 2008:71-80.

10. Auvinet B, Berrut G, Touzard C, et al. Reference data for normal subjects obtained with an accelerometric device. *Gait Posture.* 2002;16:124-134.

11. Murray MP. Gait as a total pattern of movement. *Am J Phys Med.* 1967;46:290-333.

12. Vaughn CL, O'Malley MJ. Froude and the contribution of naval architecture to our understanding of bipedal locomotion. *Gait Posture.* 2005;21:350-362.

13. Orendorff MS, Schoen JA, Bernatz GC, et al. How humans walk: bout duration, steps per bout, and rest duration. *J Rehabil Res Dev.* 2008;45:1077-1090.

14. Malanga G, DeLisa JA. Clinical observation. In: DeLisa JA, ed. *Gait Analysis in the Science of Rehabilitation.* Baltimore, MD: Department of Veterans Affairs; 1998:1-10.

15. Soutas-Little RW. Motion analysis and biomechanics. In: DeLisa JA, ed. *Gait Analysis in the Science of Rehabilitation.* Baltimore, MD: Department of Veterans Affairs; 1998:49-68.

16. Jenkyn TR, Anas K, Nichol A. Foot segment kinematics during normal walking using a multisegment model of the foot and ankle complex. *J Biomech Eng.* 2009;131:034504.

17. Gonzalez E, Edelstein JE. Energy expenditure during ambulation. In: Gonzalez E, Myers S, Edelstein JE, et al, eds. *Downey and Darling's Physiological Basis of Rehabilitation Medicine.* 3rd ed. Boston, MA: Butterworth-Heinemann; 2001:417-447.

18. Saunders JB, Inman VT, Eberhart HD. The major determinants in normal and pathological gait. *J Bone Joint Surg.* 1953;35A:543-558.

19. Gordon KE, Ferris DP, Kuo AD. Metabolic and mechanical energy costs of reducing vertical center of mass movement during gait. *Arch Phys Med Rehabil.* 2009;90:136-144.

20. Murray MP, Drought AB, Kory RD. Walking patterns of normal men. *J Bone Joint Surg.* 1964;46A:335-360.

21. Gard SA, Childress DS. What determines the vertical displacement of the body during normal walking? *J Prosthet Orthot.* 2001;13:64-67.

22. Ivanenko YP, Dominici N, Cappellini G, Lacquaniti F. Kinematics in newly walking toddlers does not depend upon postural stability. *J Neurophysiol.* 2005;94:754-763.

23. Kubo M, Ulrich BD. Early stages of walking: development of control in mediolateral and anteroposterior directions. *J Mot Behav.* 2006;38:229-237.

24. Sutherland DH, Olshen R, Cooper L, Woo SL-Y. The development of mature gait. *J Bone Joint Surg Am.* 1980;62:336-353.

25. Keen M. Early development and attainment of normal mature gait. *J Prosthet Orthot.* 1993;5:35-38.

26. Ganley KJ, Powers CM. Gait kinematics and kinetics of 7-year-old children: a comparison to adults using age-specific anthropometric data. *Gait Posture.* 2005;21:141-145.

27. Knoblauch RL, Pietrucha MT, Nitzburg M. Field studies of pedestrian walking speed and start-up time. *Transportation Res Rec.* 1996;1538:27-38.

28. Baloh RW, Ying SH, Jacobson KM. A longitudinal study of gait and balance dysfunction in normal older people. *Arch Neurol.* 2003;60:835-839.

29. Boyer KA, Beaupre GS, Andriacchi TP. Gender differences exist in the hip joint moments of healthy older walkers. *J Biomech.* 2008;41:3360-3365.

30. Prince F, Corriveau H, Hebert R, Winter DA. Gait in the elderly. *Gait Posture.* 1997;5:128-135.

31. Langhammer B, Lindmark B. Performance-related values for gait velocity, timed up-and-go and functional reach in healthy older people and institutionalized geriatric patients. *Phys Occup Ther Geriatr.* 2007;25:55-59.

32. Steffen TM, Hacker TA, Mollinger L. Age- and gender-related test performance in community-dwelling elderly people: six-minute walk test, Berg Balance Scale, timed up & go test, and gait speeds. *Phys Ther.* 2002;82:128-137.

33. Hernandez A, Silder A, Heiderscheit BC, Thelen DG. Effect of age on center of mass motion during human walking. *Gait Posture.* 2009;30:217-222.

34. Murray MP, Kory RC, Sepic SB. Walking patterns of normal women. *Arch Phys Med Rehabil.* 1970;51:637-650.

35. Blanc Y, Balmer C, Landis T, Vingerhoets F. Temporal parameters and patterns of the foot roll over during walking: normative data for healthy adults. *Gait Posture.* 1999;10:97-108.

36. Kerrigan DC, Todd MKL, Della Croce U. Gender differences in joint biomechanics during walking: normative study in young adults. *Am J Phys Med.* 1998;77:2-7.

37. Anders C, Wagner H, Puta C, et al. Healthy humans use sex-specific co-ordination patterns of trunk muscles during gait. *Eur J Appl Physiol.* 2009;105:585-594.

38. Wall-Scheffler C, Heiderscheit BC. Gender differences in walking and running on level and inclined surfaces. *Clin Biomech (Bristol, Avon).* 2008;23:1260-1268.

39. Hong WH, Lee YH, Chen HC, et al. Influence of heel height and shoe insert on comfort perception and biomechanical performance of young female adults during walking. *Foot Ankle Int.* 2005;26:1042-1048.

40. Yung-Hui L, Wei-Hsien H. Effects of shoe inserts and heel height on foot pressure, impact force, and perceived comfort during walking. *Appl Ergon.* 2005;36:355-362.

41. Wang YT, Pascoe DD, Kim CK, Xu D. Force patterns of heel strike and toe off on different heel heights in normal walking. *Foot Ankle Int.* 2001;22:486-492.

42. Shiomi T. Effects of different patterns of stair climbing on physiological cost and motor efficiency. *J Hum Ergol (Tokyo).* 1994;23:111-120.

43. Beaulieu FG, Pelland L, Robertson DG. Kinetic analysis of forwards and backwards stair descent. *Gait Posture.* 2008;27:564-571.

44. Stacoff A, Diezi C, Luder G, et al Ground reaction forces on stairs: effects of stair inclination and age. *Gait Posture.* 2005;21:24-38.

Chapter 2

Early Management

Richard A. Frieden, MD

THE CONTINUUM OF CARE

Amputation of the lower limb should be part of a continuum of care for the patient with a threatened leg. In the case of peripheral arterial disease (the major cause of limb loss, often in association with diabetes mellitus), the continuum begins with patient and caregiver education in risk factor modification, such as meticulous care of the feet, smoking cessation, and diabetes control, as well as screening efforts in the office. Medical and rehabilitative procedures are the next steps in the process, usually within a hospital setting. Surgical revascularization may occur farther along the pathway. Amputation then leads to postoperative care and rehabilitation to restore maximum function.[1] Care continues in the community, either at an outpatient facility or at home.

The decision to amputate a limb is based primarily upon the need to remove diseased tissue at a level that will heal most rapidly and permit fastest return of the patient to optimal health and function.[2] In this context, pain, disability, and cost of multiple revascularization attempts must be weighed against the impact of amputation and prosthetic rehabilitation.

PREOPERATIVE EVALUATION

The first principle of amputation rehabilitation is the potential involvement of the physiatrist before amputation. The specialist in physical medicine and rehabilitation can predict function, advise the surgeons, and interact with the patient and family as well as other members of the rehabilitation team. In addition, the physiatrist can initiate discharge planning, resulting in a shorter hospital stay and a faster rehabilitation course. One should start thinking about setting goals for future function at the first patient encounter.

When interviewing and examining a patient who may potentially require lower-limb amputation, the physician should consider the following.

General Health and the Presence of Comorbidities

Any person's ability to participate in a rehabilitation program depends primarily upon the individual's general health. The presence of comorbidities should be noted, especially whether these conditions are likely to be controlled at the time of surgery. Cardiovascular and cerebrovascular disorders, diabetes, and hypertension must be managed because they impact negatively upon all phases of rehabilitation, including energy expenditure. Diabetes can lead to visual loss due to retinopathy and loss of proprioception due to peripheral neuropathy. Sensory loss in the residual and the intact limbs hampers prosthetic use. Nutrition and hydration are also important to assess.

Functional Status

Knowledge of the patient's functional status prior to the development of the need for amputation is based upon the patient's and the caregiver's input. It is also important to assess whether amputation and prosthetic replacement will improve the person's functional status. The patient's goals must be clarified so that discussion can occur before surgery as to the potential extent of functional restoration.

Socioeconomics and Support System

Socioeconomic status and access to a support system have considerable impact upon the patient's ability to pursue postamputation rehabilitation.

Edelstein JE, Muroz A.
Lower-Limb Prosthetics and Orthotics: Clinical Concepts (pp 11-18).
© 2011 Taylor & Francis Group.

Psychological Preparation

Motivation to proceed with amputation and rehabilitation must be assessed before surgery. For many people, limb loss means a combination of altered self-image, grief over both the lost limb and the anticipated loss of function, and fear of how their community will react to their altered situation.[3-5] The family's reaction should be gauged as well; group counseling may be beneficial. Some people look ahead to prosthetic fitting as a "restoration" of social status as well as functional status. As such, discussion of the process of acquiring a prosthesis may arise early in the preoperative phase.

Condition of Other Leg

The contralateral leg must be assessed preoperatively, due to its critical importance as the major single-stance support. It is imperative to understand its neurological and vascular status. If it has been weakened by stroke, other neuropathy, or prior injury or surgery, then it will be less able to support body weight for transfers and self-care, both before and after prosthesis use. Compromised circulation, as evidenced by dependent rubor, skin atrophy or ulceration, delayed venous filling, intermittent claudication, and hair loss with or without nail hypertrophy, has a negative impact on future function. Skin condition, joint range of motion, muscle strength, and sensation must also be assessed.

Surgical Considerations

The principles of lower-limb amputation start with the removal of diseased tissue, allowing for the best healing opportunity, and fashioning of a good weight-bearing structure that will tolerate a prosthesis with minimal difficulty.[6,7]

Historically, determining the level of amputation depended upon clinical examination, noting skin and muscle condition, presence of ischemia with or without infection, and the presence or absence of pulses. This information was used by the surgeon to predict the best site of incision and shape of muscle flaps for coverage of the amputation site.

Currently, various laboratory tests assist in the decision-making process. These include the ankle-brachial index, pulse-volume recordings, assessment of segmental pressures, transcutaneous oxygen partial pressure measurement, radioisotope clearance from the skin, Doppler by both ultrasound and laser light, and thermography. Angiography remains the "gold standard" to determine circulation.

Of course, the ultimate decision on the level of amputation is made by the surgeon when the patient is "on the table." Assessment of the condition of the tissues, particularly the presence and quality of bleeding, are among the most pertinent signs observed during the procedure. Surgeons who regard amputation as a "failure" of treatment may leave its performance to junior members of the team. The best chance of healing and retaining a well-shaped residual limb is in the hands of the more experienced surgeons. Consequently, it is most appropriate that higher levels of training and expertise are brought to bear upon amputation surgery.

POSTOPERATIVE EVALUATION

If the rehabilitation physician meets the patient for the first time after amputation surgery, the issues discussed earlier as part of the preoperative assessment need to be addressed. Historical elements to be reviewed include premorbid functional status and the presence and management of comorbidities. The most relevant physical examination issues include assessment of the patient's general condition and that of the remaining leg and residual limb.

As part of the examination, recognize the signs of good circulation in the residual limb, including good capillary refill on *both* sides of the surgical wound. The limb must be checked for the qualities that promote prosthetic use (eg, full range of motion in all joints, a shape that will provide maximal contact area within the socket, nonadherent scars, sufficient length of bony lever arm, intact sensation, maximal muscle power, firm musculature, and full-thickness skin). If the desired shape was not obtained by surgery, the shape of the residual limb can be modified later by postoperative dressings. A transtibial residual limb is more likely than a transfemoral limb to have adherent scars and other lesions. Firm musculature will decrease shifting and thereby resist shear forces caused by the socket. If a bony lever arm of sufficient length is not provided, power must be supplied by the next proximal joint, and energy expenditure will rise. For example, the patient with a very short transtibial residual limb will have to supplement knee power with hip force. Inspection and palpation will enable the clinician to assess the amount of edema and the condition of the healing wound, including skin temperature and the presence of any drainage. If the posterior flap of the transtibial limb is sagging, this suggests that underlying muscle layers are not well approximated.

Psychological aspects include how the patient copes with limb loss, the alteration in body image, and expectations for the future. One means of helping the patient and family deal with the changed circumstances is through education. Clinicians need to clarify terminology unique to rehabilitation and prosthetics, which can be confusing to laypeople, and explain the planned program of rehabilitation. Another means of assisting family members in dealing with the situation is by asking them to take an active role in the rehabilitation process. For example, they could assist the occupational therapist in assessing the patient's learning ability. Visual cues and other forms of sensory feedback can be taught to the relatives in order to assist with the patient's learning. The family can also facilitate the patient's transition from the hospital back to the home. Increasing the safety of the home environment should be detailed prior to the patient's discharge from the hospital.

POSTOPERATIVE CARE OF THE AMPUTATION LIMB

Dressings

Approaches to initial wrapping of the postoperative residual limb include soft elastic dressings, semirigid Unna dressings or air splints, and rigid plaster dressings. Rigid dressings were developed to control swelling and edema and to resist the development of knee flexion contractures after transtibial amputation. Semirigid dressings were designed to control edema and provide ease of removal, so that the wound could be checked periodically.

The immediate postoperative prosthesis (IPOP) and the rigid removable dressing (RRD) allow for rapid remobilization of patients, lessening the need for analgesics and reducing the length of hospital stay.

IPOP fitting usually consists of wrapping the residual limb with plaster over a thin wound covering and a snugly-fitting limb sock, forming a rigid dressing, then applying a pylon with a foot. The rigid dressing reduces swelling, allays patient anxiety about limb loss, and permits earlier ambulation. It requires accurate application after surgery, ideally by a prosthetist in the operating room; training the on-call surgical residents in removal and reapplication if needed; and a high degree of compliance on the part of the patient, who must be monitored to make certain that the suspension belt or harness is sufficiently taut and that he or she adheres to weight-bearing restrictions.

The RRD protects the suture line yet allows for easy inspection. It can hasten limb volume stabilization and shaping without weight bearing and can be more easily reapplied.

Other options for postoperative dressings include the Unna semirigid dressing and an air splint. Both are easier to apply and remove than plaster dressings and have demonstrated ability to control edema and foster healing. Unna dressings adhere to the skin and are removed with bandage scissors. The commercially available air splint is zipped around the limb and then inflated.

Wound Care

Surgeons vary as to their preference for the frequency of wound monitoring. If the site was clean at the time of surgery, it may be acceptable to change the dressings every 3 to 5 days. If the site looked as if it were at risk of not healing or may have been infected, then it might be checked daily.

Signs of poor circulation in the residual limb include mottling, cool areas, excessive eschar, and delayed healing. After the wound has closed sufficiently, the limb may be placed in the whirlpool to loosen the eschar. Prolonged immersion in warm water, however, promotes development of edema. Increased eschar with or without cool surrounding tissue suggests that circulation is threatened. If the skin edges undergo necrosis, the suture line may be too tight or the circulation to the area may be otherwise compromised, with the risk of wound dehiscence. The presence and quality of the femoral pulse correlate with the healing potential of a transfemoral limb.

Signs of infection include unusual warmth and erythema and excessive serous or purulent drainage from the wound. A large hematoma, a retained suture, or infected bypass graft material can serve as the culture medium. The surgeon may have to open and drain the wound and then pack it.

Barring any of these problems, wound healing should occur within 3 weeks after a traumatic amputation and 4 to 6 weeks after a dysvascular amputation.

Maintaining or Improving Strength and Joint Range

In the transtibial residual limb, a long posterior flap usually results in less tension on the suture line and better muscular and subcutaneous padding over the bone ends. If the posterior flap appears to be pulling downward against the wound, with the risk of dehiscence, a posterior cast or splint can help keep the flap in place, remove tension from the surgical wound, and decrease pain.

A posterior splint also helps prevent flexion contracture of the knee, especially for those patients who are in more pain than can be controlled with analgesics. While using the splint, patients can start early exercises to counteract involuntary "protective" knee flexion. Patients are encouraged to exercise the residual limb, avoid placing pillows under either limb when in bed, lie prone for 20 to 30 minutes several times each day, avoid resting the residual limb on the hand grip of an axillary or forearm crutch, avoid excessively tight wrappings that might pull the limb into flexion, and not spend excessive time in a wheelchair. They must learn to point the limb toward the ground when standing. These measures help prevent flexion contractures of the hip and knee. The patient with a transtibial amputation should have a padded, elevated leg rest on the wheelchair to support the residual limb in the extended position.

Typical transfemoral contractures are hip flexion, abduction, and external rotation. This happens because the hip flexors and abductors are spared, whereas hip extensors and adductors are compromised by amputation. Adductor magnus and then adductor longus are sacrificed as the amputation level proceeds proximally.

Stretching exercises in the acute postoperative phase are usually not warranted. It is more important to encourage relaxation of the limb and to provide adequate pain relief to reduce the urge to draw the limb into flexion. Exercises to prevent joint contractures can start as soon as pain control is established, as can strengthening of the arms, trunk, and the intact lower limb. Strengthening the muscles in the residual limb may be delayed until sutures are removed.

Desensitization and Hygiene

Residual limb conditioning is vital to successful use of a prosthesis. To encourage tissue firmness, the patient and caregivers should knead soft tissues. For better skin mobility, massage the affected areas with cocoa butter, avoiding contact with the fresh surgical wound. Tapping and stroking the residual limb reduce hypersensitivity. Residual limb hygiene is a problem if the patient is reluctant to handle the limb. Regular cleaning and inspection are essential, especially in warm climates. The residual limb should be washed with soap and water every night. After the prosthesis is fitted, the socket should be cleaned nightly, and clean socks should be laid out for the next day's use.

Preparation for the Prosthesis

When cleared by the surgical team, the patient may be taught to wrap the residual limb with elastic bandages or apply an elastic shrinker. A 4-inch-wide bandage suffices for a transtibial limb and a 6-inch-wide bandage for a transfemoral limb. Many patients learn to bandage their transtibial limb; however, secure bandaging of a transfemoral limb requires the assistance of another person (ie, a clinician or a family member). If the bandage slips off, an elastic shrinker sock may be worn. A garter belt is needed to reduce the likelihood of having the shrinker slide down. A reasonable routine is to rewrap the limb every 4 hours while awake and to leave the wrapping off for a maximum of 10 to 15 minutes while bathing. A layered cotton stockinet provides graduated pressure and accelerates shrinking while eliminating skin abrasion that may otherwise arise along the anterior tibial surface due to motion of the edges of elastic bandage wrapping.

Postoperative Complications

Patients are at risk for renal insufficiency, atelectasis, pneumonia, and thromboembolism. One must be careful with hydration and aggressive with treatment of infection[8] and remobilization.

Surgical and Phantom Pain and Phantom Sensation

Phantom sensation is an almost universal phenomenon that causes much consternation, whether or not the patient has been warned about it. Not only is the sense of a retained limb present, but the shape or position of the phantom may be altered. The phantom limb is thought to be based upon the sensory homunculus in the brain. Even a feeling of "presence" is a hazard if the patient attempts to walk during the night and forgets about the amputation.

At some time in their postamputation experience, one-third to one-half of patients report phantom pain. Four types of phantom pain are (1) cramping sensations that resemble muscle spasms, (2) tingling or shock-like sensations that are often accompanied by rhythmic jerking motions of the residual limb, (3) squeezing or wrenching sensations, and (4) burning or lancinating pain. Most disturbing is the diffuse burning or lancinating pain that radiates proximally from the "foot" or the "toes." This type, which is severe in approximately 5% of patients, tends to be more intense for those who had painful limbs prior to amputation.

The pain experience for each person is unique. First, patients hope for relief of the preoperative pain they experienced in the ischemic, necrotic, or ulcerated leg. Next, they often have to contend with intense postsurgical pain, which fortunately usually subsides in a few days. One should never dismiss complaints of pain as being a phantom. Only after ruling out local residual limb problems should you consider the possibility of phantom limb pain. Differentiate between referred pain, the local residual limb pain from surgery and neuromas, and phantom pain and then treat them accordingly. A residual limb can experience both intermittent claudication and referred pain from a lumbar radiculopathy.[9]

The first step in dealing with the phantom limb and the phantom pain is to acknowledge that these are real, not imagined, sensations. Patients need to know that pain will fade with time. Some people report that the phantom "retracts" or gets shorter.

Frequent handling of the residual limb for inspection, massage, and desensitization is helpful. Patients can exercise the muscles of the limb by imaginary movements of the phantom (often using a mirror image of the sound limb). Using a prosthesis helps to decrease the phantom presence. Other treatments include analgesic injections, acupuncture, topical capsaicin, transcutaneous and other forms of electrical nerve stimulation, nerve blocks, and nerve severance. Oral medications, such as neuroleptics, beta blockers, and anticonvulsants, have variable success. Epidural anesthesia for several days before surgery may dampen the injury and pain response by the neural network. Psychological techniques attempt to modify stress, depression, and anxiety, which can exacerbate painful sensations. The clinician needs to help separate the experience of pain from the experience of using a prosthetic limb.[10] None of these methods, however, is totally successful.

PRINCIPLES OF INPATIENT REHABILITATION

Both physical therapy and occupational therapy are important parts of a prosthetic rehabilitation program. Ideally, people who have the medical stability, energy reserves, and motivation should be admitted to an inpatient rehabilitation unit to participate in the full multidisciplinary program. The initial postoperative phase includes 24-hour nursing care and daily physician visits, with periodic monitoring of laboratory tests and vital signs. This is important due to the possible existence of comorbidities. The stress of increased physical effort can change blood pressure readings, insulin requirements, and other parameters. Receiving rehabilitation in the acute postoperative phase is associated with a higher possibility of 1-year survival and home discharge from the hospital,[11] as well as the greater likelihood of acquiring a prosthesis and fewer subsequent amputations.[12]

The Role of Physical Therapy

Patients attending physical therapy should start with passive range of motion, leading to active-assisted and then resistive exercises. Next, they learn mobility and strengthening skills. Exercise of crutch muscles, particularly shoulder depressors and the elbow extensors (eg, pectoralis minor and major, serratus anterior, lower trapezius, latissimus dorsi, rhomboids, and triceps), as well as wrist extensors and finger flexors, is important for use of assistive devices and transferring from one chair to another.

Exercising the remaining limb is vital for single-support activities. Hip extensors must be strengthened to help stabilize a transfemoral prosthesis. The patient with transtibial amputation must strengthen the knee extensors to control the prosthesis.

The physical therapist checks for range of motion of the hip and knee joints bilaterally. Residual limb handling and hygiene are addressed. After the prosthesis is delivered, the physical therapist teaches the patient to don and doff it and to use it for gait and other ambulatory activities.[13]

The Role of Occupational Therapy

Occupational therapists assess learning ability and the home situation. In addition, they teach patients self-care skills, including bathing, toileting, and dressing. These must be relearned because they are disturbed by the change in body configuration with the loss of bipedal support. Many other daily activities are also affected by wearing a prosthesis.

The patient must first become as independent as possible without a prosthesis.[14] Then, prosthetic fitting should be considered. Some people with limb loss adapt to other mobility methods while waiting for the prosthesis to be provided, including crutch use and crawling on the floor.[15]

THREE PHASES OF PROSTHETIC REHABILITATION

Simply stated, the period of preprosthetic training should be directed first toward assessing patients and their goals; second, to training them to be as independent as possible; and last, to prescribing, fitting, and training them to use a prosthesis. If a person demonstrates difficulty during the first two phases, then it is unlikely that the individual will make functional use of a prosthesis.

Phase I—Assessment and Prevention of Complications

In addition to the previous discussion, education in the care of the remaining foot is vital and is usually conducted by the nursing staff. Emotional adjustment can be facilitated by staff psychologists who are trained in the management of body-image issues and grief reactions, as well as by encouraging patient and family access to peer support groups.

Phase II—Conditioning and Training

Patients should be instructed in breathing exercises as well as limb strengthening exercises. Bed mobility is a key component, considering the effort needed to roll to the side of the bed. As soon as feasible, patients should get out of bed, standing with assistance to perform a pivot transfer to a bedside chair or commode. Other skills include rising from the floor and transitions from sitting to standing. They progress to standing within the parallel bars, then with a walker or crutches, and finally ambulation and elevation activities. New techniques may be needed to accomplish self-care while standing on one leg.

Phase III—Receiving a Prosthesis
Prescribing and Fitting a Prosthesis

Prediction of function after amputation and deciding who should receive a prosthesis depends, first, on consideration of the whole patient, as we would with any other disability. In relation to the prosthesis, one must be conscious of what is being fitted and who is being fitted. Means of checking the status of both the residual limb and the sound leg have already been discussed.

The key to prescription and training for successful use of a prosthesis is the ability to set realistic goals, which is important for both the patient and the members of the rehabilitation team. Goals depend on the patient's emotional status and the degree of financial, social, and educational support services available. Attitudes and expertise of the team members are factors in this process.

One strategy for prediction and classification of function with a prosthesis takes the personal, residual limb, sound limb, and socioeconomic factors and fits them into a framework of "functional objectives." Functional objectives are full restoration, partial restoration, self-care plus, self-care minus, cosmesis plus, and not feasible.[16]

> *Full restoration* describes the patient who wears the prosthesis full-time and resumes all ambulatory activities, often including athletics.

> *Partial restoration* is the state of the individual who wears the prosthesis for walking relatively short distances on level surfaces and limited stair climbing and relies on a wheelchair for traversing longer distances.

> *Self-care plus* is the rating of one who can don and doff the prosthesis with minimal assistance and uses it to walk at home.

> *Self-care minus* describes a person who requires minimal assistance with donning the prosthesis and transferring from a wheelchair to standing and walking short distances at home.

> *Cosmesis plus* refers to someone who needs considerable assistance with donning the prosthesis and wears it to improve the individual's appearance while sitting in the wheelchair.

> *Not feasible* describes those patients for whom a prosthesis is contraindicated, most especially those with advanced cardiopulmonary disease with or without dementia.

Determining the appropriate functional level is made easier if the patient is fitted with a preparatory device, also known as a *temporary prosthesis*. It provides the opportunity for ambulation training and shaping of the residual limb, as well as testing the learning ability and exercise tolerance of the patient. The preparatory limb is usually not aesthetically pleasing and is used only for a brief training period. It is prescribed by the physician, after discussion with the patient, surgeon, therapists, and prosthetist who will make it. Cost is variable. Time and skills of the prosthetist, as well as the price of materials and prosthetic components, are factors involved in the cost. Insurance companies compute costs differently from equipment providers and use specialized terminology for components. Medicare will pay for 80% of what it deems is the appropriate cost. This can leave the patient with a fairly large bill, depending upon the device being provided.

In 1995, Medicare promulgated rules designating "K-levels." These functional levels, which apply only to prescription of unilateral transtibial and transfemoral prostheses, include the following:

> K0—Not a candidate
> K1—Household ambulation
> K2—Limited community ambulation
> K3—Community ambulation (and the ability to vary cadence) with vocational, therapeutic, or exercise needs
> K4—High levels of activity such as demonstrated by active adults and athletes

K-levels are used to determine the medical necessity of knee and ankle-foot units. Documentation must be provided to justify the use of certain devices at each level. For example, patients should be at least K2 to qualify for flexible-keel and multiaxial ankle and foot-ankle units. Patients at K3 and above can be funded for energy-storing, dynamic response, and Flex-Foot (Ossur, Alsio Viejo, California); they can also receive hydraulic and pneumatic knees. Medicare also imposes strict requirements for the justification of test sockets, adjustments, repairs, and component replacement.

Before the first prosthesis is delivered, patients should be made familiar with the basic terminology. The prosthesis is checked for accuracy, fit, and comfort, as detailed in Chapters 5 and 9. Training begins with donning and doffing the limb. Patients learn to control the position of the body's center of gravity and how to maintain balance while standing. They gain proprioceptive awareness by wearing the prosthesis and feeling the ground by variations in socket pressure as they move the residual limb. Transfer techniques and gait training come next. They require instruction regarding the care and cleaning of the prosthesis and the residual limb. Chapter 14 presents a comprehensive prosthetic training program.

During training, the physician, physical therapist, and prosthetist periodically review the patient's status. The speed of training depends on the patient's learning ability and motivation, the skills of the therapist and prosthetist, and the presence of any complications related to the amputation and to any other systemic illnesses.

Complications at this stage include the following:

> Blisters and abrasions occur with difficulties with socket fit, which may be reduced by use of a nylon or silicone sheath.

> Hypersensitivity or allergy to socket or sock material requires substituting materials or shielding the skin from the original materials.

> Infections of the wound site or hair follicles in the groin due to poor hygiene may require antibiotics and surgical drainage.

> Perspiration can macerate the skin if nonporous socket materials are used and hygiene is inadequate. Skin disorders may resolve by using prosthetic socks made of porous, natural materials and by iontophoresis with a dilute copper sulfate solution.

➢ *Verrucous hyperplasia,* or warty induration of the distal end of the residual limb, is caused by a loss of distal contact and exacerbated by edema and proximal compression. This results in a pressure gradient from proximal to distal. Squamous cell carcinoma has been associated with verrucous hyperplasia.[17]

Training With a Prosthesis

The schedule of training and the overall time needed for a patient to learn to walk with a prosthesis varies from one person to the next. An outpatient program of prosthetic and daily activity training will take longer than an inpatient stay and is most feasible for the individual having a unilateral transtibial prosthesis. Persons with additional disabilities, such as cerebrovascular accident or fragile cardiac status, often require admission to an inpatient rehabilitation unit for close monitoring. While at first glance inpatient rehabilitation may seem ideal for more rapid training, the patient's medical instability will delay prosthetic training.

It is advisable to let the patient and the therapists work with the new prosthesis for several weeks to evaluate the prosthesis as a whole before starting to correct gait problems, which reflect many factors contributing to their development. It should be emphasized that safety and patient comfort must be balanced against efforts to reduce gait deviations. Remember that no prosthetic gait is "normal." Chapters 6 and 10 describe typical prosthetic gaits and common deviations.

SUMMARY

Rehabilitation of the person undergoing amputation is a process that begins with the preoperative assessment and proceeds to surgical care, postoperative management, preprosthetic and prosthetic management, and continuous follow-up.

REFERENCES

1. Bates B, Stineman MG, Reker DM, et al. Risk factors associated with mortality in veteran population following transtibial or transfemoral amputation. *J Rehabil Res Dev.* 2006;43:917-928.

2. Smith DG. General principles of amputation surgery. In: Smith DG, Michael JW, Bowker JH, eds. *Atlas of Amputation and Limb Deficiencies: Surgical, Prosthetic, and Rehabilitation Principles.* 3rd ed. Rosemont, IL: American Academy of Orthopaedic Surgeons; 2004:21-30.

3. Atherton R, Robertson N. Psychological adjustment to lower limb amputation amongst prosthesis users. *Disabil Rehabil.* 2006;15:1201-1209.

4. Grobler I. Re-defining self after limb loss: a psychological perspective. *Prosthet Orthot Int.* 2008;32:337-344.

5. Mayer A, Kudar K, Bretz K, Tihanyi J. Body schema and body awareness of amputees. *Prosthet Orthot Int.* 2008;32:363-382.

6. Bowker JH. Transtibial amputation: surgical management. In: Smith DG, Michael JW, Bowker JH, eds. *Atlas of Amputation and Limb Deficiencies: Surgical, Prosthetic, and Rehabilitation Principles.* 3rd ed. Rosemont, IL: American Academy of Orthopaedic Surgeons; 2004:483-501.

7. Gottschalk F. Transfemoral amputation: surgical management. In: Smith DG, Michael JW, Bowker JH, eds. *Atlas of Amputation and Limb Deficiencies: Surgical, Prosthetic, and Rehabilitation Principles.* 3rd ed. Rosemont, IL: American Academy of Orthopaedic Surgeons; 2004:533-540.

8. McIntosh J, Earnshaw JJ. Antibiotic prophylaxis for the prevention of infection after major limb amputation. *Eur J Vasc Endovasc Surg.* 2009;37:696-703.

9. Ehde DM, Smith DG. Chronic pain management. In: Smith DG, Michael JW, Bowker JH, eds. *Atlas of Amputation and Limb Deficiencies: Surgical, Prosthetic, and Rehabilitation Principles.* 3rd ed. Rosemont, IL: American Academy of Orthopaedic Surgeons; 2004:711-720.

10. Desmond D, Gallagher P, Henderson-Slater D, Chatfield R. Pain and psychosocial adjustment to lower limb amputation amongst prosthesis users. *Prosthet Orthot Int.* 2008;32:244-252.

11. Stineman MG, Kwong PL, Kurichi JE, et al. The effectiveness of inpatient rehabilitation in the acute postoperative phase of care after transtibial or transfemoral amputation: study of an integrated health care delivery system. *Arch Phys Med Rehabil.* 2008;89:1863-1872.

12. Dillingham TR, Pezzin LE. Rehabilitation setting and associated mortality and medical stability among persons with amputations. *Arch Phys Med Rehabil.* 2008;89:1038-1045.

13. Gailey RS, Clark CR. Physical therapy. In: Smith DG, Michael JW, Bowker JH, eds. *Atlas of Amputation and Limb Deficiencies: Surgical, Prosthetic, and Rehabilitation Principles.* 3rd ed. Rosemont, IL: American Academy of Orthopaedic Surgeons; 2004:589-619.

14. Edelstein JE. Rehabilitation without prostheses. In: Smith DG, Michael JW, Bowker JH, eds. *Atlas of Amputation and Limb Deficiencies: Surgical, Prosthetic, and Rehabilitation Principles.* 3rd ed. Rosemont, IL: American Academy of Orthopaedic Surgeons; 2004:745-756.

15. Stokes D, Curzio J, Berry A, et al. Pre prosthetic mobility: the amputees' perspectives. *Disabil Rehabil.* 2009;31:138-143.

16. Russek AS. Management of lower extremity amputees. *Arch Phys Med Rehabil.* 1961;42:687-703.

17. Levy SW. Skin problems in the amputee. In: Smith DG, Michael JW, Bowker JH, eds. *Atlas of Amputation and Limb Deficiencies: Surgical, Prosthetic, and Rehabilitation Principles.* 3rd ed. Rosemont, IL: American Academy of Orthopaedic Surgeons; 2004:701-710.

Chapter 3

Transtibial Prostheses

The permanent (also known as *definitive*) transtibial prosthesis consists of 4 major components (Figure 3-1):

1. Foot-ankle assembly
2. Shank
3. Socket
4. Suspension

Prescription of components in a given prosthesis depends on the clinical status of the patient, the individual's anticipated functional capacity and applicable financial resources, as well as the person's concern regarding the appearance of the prosthesis.[1] Some activities, such as running or swimming, may require special components; these will be described in Chapter 14. Individuals who wear sports prostheses also have a basic prosthesis, which will be described here.

Although contemporary rehabilitation aims for evidence-based practice, this goal is yet to be realized with regard to prosthetics and orthotics. Double-blind placebo-controlled research conducted with validated outcome measures is virtually absent.[2] Human studies cited in this chapter and elsewhere in the book involve small, diverse samples and have other methodological shortcomings,[3] hampering generalization to other patients. Most published research is conducted in laboratories rather than in the complex real world.[4] Another deficiency is the paucity of research relating to wearers' subjective perceptions.[5] Finally, few studies test the mechanical properties of components.[6] These deficiencies will be reduced when more practitioners are trained in conducting research and when time and resources are devoted to establishing evidence-based practice.[7]

FOOT-ANKLE ASSEMBLY

The distal portion of the transtibial prosthesis is the foot-ankle assembly. All prosthetic feet are mass produced and serve the following functions:

➢ Resembles the shape of a normal foot, at least the length of the foot. Many assemblies have an exterior cover similar to the color and contour of the human foot. Patients can wear a wide variety of shoes. All shoes, however, must have the same heel height, unless the foot-ankle assembly has an adjustment mechanism.

➢ Provides a stable base when the wearer stands.

➢ Absorbs shock during early stance when the wearer walks.

➢ Plantar flexes during early stance, enabling the wearer to proceed from heel contact to foot flat position.

➢ Provides toe break action (ie, hyperextension of the distal portion of the foot, during late stance).

➢ Maintains a neutral ankle position during swing phase.

Most prosthetic feet also provide slight frontal and transverse plane motion.

No commercially available prosthetic foot provides certain basic functions:

➢ No sensory feedback from the foot itself.

➢ Much less excursion than the comparable anatomic joint.

➢ Usually does not plantar flex unless the wearer applies full body weight.

➢ Does not permit tip-toe walking.

Two broad categories of foot-ankle assemblies are nonarticulated and articulated. Within both categories are units that store and return energy, sometimes termed *dynamic feet*.

Nonarticulated Feet

These components have no separation between the upper and lower parts of the foot at a point corresponding to the anatomic ankle joint. The relatively simple

Edelstein JE, Muroz A.
Lower-Limb Prosthetics and Orthotics: Clinical Concepts (pp 19-32).
© 2011 Taylor & Francis Group.

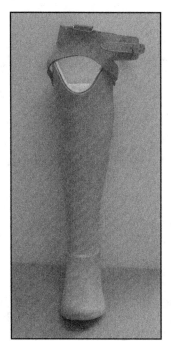

Figure 3-1. Transtibial prosthesis

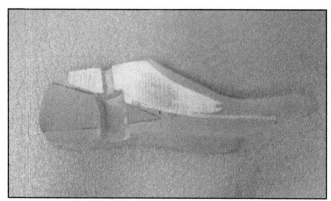

Figure 3-2. Cross section of SACH foot.

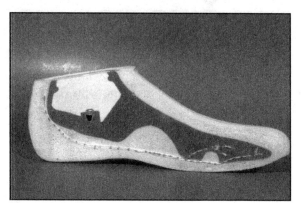

Figure 3-3. Cross section of SAFE foot.

construction with few or no moving parts means that the foot is generally more durable, lighter in weight, and less expensive than articulated units. Nonarticulated feet permit some passive motion in all directions, depending on the direction of load applied by the wearer.

The most basic example of a nonarticulated foot is the SACH foot (Otto Bock, Minneapolis, Minnesota; Kingsley, Costa Mesa, California; Figure 3-2). The name refers to its solid ankle cushion heel design. The solid ankle is made of wood or other rigid material. It forms the posterior portion of the keel, the longitudinal support of the foot. The keel extends proximally from the portion of the foot adjacent to the distal aspect of the shank to a distal curvature in the vicinity of the foot corresponding to the metatarsal heads. The cushion heel is made of resilient rubber or similar material. The SACH foot is covered with synthetic rubber, creating a life-like appearance in the dorsum of the foot. The junction between the flexible rubber cover and the rigid distal portion of the keel enables the wearer to simulate metatarsophalangeal hyperextension during late stance.

The distal rubber portion may be molded to suggest toes with toenails; some wearers paint the toenails with nail polish to increase the life-like appearance, especially when the foot is worn with an open-toe sandal or shoe. SACH feet are manufactured in several skin tones; the feet may also be custom painted to match the color of the wearer's skin.

When the wearer applies sufficient body weight to the rear portion of the SACH foot at the time of heel contact, the component moves from neutral position to plantar flexion to provide the stability afforded by the foot flat position. For the patient who hesitates to step vigorously onto the prosthesis, a softer heel cushion facilitates plantar flexion.

Unlike the rigid keel of the SACH foot, several nonarticulated feet have a flexible keel including the SAFE foot (Campbell-Childs, White City, Oregon; Figure 3-3). The stationary attachment flexible endoskeleton foot has a keel make of semirigid plastic. Consequently, when the wearer walks on cobblestones or other uneven terrain, the SAFE foot yields to provide more sole contact than possible with a SACH foot. During late stance, the SAFE foot provides slight dorsiflexion. This foot is heavier and more expensive than a SACH foot and is only available in adult sizes.

Some nonarticulated feet store and release energy. They have a flexible keel that bends during early or midstance and then recoils as the wearer transfers weight from the prosthesis to the opposite leg. The potential energy stored in the keel as it bends changes to kinetic energy during late stance and early swing phase as the keel recoils, enabling the wearer to walk with greater propulsive force than possible with

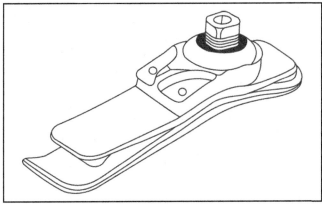

Figure 3-4. Quantum Truestep.

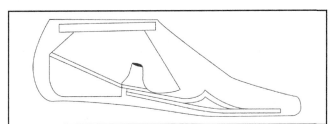

Figure 3-5. Carbon Copy 2.

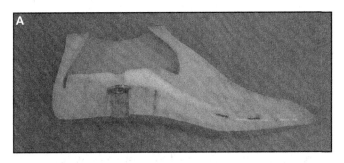

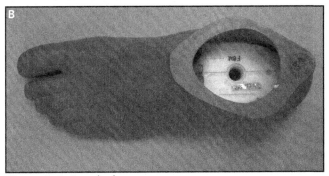

Figure 3-6. Seattle foot.

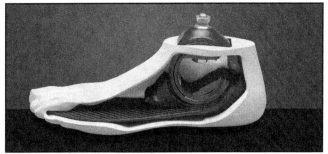

Figure 3-7. C-Walk. (Reprinted with permission from Otto Bock HealthCare.)

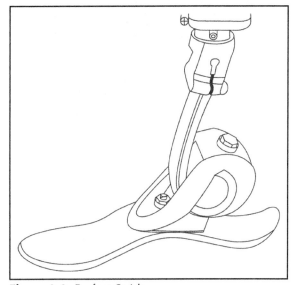

Figure 3-8. Perfect Stride.

the basic SACH foot. Energy storage in a prosthetic foot attempts to imitate the action of the gastrocnemius soleus muscle group. Examples of energy storing, dynamic feet include Quantum Truestep (Fillauer, Chattanooga, Tennessee; Figure 3-4), Carbon Copy 2 (Ohio Willow Wood, Sterling, Ohio; Figure 3-5), Seattle (Trulife, Poulsbo, Washington; Figure 3-6), C-Walk (Otto Bock; Figure 3-7), Perfect Stride (BioQuest, Bakersfield, California; Figure 3-8), and Flex-Foot (Ossur, Aliso Viejo,

California; Figure 3-9). Energy-storing feet are appropriate for individuals at K3-4 levels who are capable of applying substantial force to the foot causing the keel to change shape and those at K2 who need to walk rapidly, as when crossing a street.

The keel of the Quantum foot is made of 2 slender plates that the prosthetist can adjust to suit the walking characteristics of the wearer. The foot is covered with a flexible rubber cover. It is particularly suitable for someone with a narrow foot.

The distal portion of the keel of the Carbon Copy 2 foot consists of 2 carbon fiber plates. When the wearer walks at normal pace, during mid- and late stance, the lower plate, known as the *primary plate*, bends, storing energy. When the wearer runs, the additional force causes both the primary and the secondary (upper) plates to bend, storing more energy, which is released during early swing phase.

The basic Seattle foot has a nylon keel with a posterior angle. When the wearer initiates stance phase with this foot, the angle of the keel becomes more acute, storing potential energy. Upon transferring weight to the distal portion of the foot in late stance, the keel recoils,

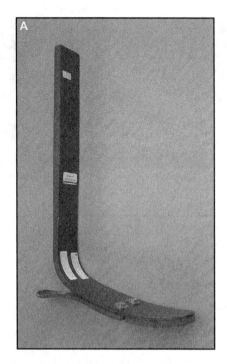

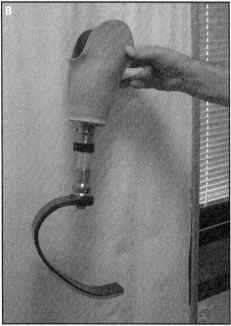

Figure 3-9. (A) Flex-Foot. (B) Flex-Run.

Flex-Foot has several models. The original design consists of a carbon fiber band extending from the foot section to the midshank; a second carbon fiber portion comprises the posterior portion of the foot. Ordinarily, the unit is covered with a life-like cosmetic cover. The long, flexible keel enables the Flex-Foot to store appreciable energy, allowing the wearer to walk with a springy gait. A longitudinal split in the foot section allows the foot to accommodate to irregular terrain. Another model of the Flex-Foot is one that omits the posterior foot section, making the foot suitable for sprinters (Figure 3-9B). One Flex-Foot design has a telescoping shank section with an exterior leaf spring, making the component particularly adept at absorbing shock.

Limited research is inconclusive regarding the clinical effectiveness of these feet. Benefits appear to be present when the patient increases walking speed or walks on ramps.[8] Some wearers exhibited reduced heart rate and rate of perceived exertion,[9] while another study group preferred energy-storing units to assemblies that did not store energy.[10] A third study demonstrated that wearing energy-storing units reduced compensations in the sound lower limb.[11] In contrast, other investigators[12,13] found no appreciable difference between wearers' function with and without energy-storing feet.

Articulated Feet

The defining characteristic of all articulated foot-ankle units is a space above the foot section. When the prosthesis is cosmetically finished, the space is covered with a leather or similar flexible material. As a group, these feet provide greater range of motion, enabling the wearer to accommodate the foot more readily to sloped terrain. Drawbacks of articulated feet are their greater number of moving parts and discontinuity between foot and shank, thus making these units vulnerable to infiltration by debris and loosening of the mechanism, as well as presenting a less attractive appearance.

The most common example of an articulated foot is the single-axis foot (Kingsley; Otto Bock; Figure 3-10). The foot section moves on the proximal portion via a transverse bolt. The mechanism permits passive plantar flexion and dorsiflexion. These motions are controlled by resilient bumpers. A relatively large plantar bumper is in the rear and a thin dorsiflexion stop lies in front of the ankle bolt. The single-axis foot moves into plantar flexion as soon as the wearer applies minimal weight to the heel, thus providing a stable foot flat position. This action is particularly useful for patients who hesitate to put much load on the prosthesis.

The single-axis foot does not accommodate to transverse irregularities of the walking surface. Consequently, when the wearer walks on a side slope, additional force is transmitted to the proximal portion of the prosthesis, particularly the socket.

fostering a dynamic, springy gait. One model of the Seattle foot features a life-like cover with molded toes and a space between the hallux and the second toe. This design enables the individual to wear a thong sandal.

C-Walk and Perfect Stride feet include a carbon fiber circular unit in the rear foot; the circle stores energy in early stance and, when the rear foot is unloaded in late stance, releases the stored energy.

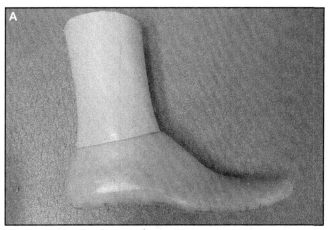

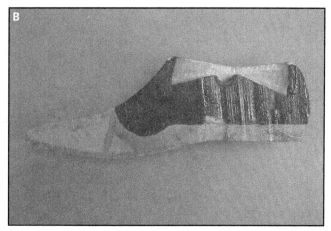

Figure 3-10. Single-axis foot. (A) Exterior. (B) Cross section.

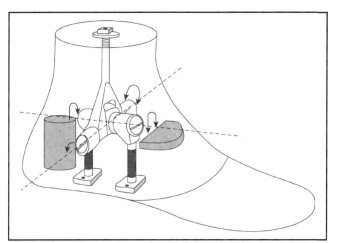

Figure 3-11. Greissinger foot.

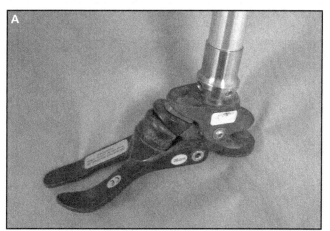

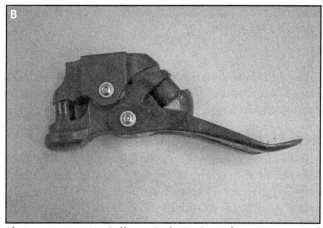

Figure 3-12. (A) College Park TruStep foot. (A) Frontal view. (B) Side view.

Multiple-axis feet provide slight passive motion in all planes. The range of motion is usually controlled by resilient bumpers or flexible material in the rear of the foot. These feet accommodate to uneven surfaces; however, they are heavier and more expensive than the basic single-axis foot.[14]

The Greissinger foot (Otto Bock; Figure 3-11) has a foot-ankle unit that includes anterior, posterior, and mediolateral bumpers as well as a resilient portion that allows motion in the transverse plane, simulating intertarsal action. Wearers demonstrated improved symmetry of hip and ankle motion with this foot.[15] Newer examples of multiple-axis feet include various College Park models (College Park, Fraser, Michigan; Figure 3-12). They provide greater triplanar passive excursion.

A single-axis foot with a longitudinal split in the forefoot will also permit inversion and eversion. The ProprioFoot (Ossur; Figure 3-13) includes an electronic motor that responds to input from accelerometers that sample the wearer's movements 1000 times per second, detecting the walking terrain and the wearer's activity (eg, sitting or stair climbing). The single-axis mechanism allows substantial plantar flexion and dorsiflexion and results in higher symmetry between the intact and prosthetic limbs.[16] The forefoot split permits triplanar motion. ProprioFoot is bulkier and much heavier than other prosthetic feet. Other electronic feet are in the advanced stages of development.

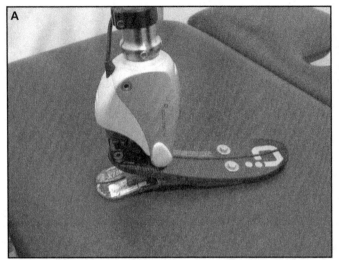
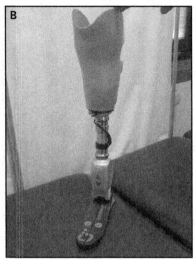
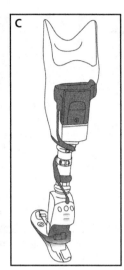

Figure 3-13. ProprioFoot. (A) Lateral view. (B) Anterior view. (C) Posterior view.

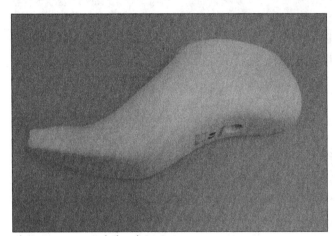

Figure 3-14. High-heel SACH.

In addition to foot design, the alignment of the foot relative to the rest of the prosthesis affects the wearer's comfort and function.[17]

Heel Height Accommodation

Individuals who wish to wear various styles of shoes differing in the height of the heel usually are unable simply to don the desired shoe because the alignment of the prosthesis would be disturbed. Consequently, several options that will allow appropriate alignment exist.

➢ Two or more prostheses. Each prosthesis includes a foot that accommodates a specific heel height. Some models of feet are manufactured to suit shoes of various heel height, typically a 2-inch high heel. Although this is the most expensive option, the cosmetic and functional effects are optimal.

➢ One prosthesis plus 2 or more feet. The wearer unbolts the original foot and installs the foot with the desired heel height accommodation (Figure 3-14).

➢ One prosthesis with an adjustable foot. Several prosthetic feet incorporate a mechanism that the wearer can adjust to match the height of the shoe. These mechanisms add weight, cost, and fragility to the prosthesis.

SHANK

The component located between the proximal aspect of the foot-ankle assembly and the distal portion of the socket is the *shank*. All shanks transmit the wearer's weight from the socket to the foot. Most shanks are shaped and colored to match the individual's leg. The 2 types of shank are endoskeletal and exoskeletal.

The *endoskeletal* shank has a central support structure, sometimes called the *pylon* (Figure 3-15), that is mass-produced. Screws on the proximal portion of the pylon permit the prosthetist to make slight alterations of the tilt of the pylon in the frontal and sagittal planes, contributing to the comfort and ease of walking with the prosthesis. Most endoskeletal shanks are covered with a resilient cosmetic cover that contributes to the life-like appearance of the prosthesis.

Exoskeletal shanks (see Figure 3-1) are custom made of rigid material, usually plastic or wood. Although they are shaped and colored to harmonize with the wearer's contralateral leg, exoskeletal shanks seldom achieve a truly natural appearance because, in most instances, the exterior has a shiny finish. Exoskeletal shanks are more durable and less expensive than endoskeletal shanks.

Some shanks incorporate a shock-absorbing unit. Both exo- and endoskeletal shanks may include a transverse rotator that absorbs shock as the wearer twists the torso (Figure 3-16). Rotators reduce rotational force to the amputation limb.[18] This action is especially useful during golfing.

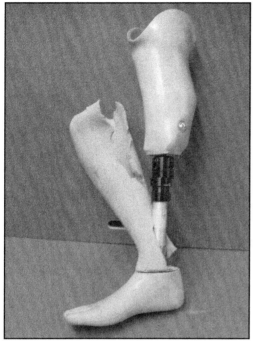

Figure 3-15. Endoskeletal shank with cover.

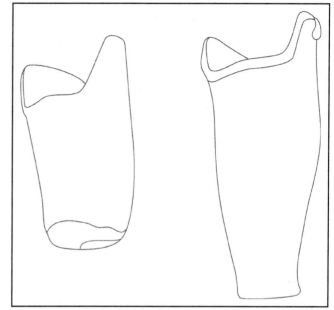

Figure 3-17. Liner and socket.

socket is custom made of plastic molded over a plaster model of the patient's amputation limb.

Although each socket reflects the unique characteristics of the intended wearer, several basic shapes are common. The patellar tendon bearing (PTB) socket is noteworthy for a prominent indentation in the antero-proximal aspect. The total surface bearing socket has smoother contours. The hydrostatic socket has a relatively large distal portion, intended to enhance cushioning of the amputation limb. Details of socket contours are presented in Chapter 4.

Most transtibial prostheses are furnished with some combination of insert (Figure 3-17) and liner or sheath and are usually worn with socks. These terms, sometimes used interchangeably or termed *interface*, refer to soft material worn between the socket and the skin. *Sock* generally connotes woven fabric.

Socks

Most people wear one or more socks in addition to an insert. Socks are manufactured in various sizes to fit people with different limb circumferences and lengths. Socks permit the wearer to adjust the fit of the socket, adding one or more socks when the socket feels loose and removing socks when the amputation limb is edematous, causing the socket to be tight.

The simplest sock is cotton, woven in 1- and 3-ply thicknesses. *Ply* refers to the number of threads in the weave. Cotton is hypoallergenic, inexpensive, and absorbent; however, it may not provide sufficient cushioning of the amputation limb.

Another popular material is wool, woven in 5-ply thickness. Wool provides excellent resilience but is more expensive than cotton and requires special laundering to avoid shrinkage.

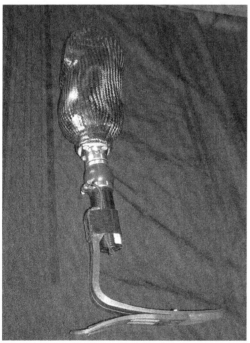

Figure 3-16. Rotator installed in pylon.

Endoskeletal shanks may also have a vertical shock absorber. Units that combine vertical and transverse shock absorbers can be fitted to endoskeletal shanks. Shock absorbers may be beneficial for those who walk rapidly.[19,20]

SOCKET

The most important part of the prosthesis is the socket because this is the part of the prosthesis that contacts the wearer's skin. In the permanent prosthesis, the

Ordinarily, the combination of socks should not exceed 15 ply. A thicker layer of socks obscures the contours of the socket, interfering with precise fit.

A 2-part sock is another option manufactured in lengths and girths for transtibial and transfemoral amputation limbs. The inner nylon sock minimizes friction against the skin, and the outer sock, made of acrylic fiber and wool for resilience and ease of laundering, cushions the amputation limb.

Insert

An insert is a custom-made concentric version of the socket. Typically molded of polyethylene foam, the insert cushions the amputation limb. When the socket requires alteration to accommodate atrophy of the amputation limb, the prosthetist may add plastic to the socket interior at the required location; the insert provides a smooth interface between the altered socket and the wearer's skin. Because nearly all new prosthesis wearers experience pressure atrophy with the first prosthesis, an insert is highly desirable.

For subsequent prostheses, the insert is optional. Some people prefer to wear an insert permanently. Others dislike the added bulk of the insert, which interferes with wearing snug trousers. For individuals who live in a hot, humid climate, the insert may be uncomfortable because it tends to retain body heat.

Liner

Many manufacturers offer liners, also known as *sheaths*, intended to reduce skin abrasion and, in some instances, to contribute to suspension of the prosthesis. Liners are usually made of silicone, urethane, or mineral oil-based gel. Some liners have vertical channels filled with mineral oil or other viscous fluid, to distribute pressure uniformly. Several liners can be custom-shaped to fit a given patient. Snug-fitting liners may be unrolled onto the amputation limb.

Liners create a smooth interface between the patient's skin and the socket or insert, reducing the likelihood of skin abrasion. If the prosthesis is to be suspended with a distal pin, a silicone liner is customary. Nevertheless, silicone is difficult to reshape, tends to stretch distally during swing phase, retains body heat, and is expensive. Wearing a liner is associated with better suspension and more comfortable walking,[21] although patients may complain about poor material durability[22] and, with silicone liners, itching, perspiration, rashes, and odor.[23]

SUSPENSION

Suspension is a component that prevents the prosthesis from slipping off the amputation limb during the swing phase of walking and when the wearer climbs stairs and ladders and engages in similar pursuits during which the prosthesis is not on the ground.

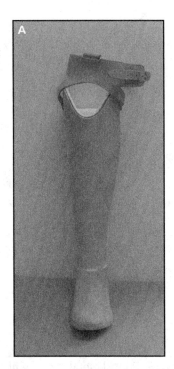

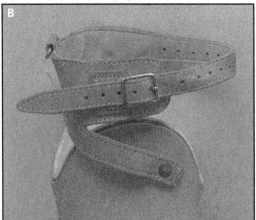

Figure 3-18. Cuff suspension. (A) Anterior view. (B) Lateral view.

The simplest suspension is a supracondylar cuff (Figure 3-18) usually made of leather. The cuff is attached to the medial and lateral sides of the upper portion of the socket. It is fastened with hook and pile tape or a buckle around the distal thigh. The cuff should be reasonably snug when the wearer extends the knee and should become slack when the knee is flexed. The wearer can adjust cuff fit readily; however, when the individual sits, the contour of the cuff may be apparent through the trouser leg.

A waist belt and elastic fork strap (Figure 3-19) may be added to the cuff to augment suspension, especially if the wearer engages in activities such as climbing ladders or rock climbing. The user can attach and detach the waist belt and fork strap when not needed.

For the individual with a relatively slender thigh and strong hands, sleeve suspension (Figure 3-20) is

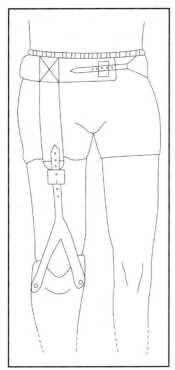

Figure 3-19. Fork strap suspension.

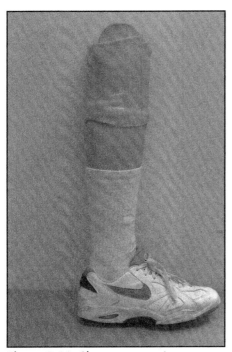

Figure 3-20. Sleeve suspension.

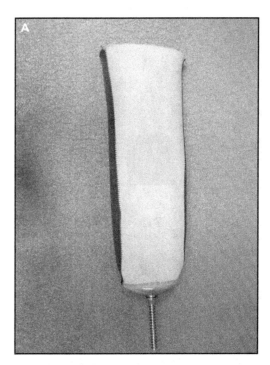

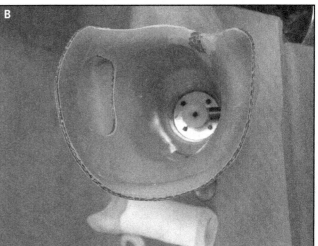

Figure 3-21. (A) Liner. (B) Icelock pin retention fixture in bottom of socket, superior view.

excellent. An elastic sleeve extends from the distal thigh to the midportion of the shank. Suspension is secure when the wearer sits and the contour closely matches the sound side. Sleeve suspension is unsuitable for obese patients and those who do not have good bimanual strength.

Several modes of suspension through the distal end of the socket are available. The distal pin is a metal projection from the end of a silicone liner; the pin engages a locking mechanism (Figure 3-21) in the base of the socket. Pin suspension provides very secure suspension; however, some patients have difficulty fitting the pin into the relatively small hole in the socket and others experience chronic skin changes attributable to the relatively high negative pressure during swing phase.[24] Subjects in a randomized crossover trial using elastomeric liners with distal pins compared with polyethylene foam liners with neoprene sleeve suspensions generally preferred the sleeve.[25]

A lanyard is a similar mode of suspension. A fabric cord or tape is attached to the distal end of the socket

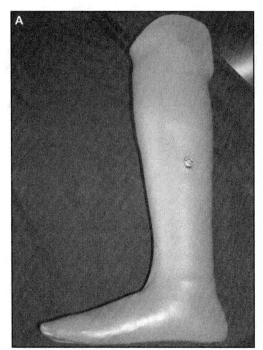
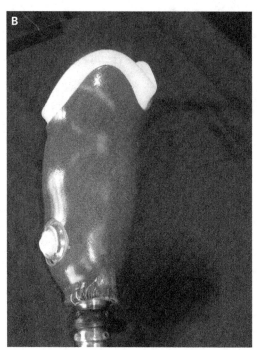

Figure 3-22. Suction release valve on exterior of socket. (A) Medial view. (B). Anteromedial view.

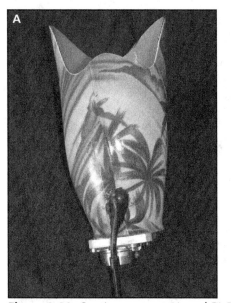
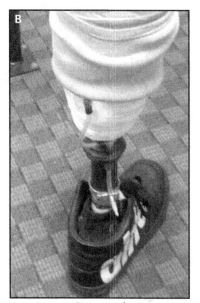
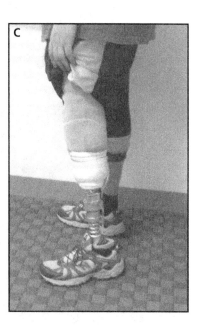

Figure 3-23. Suction system. (A and B) Posterior views. (C) Lateral view.

liner. The patient guides the free end of the cord or tape through an opening in the distal socket and secures the cord or tape on the outside of the socket.

Suction suspension can be achieved with a liner that has one or more exterior ridges in the distal third and an air expulsion valve (Figure 3-22). When the user dons the liner, the amputation limb displaces air through the valve, creating a suction seal. To doff the liner, the patient presses a release button on the valve, breaking the suction. The dual-suspension system combines suction with a distal pin. Suction suspension

tends to stabilize the volume of the amputation limb,[26] increase proprioception, and decrease the perception of heaviness of the prosthesis.

Another way to achieve suction suspension is with a miniature electric pump in the distal socket, such as the Harmony (Otto Bock) or LimbLogic VS (Ohio Willow Wood; Figure 3-23). The prosthesis is worn with a liner and a suspension sleeve which maintains negative pressure between the liner and the socket.

Alternate suspension may involve the brim of the socket. Supracondylar suspension (Figure 3-24) is

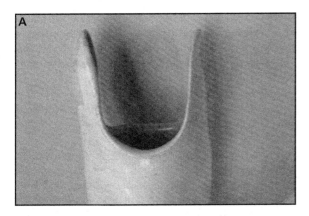

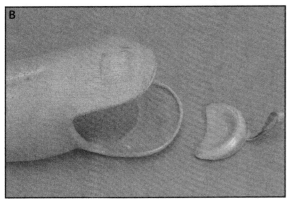

Figure 3-24. Supracondylar suspension. (A) Anterior view. (B) Lateral view with epicondylar insert.

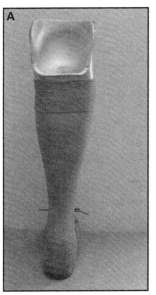
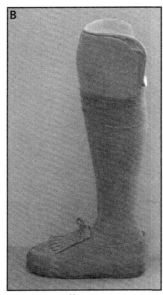

Figures 3-25. Supracondylar-suprapatellar suspension. (A) Posterior view. (B) Lateral view.

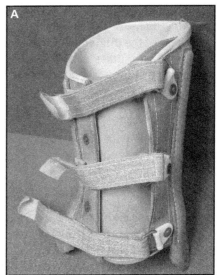

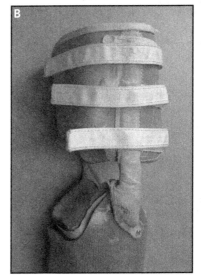
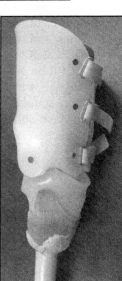

Figure 3-26. Corset suspension. (A) Leather-metal corset, anterior view. (B) Leather-metal corset, lateral view. (C) Plastic corset.

achieved with a socket that encompasses the medial and lateral femoral epicondyles. Mediolateral stability is enhanced, no fastenings are required, and, when the user sits, the silhouette at the knee almost resembles that of the sound knee. Supracondylar suspension, however, cannot be adjusted by the patient; if socket fit is too loose or tight, the prosthetist must make the necessary adjustment. A variation is supracondylar/suprapatellar suspension (Figure 3-25). The medial, lateral, and anterior margins of the socket are relatively high. This suspension is indicated for the person with a very short amputation limb; otherwise, during swing phase, the amputation limb might withdraw from the socket. The drawbacks of the supracondylar/suprapatellar suspension are its unnatural contour when the user sits and the need for the prosthetist to make any adjustments if the socket no longer fits.

The oldest mode of suspension is the thigh corset with side joints (Figure 3-26). The leather or flexible plastic thigh corset is fastened with laces or straps and is attached to the socket by a pair of metal side bars with single-axis hinges. The thigh corset provides maximum mediolateral stability and transfers some weight to the thigh. The disadvantages of this suspension are many. It promotes atrophy of the thigh muscles, is warm, adds weight to the prosthesis, takes extra time to don, and presents an unnatural contour when the wearer sits.

PROSTHETIC DURABILITY

Over a 10-year period, patients required an average of 1.4 new prostheses, 2.9 new sockets, and 17.3 repairs.[27]

PRESCRIPTION GUIDELINES

Lacking conclusive scientific evidence regarding the suitability of given components, clinicians rely on clinical consensus among experts.[28] Current practice suggests that a patient who is classified at the K1-2 level may benefit from a prosthesis that includes a SACH foot, endoskeletal shank, socket with liner and a supply of cotton and wool socks, and cuff suspension. The person rated as K2 may perform better with an energy-storing foot if he or she frequently needs to cross busy streets.[29] At K3-4 levels, the prosthesis should have an energy-storing foot, endoskeletal shank with vertical and transverse shock absorbers, socket with silicone liner, and suction suspension.

REFERENCES

1. Versluys R, Beyl P, Van Damme M, et al. Prosthetic feet: state-of-the-art review and the importance of mimicking human ankle-foot biomechanics. *Disabil Rehabil Assist Technol.* 2009;4:65-75.

2. Czerniecki JM. Research and clinical selection of foot-ankle systems. *J Prosthet Orthot.* 2005;17:S35-S37.

3. Hafner BJ. Clinical prescription and use of prosthetic foot and ankle mechanisms: a review of the literature. *J Prosthet Orthot.* 2005;17:S5-S11.

4. Hafner BJ. Perceptive evaluation of prosthetic foot and ankle systems. *J Prosthet Orthot.* 2005;17:S42-S46.

5. Rietman JS, Postema K, Geertzen JHB. Gait analysis in prosthetics: opinions, ideas and conclusions. *Prosthet Orthot Int.* 2002;26:50-57.

6. Hofstad C, Linde H, Limbeek J, Postema K. Prescription of prosthetic ankle-foot mechanisms after lower limb amputation [serial on CD-ROM]. *Cochrane Database Syst Rev.* 2004:2004;1:CD003978.

7. Geil MD. Assessing the state of clinically applicable research for evidence-based practice in prosthetics and orthotics. *J Rehabil Res Dev.* 2009;46:305-314.

8. Hansen AH. Scientific methods to determine functional performance of prosthetic ankle-foot systems. *J Prosthet Orthot.* 2005;17:S23-S29.

9. Hsu MJ, Nielsen DH, Lin-Chan SJ, Shurr D. The effects of prosthetic foot design on physiologic measurements, self-selected walking velocity, and physical activity in people with transtibial amputation. *Arch Phys Med Rehabil.* 2006;87:123-129.

10. Hafner BJ, Sanders JE, Czerniecki J, Fergason J. Energy storage and return prostheses: does patient perception correlate with biomechanical analysis? *Clin Biomech.* 2002;17:325-344.

11. Underwood HA, Tokuno CD, Eng JJ. A comparison of two prosthetic feet on the multi-joint and multi-plane kinetic gait compensations in individuals with unilateral trans-tibial amputation. *Clin Biomech (Bristol, Avon).* 2004;19:609-616.

12. Schmalz T, Blumentritt S, Jarasch R. Energy expenditure and biomechanical characteristics of lower limb amputee gait: the influence of prosthetic alignment and different prosthetic components. *Gait Posture.* 2002;16:255-263.

13. Zmitrewicz RJ, Neptune RR, Sasaki K. Mechanical energetic contributions from individual muscles and elastic prosthetic feet during symmetric unilateral trans-tibial amputees walking: a theoretical study. *J Biomech.* 2007;40:1824-1831.

14. Zmitrewicz RJ, Neptune R, Walden JG, et al. The effect of foot and ankle prosthetic components on braking and propulsive impulses during transtibial amputee gait. *Arch Phys Med Rehabil.* 2006;87:1334-1339.

15. Marinakis GN. Interlimb symmetry of traumatic unilateral transtibial amputees wearing two different prosthetic feet in the early rehabilitation stage. *J Rehabil Res Dev.* 2004;41:581-590.

16. Agrawal V, Gailey R, O'Toole C, et al. Symmetry in external work (SEW): a novel method of quantifying gait differences between prosthetic feet. *Prosthet Orthot Int.* 2009;33:146-156.

17. Stark G. Perspectives on how and why feet are prescribed. *J Prosthet Orthot.* 2005;17:S18-S22.

18. Segal AD, Orendurff MS, Czerniecki JM, et al. Transtibial amputee joint rotation moments during straight-line walking and a common turning task with and without a torsion adapter. *J Rehabil Res Dev.* 2009;46:375-384.

19. Gard SA, Konz RJ. The effect of a shock-absorbing pylon on the gait of persons with unilateral transtibial amputation. *J Rehabil Res Dev.* 2003;40:109-124.

20. Berge JS, Czerniecki JM, Klute GK. Efficacy of shock-absorbing versus rigid pylons for impact reduction in transtibial amputees based on laboratory, field, and outcome metrics. *J Rehabil Res Dev.* 2005;42:795-808.

21. Baars ECT, Geertzen JHB. Literature review of the possible advantages of silicon liner socket use in trans-tibial prostheses. *Prosthet Orthot Int.* 2005;29:27-37.

22. van de Weg FB, van der Windt DAWM. A questionnaire survey of the effect of different interface types on patient satisfaction and perceived problems among trans-tibial amputees. *Prosthet Orthot Int.* 2005;29:231-239.

23. Hachisuka K, Nakamura T, Ohmine S, et al. Hygiene problems of residual limb and silicone liners in transtibial amputees wearing the total surface bearing socket. *Arch Phys Med Rehabil.* 2001;82:1286-1290.

24. Beil TL, Street GM. Comparison of interface pressures with pin and suction suspension systems. *J Rehabil Res Dev.* 2004;41:821-828.

25. Coleman KL, Boone DA, Laing LS, et al. Quantification of prosthetic outcomes: elastomeric gel liner with locking pin suspension versus polyethylene foam liner with neoprene sleeve suspension. *J Rehabil Res Dev.* 2004;41:591-602.

26. Board WJ, Street GM, Caspers C. A comparison of transtibial amputee suction and vacuum socket conditions. *Prosthet Orthot Int.* 2001;25:202-209.

27. Nair A, Hanspal RS, Zahedi MS, et al. Analyses of prosthetic episodes in lower limb amputees. *Prosthet Orthot Int.* 2008;32:42-49.

28. van der Linde H, Hofstad CJ, Geurts AC, et al. A systematic literature review of the effect of different prosthetic components on human functioning with a lower-limb prosthesis. *J Rehabil Res Dev.* 2004;41:555-570.

29. Supan TJ. Clinical perspectives on prosthetic ankle-foot designs. *J Prosthet Orthot.* 2005;17:S33-S34.

Chapter 4

Transtibial Biomechanics

Biomechanics is the branch of physics that concerns forces applied to biological tissues. *Force* is a push or pull that causes an object to change shape or state of movement. *Kinesiology* is the study of forces causing movement. In the case of prostheses, biomechanics refers to socket design and alignment (ie, the spatial placement of the socket in relation to other parts of the prosthesis).

The twin concerns of biomechanics in prosthetics are comfort and ease of walking. Comfort results from minimizing pressure, the amount of force applied per unit of surface area. Pressure is reduced both by increasing the area of the body in contact with the prosthesis (socket design) and by reducing the force applied to the body (alignment). Comfort also requires that the area that is covered not be overly sensitive.

GOALS

Every prosthesis should afford the wearer maximum comfort and should enable the individual to function to the highest extent permitted by his or her physical status. Comfort is achieved by rational socket design and strategic alignment of the socket relative to the prosthetic foot. Alignment also has a great influence on the wearer's function.

SOCKET DESIGNS

All sockets for permanent prostheses are custom-made over a model of the patient's amputation limb. Several methods of manufacture and various socket shapes are in current use.

The limb may be wrapped in a plaster bandage. The resulting hollow cast is filled with liquid plaster to form a solid model. The prosthetist then alters the model to exaggerate loading on tissue that tolerates pressure well. The model is also altered to reduce loading on more sensitive tissues. Plastic is then molded over the modified model. An alternative approach is computer-aided design and computer-aided manufacture (CAD-CAM). The contours of the amputation limb are recorded electronically so that the prosthetist can alter the resulting image of the limb shape in accordance with the same principles used in plaster fabrication. The modified computer image is then used to carve a solid model that will be used for plastic molding.

Sockets are designed to contact all portions of the amputation limb so that load can be distributed over the maximum area, thus minimizing pressure. Contact, however, should not be uniform. The socket has build-ups (interior convexities) over tissues that tolerate pressure easily, such as the flat patellar ligament, the gastrocnemius belly, and, to a lesser extent, the proximomedial aspect of the leg (also known as the *medial tibial flare* or *pes anserinus*) and the anterolateral portion of the leg (Figures 4-1 to 4-3). Tissues that are pressure sensitive (eg, the head of the fibula, tibial crest, tibial condyles, and distal ends of the fibula and tibia) receive less pressure from a socket that has reliefs (interior concavities) in these areas (Figures 4-4 to 4-6). The distal end of the amputation limb should contact the end of the socket, without sustaining the full weight-bearing load. Failure to achieve distal contact can reduce the pressure distribution and can lead to verrucous hyperplasia, a warty thickening of the distal tissue caused by venous pooling.

The posterior margin of the socket should not be horizontal. Rather, the posterior wall should have a medial and a lateral lower area, slightly lower than the midportion (Figure 4-7). The lower areas lie over the pressure-sensitive hamstring tendons. Because the medial hamstring tendon inserts more distally, the medial portion should be lower than the lateral portion to avoid impingement on these tender tendons.

Edelstein JE, Muroz A.
Lower-Limb Prosthetics and Orthotics: Clinical Concepts (pp 33-38).
© 2011 Taylor & Francis Group.

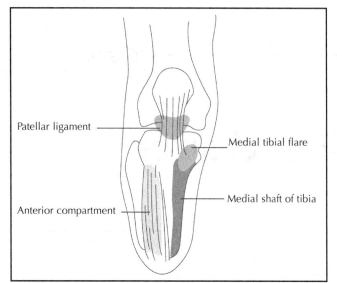

Figure 4-1. Anterior view of the amputation limb, showing pressure-tolerant areas.

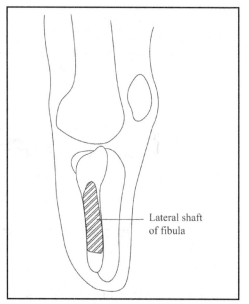

Figure 4-2. Lateral view of the amputation limb, showing pressure-tolerant areas.

The oldest contemporary transtibial socket design is the patellar tendon bearing (PTB), introduced in the 1960s. This socket features a pronounced buildup over the patellar ligament (patellar tendon; Figures 4-7 to 4-9).

A newer design is the total surface bearing (TSB; Figure 4-10), which resembles the PTB socket, although the anterior buildup is reduced, avoiding the skin irritation experienced by some PTB wearers. Other buildups and reliefs are similar to those in the PTB socket. In comparison with prostheses with PTB sockets, those with TSB sockets are lighter and more securely suspended; wearers also applied greater load to the prosthesis.[1] Subjectively, wearers preferred the TSB design for its greater comfort, ease of flexing the knee, reduced slippage, less skin irritation, better appearance, and greater durability.[2] Other investigators reported no significant difference between prostheses with PTB and with TSB sockets with regard to patient satisfaction, extent of activity, and gait analysis.[3]

The hydrostatic socket is molded over a model of the patient's amputation limb and is made as the prosthetist applies downward pressure over the distal tissues. The hydrostatic socket thus has more distal soft tissue cushioning than the PTB or TSB sockets.

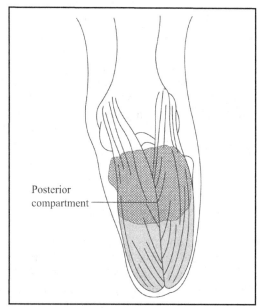

Figure 4-3. Posterior view of the amputation limb, showing pressure-tolerant areas.

ALIGNMENT

Placement of the socket relative to the foot is important in enhancing the wearer's comfort beyond that achieved by socket design and fit. The patient's walking ease is also influenced by alignment. After the socket is made, it is placed on a block of wood, the bottom of which is level with the floor. Strategic angulation of the socket on the block influences comfort and gait. The socket and block are then placed on an adjustable leg, an apparatus consisting of plates that can slide and rotate over a rather large range. The distal end of the adjustable leg is fitted to the prosthetic foot with its shoe. *Bench alignment* refers to placement of the components according to established standards. Dynamic alignment occurs when the patient wears the adjustable leg, standing and walking on it. The prosthetist achieves optimal alignment by observing the patient's performance and by responding to the patient's comments. Alignment

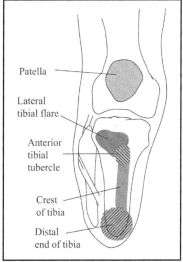

Figure 4-4. Lateral view of the amputation limb, showing pressure-sensitive areas.

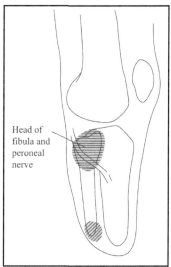

Figure 4-5. Medial view of the amputation limb, showing pressure-sensitive areas.

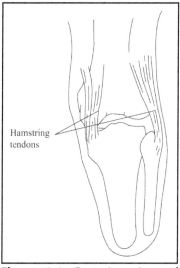

Figure 4-6. Posterior view of the amputation limb, showing pressure-sensitive areas.

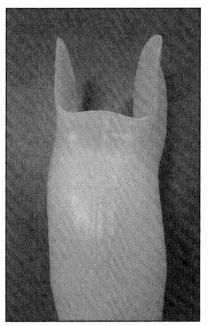

Figure 4-7. Patellar tendon bearing socket, posterior view.

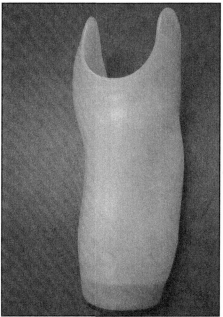

Figure 4-8. Patellar tendon bearing socket, anterior view.

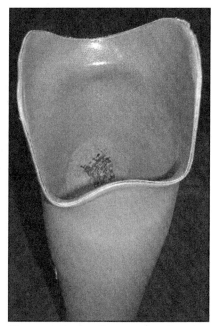

Figure 4-9. Patellar tendon bearing socket, interior view.

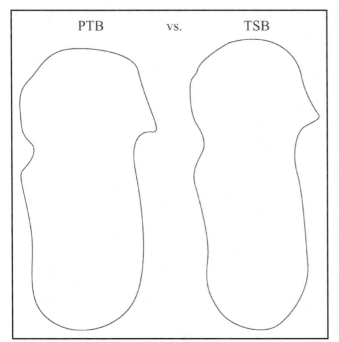

Figure 4-10. Patellar tendon bearing socket compared with total surface bearing socket.

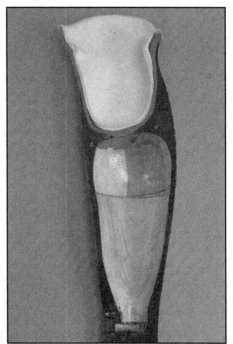

Figure 4-11. Sagittal alignment, socket on shank.

should aim to equalize vertical ground reaction force, stance duration, step length, and the time to full knee flexion during swing phase between the amputated and intact legs.[4] Alignment appears to have a greater effect on patient performance than does prosthetic foot selection.[5] Alignment also affects the duration of pressure application.[6] In addition to level walking, the patient should try the prosthesis on stairs, ramps, and irregular terrain; walking on these surfaces increases force on the patellar ligament.[7]

Sagittal Plane

The goal of sagittal alignment is to reduce the tendency of the amputation limb to slide downward in the socket, which would overstress the distal end of the limb, as well as permit the wearer optimal control of the anatomic knee.

The socket is tilted approximately 5 degrees to enhance loading on the pressure-tolerant patellar ligament and reduce the vertical angulation of the amputation limb (Figure 4-11). Dynamic alignment is performed with the shoe on the prosthetic foot; heel height markedly influences walking comfort and performance. Ordinarily, the socket is placed directly over the foot. If, however, the patient has poor control of the knee, the socket will be placed slightly posterior to the foot. Such alignment shifts the line of gravity anterior to the anatomic knee, thus increasing knee stability. Conversely, if the patient is exceptionally strong and active, the socket may be aligned slightly anterior to the foot, so that the individual can flex the knee easily (Figure 4-12).

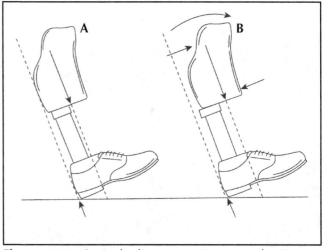

Figure 4-12. Sagittal alignment. (A) Normal. (B) Foot posterior.

Heel wedging reduces pressure on the patellar ligament while increasing pressure on the distal tibia when wearers stand and walk.[8] Alignment also influences the wearer's ability to walk on sloped surfaces.[9]

Frontal Plane

Frontal alignment serves primarily to increase comfort and, secondarily, to maintain a relatively narrow walking base. The socket is placed on the wood block in about 5 degrees of adduction to diminish load on the fibular head. On the adjustable leg, the socket is generally aligned so that the prosthetic foot is slightly

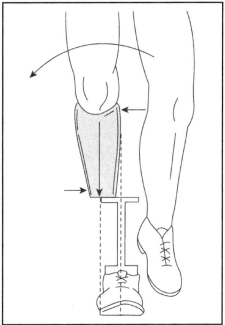

Figure 4-14. Frontal alignment, medial foot placement, and socket on shank.

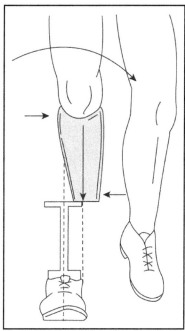

Figure 4-15. Frontal alignment, lateral foot placement.

medial to the socket (foot inset; Figure 4-14); such placement further reduces proximolateral load and keeps the walking base within the normal 2- to 4-inch range. Excessively medial placement of the prosthetic foot would increase pressure on the sensitive distal end of the fibula. Lateral foot placement (foot outset; Figure 4-15) is occasionally indicated to increase mediolateral standing stability; however, such alignment increases pressure on the fibular head.

REFERENCES

1. Yigiter K, Senar G, Bayar K. Comparison of the effects of patellar tendon bearing and total surface bearing sockets on prosthetic fitting and rehabilitation. *Prosthet Orthot Int.* 2002;26:206-212.

2. Hachisuka K, Dozono K, Ogata H, et al. Total surface bearing below-knee prosthesis: advantages, disadvantages, and clinical implications. *Arch Phys Med Rehabil.* 1998;79:783-789.

3. Selles RW, Janssens PJ, Jongenengel CD, Bussmann JB. A randomized controlled trial comparing functional outcome and cost efficiency of a total surface-bearing socket versus a conventional patellar tendon-bearing socket in transtibial amputees. *Arch Phys Med Rehabil.* 2005;86: 154-161.

4. Chow DH, Holmes AD, Lee CK, Sin SW. The effect of prosthesis alignment on the symmetry of gait in subjects with unilateral transtibial amputation. *Prosthet Orthot Int.* 2006;30:114-128.

5. Schmalz T, Blumentritt S, Jarasch R. Energy expenditure and biomechanical characteristics of lower limb amputee gait: the influence of prosthetic alignment and different prosthetic components. *Gait Posture.* 2002;16:255-263.

6. Jia X, Suo S, Meng F, Wang R. Effects of alignment on interface pressure for transtibial amputee during walking. *Disabil Rehabil Assist Technol.* 2008;3:339-343.

7. Dou P, Jia X, Suo S, et al. Pressure distribution at the stump/socket interface in transtibial amputees during walking on stairs, slope and non-flat road. *Clin Biomech (Bristol, Avon).* 2006;21:1067-1073.

8. Seelen HA, Anemaat S, Janssen HM, Deckers JH. Effects of prosthesis alignment on pressure distribution at the stump/socket interface in transtibial amputees during unsupported stance and gait. *Clin Rehabil.* 2003;17:787-796.

9. Sin SW, Chow DH, Cheng JC. Significance of non-level walking on transtibial prosthesis fitting with particular reference to the effects of anterior-posterior alignment. *J Rehabil Res Dev.* 2001;38:1-6.

Chapter 5

Transtibial Static Evaluation

Evaluation, sometimes referred to as *checkout*, of the fit and construction of the prosthesis and the patient's function while wearing it is essential to rehabilitation. The goal of evaluation is to ensure that the patient has the best possible prosthesis so that the individual can achieve the maximum benefit from prosthetic rehabilitation and enjoy optimal function after rehabilitation is completed.

Ideally, the evaluation is performed by the key members of the prosthetic clinic team (ie, the physician, physical therapist, and prosthetist). In the busy clinic, however, the therapist often examines each aspect of prosthetic fit and function and summarizes the results for the other personnel. Each department is apt to have some variation in role for each staff member.

For the patient who receives his or her first prosthesis, a comprehensive evaluation should be conducted twice. Initial evaluation is performed when the prosthesis is delivered and the patient has achieved wound healing and has regained sufficient strength and joint flexibility to make good use of the prosthesis. If all items in the evaluation are found to be satisfactory, the rating is *pass* and the patient proceeds to prosthetic training. If 1 or more items are unsatisfactory and if these unsatisfactory items will not interfere with gait training, the rating is *provisional pass* (eg, if the stitching on the supracondylar cuff is faulty, this fault will not compromise balance and walking). In contrast, if one or more items are unsatisfactory and will interfere with the patient's comfort or function, the appropriate rating is *fail*. If, for example, the socket is so tight that the patient cannot don it, the socket must be adjusted before the individual proceeds to gait training.

Final evaluation should occur when the patient has completed basic rehabilitation (ie, donning, transfers, and walking on level surfaces). The procedure is the same as for the initial evaluation, although additional attention should be directed at the individual's gait. If all items in the evaluation are found to be satisfactory,

the rating is pass, and the patient can be discharged. If any items, whether pertaining to socket fit and prosthetic alignment or referable to construction of the prosthesis, are found to be unsatisfactory, the rating is fail. Ideally, the patient would not be discharged from active training until all problems are resolved.

At both evaluations, the patient should wear the number of socks or liners provided by the prosthetist and should wear the same style of shoes for which the prosthesis was made. Shoes should match and be in good repair. Prior to prosthetic evaluation, examine the skin of the amputation limb, noting any scars or other discolored areas.

To expedite the evaluation, the clinician should have a checklist listing the following questions, as well as 2 sheets of paper, several pieces of plywood approximately 9 × 12 × 0.5-inch, a ruler, a piece of colored chalk, modeling clay, an armless chair, and a table.

The following evaluation is intended for the person wearing a unilateral prosthesis. If the patient wears bilateral prostheses, the items comparing the prosthesis with the sound limb should be modified to compare the right with the left prosthesis.

1. Is the prosthesis as prescribed? Verify that the foot, shank, socket, and suspension are the same as in the prescription. Occasionally, the clinical team determines that the patient would benefit from different components; if the change is reflected in an amended prescription, then the prosthesis is satisfactory. If not, the prosthesis must include the prescribed components.

2. Can the patient don the prosthesis easily? Although the patient has not been trained to don the prosthesis, the individual should be able to insert the amputation limb into the socket with minimal difficulty. At the time of the final evaluation, the person should be able to don the prosthesis accurately, independently, and rapidly.

Edelstein JE, Muroz A.
Lower-Limb Prosthetics and Orthotics: Clinical Concepts (pp 39-44).
© 2011 Taylor & Francis Group.

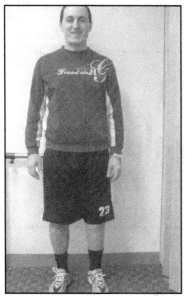

Figure 5-1. Man standing facing forward.

> If the patient cannot don the prosthesis easily, the socket may need adjustment.

STANDING

3. Is the patient comfortable when standing with the heel midlines 6 inches (15 cm) apart? The patient should stand in the best obtainable posture with minimal support facing forward (Figure 5-1). Feet should be on a line parallel with the shoulders. Feet may be separated so that the midlines are approximately 6 inches, representing a compromise between the normal walking base of 2 to 4 inches and a standing at ease position with feet in line with the shoulders. Record the patient's comments about overall comfort.

> If the individual complains of discomfort, note specific painful areas. Responses to other items in the evaluation, including examination of the amputation limb when the prosthesis is removed, will confirm or refute the response to this item.

> Anterodistal pain may be caused by a loose socket, allowing the amputation limb to bear too much load distally. Have the patient remove the prosthesis. Examine the distal end of the amputation limb (redness indicates pressure), then place a pea-sized ball of clay in the bottom of the socket, reapply the prosthesis, and ask the patient to stand for a few minutes. Remove the socket a second time to determine whether the clay has been flattened, indicating high distal force. Adding a sock will reduce socket looseness. Paradoxically, an unduly snug socket can also cause anterodistal pain if the amputation limb cannot fit fully into the socket; either a sock should be removed or the socket interior adjusted.

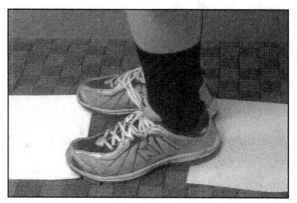

Figure 5-2. Side view of man standing with paper slid under the anterior and posterior portions of the shoe on the prosthesis.

> Anteroproximal pain over the patellar ligament may result from a patellar bulge that is excessively prominent. Anterior pain over the tibial crest can result from insufficient relief for this sensitive structure.

> Proximolateral pain suggests an insufficient relief for the head of the fibula or outset of the prosthetic foot.

4. Is the anterior-posterior alignment satisfactory? The patient should remain in the same position as for item #3. Place a piece of paper under both heels and note whether the paper can be slid an equal distance forward (Figure 5-2). Place a sheet of paper under both forefeet and note whether the paper can be slid an equal distance posteriorly. Ideally, the wearer should place equal weight on both feet. If the individual has a knee flexion contracture, the heel on the prosthetic side will be slightly raised.

> If, in the absence of contracture, the heel is raised, then the patient is bearing excessive weight anteriorly, jeopardizing knee stability and the alignment should be adjusted. If the prosthetic forefoot is raised, weight has shifted posteriorly, making it difficult for the wearer to flex the knee during walking; therefore, the alignment may be faulty.

5. Is the medial-lateral alignment satisfactory? The patient should remain in the same position as for item #3. Slide one sheet of paper under the medial border of the foot on the amputated side and the other sheet under the lateral border (Figure 5-3). The patient should bear weight equally on both shoe borders.

> If paper can be slid under the lateral border, the patient is bearing excessive weight on the medial shoe border and may complain of proximolateral pain in the amputation limb. Conversely, if paper can be slid under the medial border, the lateral border is bearing too much weight. This condition may be associated with distolateral pain. Alignment should be altered.

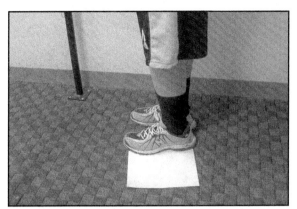

Figure 5-3. Front view of man standing with paper slid under the medial and lateral borders of the shoe on the prosthesis.

6. Do the contours and color of the prosthesis match the opposite limb? Compare the shape and color of the prosthesis with that of the sound limb and note any marked disparity.

➢ If there is a considerable difference, reserve judgment until item #18, which pertains to the patient's appraisal of the prosthesis.

7. Is the prosthesis the correct length? The patient should stand in the same position as specified for item #3. Ask the individual to bend forward, then assess the symmetry of the torso. If the person does not have a fixed scoliosis, compare the heights of the anterior superior iliac spines, the iliac crests, and the posterior superior iliac spines. If both spines are not parallel with the floor, place as many pieces of plywood under the shorter leg as needed to place the pelvis in the level position.

➢ Measure the height of the plywood (Figure 5-4); if less than 0.5-inch (1 cm), the prosthesis is most likely to be the proper height.

➢ If the patient requires more than a 0.5-inch lift under the prosthesis, any of the following aspects of the prosthesis may be deficient:

  ¤ The socket is too loose, causing the amputation limb to bear excessive weight distally. Usually the patient will complain of distal pain. Additional socks may alleviate the problem; otherwise, the socket needs adjustment.

  ¤ The heel on the prosthetic foot is too soft. The prosthesis will appear too short and the patient will likely shift weight posteriorly. Verify the adequacy of the heel during gait analysis. A soft heel will cause the patient to walk with limited knee flexion.

  ¤ The shank may be too short. The clinician has no reference points to measure shank length in a cosmetically finished prosthesis. In the absence of other deficiencies, one may infer that the shank is too short.

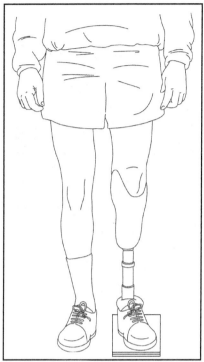

Figure 5-4. Front view of man standing on 2 plywood boards. Note the level position of iliac crests.

➢ If the patient requires more than 0.5-inch lift under the sound leg,

  ¤ The socket is too tight, preventing the amputation limb from lodging correctly in the socket. The wearer may complain of circumferential or proximal pain. If adjustment of sock thickness does not correct the problem, the socket will have to be adjusted.

  ¤ The heel on the prosthetic foot is too firm. The patient may shift weight anteriorly and will tend to walk with excessive knee flexion.

  ¤ The shank may be too long.

8. Is piston action minimal? Mark a chalk line along the posterior portion of the sock or liner along the edge of the socket (Figure 5-5). Ask the wearer to elevate the pelvis on the amputated side. Note whether the socket drops below the chalk line. If the shift is less than 0.5-inch, the prosthesis is probably satisfactory. If the prosthesis has thigh corset suspension, it is likely that the shift may be as much as 0.5-inch because the fixed single-axis side joints cannot coincide with the variable anatomic knee axis. Side joints are customarily set slightly above the anatomic knee axis to prevent the amputation limb from shifting downward when the patient sits.

➢ If the socket lowers more than 0.5-inch, check for the following deficiencies:

  ¤ (a) The socket is too loose. If additional socks do not restore adequate snugness, then the socket needs to be adjusted.

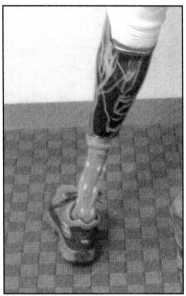

Figure 5-5. Posterior view of socket showing a chalk line on the sock along the posterior brim.

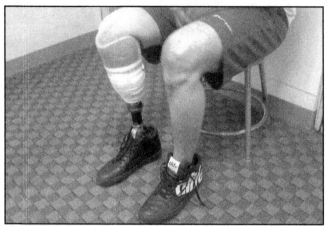

Figure 5-6. Side view of man sitting on straight chair with knee on prosthetic side flexed 90 degrees.

¤ Suspension is inadequate. The cuff may not be attached to the socket at the appropriate sites. The distal pin or lanyard may not be engaged properly.

9. Does the socket contact the amputation limb without pinching or gapping? Check the anterior margins of the socket, noting any areas of gapping or pinching. Ask the wearer whether he or she feels the socket on all areas of the amputation limb.

➢ Pinching is likely to be uncomfortable. Gapping may cause the socket to shift on the amputation limb as the user walks, impacting the opposite aspect of the limb. If the excessive or insufficient contact cannot be remedied by adjusting sock thickness, the socket needs adjustment. If the patient comments on excessive or insufficient pressure within the socket, verify the complaint with item #19: skin inspection. Socket adjustment may be required.

SUSPENSION

10. Does the thigh corset fit the thigh properly? Examine the margins of the thigh corset to determine whether there is undue soft tissue overhanging the corset. An obese patient is likely to have such overhang; however, the corset must fit comfortably.

➢ If the wearer has uncomfortable overhang, the shape of the corset or its placement on the side bars may require alteration.

11. Does the cuff, fork strap, or thigh corset have adequate provision for adjustment? Check to make certain that the patient can tighten and loosen the suspension component.

➢ If the suspension component is set at the tightest or loosest hole or end of the hook and pile strap, the component should be adjusted to provide for the user's possible future needs.

SITTING

12. Can the patient sit comfortably with hips and knees flexed 90 degrees? Ask the patient to sit in an adult-sized, unupholstered, straight chair (Figure 5-6). Posture should be symmetrical with both hips and both knees flexed 90 degrees. Feet should be flat on the floor. Record the wearer's comments about sitting comfort.

➢ If the patient complains of discomfort, ask the individual to specify the painful area(s). Anterodistal pain may be alleviated by altering the socket, increasing the relief in this area. Posteroproximal pain may be caused by impingement of the socket brim into the popliteal fossa. Sometimes, deepening the socket curvature by the medial hamstring tendons suffices. As a last resort, the entire posterior brim may have to be lowered. If the prosthesis includes a thigh corset, check to detect whether the posterodistal margin of the corset is exerting undue pressure; if so, the prosthetist may need to adjust the corset.

WALKING

13. Is the patient's performance in level walking satisfactory? Although the individual who receives his or her first prosthesis will not have had much gait training, the prosthetist will have guided the patient through a few steps in order to accomplish the alignment procedure. Judgments made at the initial evaluation are tentative; however, any gross gait abnormalities should be recorded. Chapter 3 details gait problems encountered by some people who wear transtibial prostheses.

14. Is the patient's performance on stairs and ramps satisfactory? This item can be omitted at the initial evaluation. If the patient has a marginal functional prognosis, such as K1, the item is also irrelevant. Otherwise, the patient should demonstrate confidence on stairs and ramps.

➤ The individual who is unable to traverse stairs and ramps safely may require additional training.

15. Can the patient kneel satisfactorily? (Figure 5-7) This item may be omitted for those at the K1 level. For other wearers, first ask the person to sit on a straight, armless chair and then slide to the amputated side, so that only the buttock on the intact side rests on the chair. Have the individual extend the hip and flex the knee on the amputated side simulating kneeling.

➤ If the person cannot flex the knee fully, the posterior border of the socket may be encroaching into the popliteal fossa. If so, the socket will have to be adjusted.

16. Does the suspension function properly? Observe the suspension component, particularly cuff, elastic sleeve, and thigh corset, to note any slippage as the patient walks. The person who has distal pin, supracondylar brim, or supracondylar-suprapatellar brim suspension should be able to walk without untoward shifting of the prosthesis.

➤ If the suspension appears inadequate, the component usually requires adjustment.

17. Does the prosthesis operate quietly? Listen to the prosthesis as the patient walks. If the prosthesis includes an articulated foot or a thigh corset, listen for metallic noises indicating excessive contact between joint surfaces.

➤ A prosthesis that is unacceptably noisy usually requires maintenance.

18. Does the patient consider the prosthesis satisfactory regarding comfort, function, and appearance? Solicit the patient's opinion, noting any favorable and unfavorable comments. The new wearer may be disappointed in the appearance or function of the prosthesis; however, with experience and emotional adjustment to prosthetic use, many complaints resolve spontaneously.

➤ If the patient is dissatisfied, referral to the prosthetic clinic team is indicated. Problems that are identified should be resolved.

PROSTHESIS OFF THE PATIENT

19. Is the skin free of abrasions or other discolorations attributable to this prosthesis? Compare the examination of the skin of the amputation limb after prosthetic wear with the examination conducted prior to donning the prosthesis, looking for any new color changes.

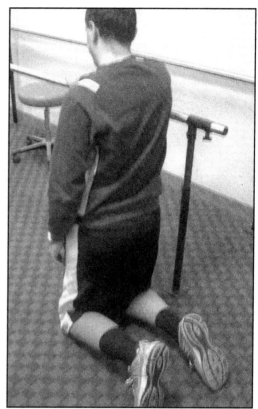

Figure 5-7. Kneeling with plantar flexion of the intact right ankle.

➤ Redness persisting for more than 10 minutes may necessitate adjustment of the socket.

20. Is the socket interior smooth? The clinician should touch all portions of the socket to determine whether any roughness exists, particularly if a suspension component has been riveted through the socket.

➤ A socket that has any coarse areas should have those areas smoothed.

21. Is the posterior wall of the socket of adequate height? Stand the prosthesis, including the shoe, on the table. Place the end of a ruler at the point of maximum indentation over the patellar ligament and rest the remainder of the ruler on the midpoint of the posterior brim. The ruler should be level with the table or slightly angled upward at the posterior brim, indicating that the anterior wall exerts adequate posteriorly directed force on the amputation limb (Figure 5-8).

➤ If the ruler is angled downward at the posterior brim, the posterior wall may be too low. The socket may need adjustment.

22. Is the construction satisfactory? Check for uniformity of stitching. Determine whether the plastic portions are uniform. If the prosthesis has an articulated foot, look for a thin leather guard surrounding the ankle. Check all rivets and other fasteners for smooth placement.

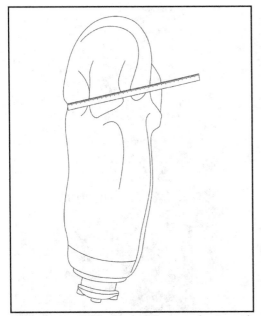

Figure 5-8. Side view of the prosthesis with the end of a ruler positioned on apex of patellar bulge and the midportion of the ruler resting on the posterior brim.

Durability is particularly important for prostheses fitted to obese patients, regardless of the person's age.[1]

➤ Any construction deficiencies should be rectified.

23. Do all components function satisfactorily? If the prosthesis has pin suspension, make certain that the pin engages the lock easily. If the foot has any adjustment feature, check that it is easy to operate.

➤ Any functional deficiencies should be rectified.

REFERENCE

1. Haboubi NHJ, Heelis M, Woodruff R, Al-Khawaja I. The effect of body weight and age on frequency of repairs in lower-limb prostheses. *J Rehabil Res Dev.* 2001;38:375-377.

Chapter 6

Transtibial Gait Analysis

In the community, some individuals walk with a transtibial prosthesis in a manner virtually undetectable from able-bodied adults. In a gait laboratory, however, prosthesis wearers exhibit kinematic and kinetic differences from nonprosthetic gait. Most of the published studies do not specify the components of the prostheses worn by research subjects since the number of subjects is usually less than 20 and their ages and overall health are diverse. Gait alterations can be attributed to asymmetrical weight of the intact and prosthetic legs and disparate function of the sound and prosthetic foot. Additionally, because the prosthetic socket surrounds the exterior of the amputation limb, soft tissue displacement within the socket reduces the normal stabilization provided by an intact skeleton. The patient with a short amputation limb, or one who has poor balance, is at a greater disadvantage than someone who has a longer amputation limb or a person who has good balance.

TYPICAL TRANSTIBIAL GAIT

Laboratory studies demonstrate that prosthesis wearers exhibit longer swing time, and shorter stance time and single support time on the prosthesis.[1] Walking with a prosthesis incurs more loading on the intact limb, prolonging the period of propulsive force production in the intact limb.[2] Wearers show hyperactive hip extensor activity to compensate for absent plantar flexor contraction.[3,4] Other asymmetries include a longer prosthetic step length[5] and reduced knee extensor activity on the amputated side.[6,7] These differences are also evident when subjects walk on a ramp.[8] People who wear transtibial prostheses walked somewhat slowly; when they walked faster, temporal asymmetry reduced but loading asymmetry increased as subjects put more stress on the sound limb.[9]

The type of prosthetic foot and material of the shoe sole affect gait. Though foot action was quite similar among prosthetic feet, rubber-soled shoes produced substantially more shock absorption than did leather shoes. Patients tended to remain on the prosthetic heel longer than normal, delaying foot flat stability; the solid ankle, cushion heel foot (SACH; Otto Bock, Minneapolis, Minnesota; Kingsley, Costa Mesa, California) demonstrated the longest heel duration, whereas the single-axis caused the briefest. Patients tend to reduce knee flexion in early stance on the amputated side for a longer than normal period, while hip flexion is slightly greater.[10] Heavier feet increase muscular effort and interface forces between the amputation limb and the socket during walking.[11]

CLINICAL GAIT ANALYSIS

Clinical gait analysis focuses on readily observable gait abnormalities, which may indicate socket discomfort, faulty alignment, inadequate balance, or any combination of these problems. Dynamic evaluation, also known as *gait analysis*, is an important part of assessing the adequacy of prosthetic rehabilitation.

The patient should have an unobstructed walkway, at least 15 feet long. Ideally, the walkway would be a raised platform at eye level to the observer. In most situations, however, this is not possible. Videotaping the walker is an excellent way of documenting performance and enables consulting with other clinicians at a later date. The examiner should view the patient from the rear, front, and amputated side.

Transtibial gait analysis focuses on the action of the knee on the prosthetic side during stance phase. Unless the prosthetic foot is in such poor condition that it fails to clear the floor, swing phase should not be impeded.

Edelstein JE, Muroz A.
Lower-Limb Prosthetics and Orthotics: Clinical Concepts (pp 45-48).
© 2011 Taylor & Francis Group.

ABNORMAL TRANSTIBIAL GAIT

Sagittal Plane Analysis

Ordinarily, the knee on the prosthetic side should flex slightly in early stance and then move to nearly full extension at midstance, followed by slight flexion in late stance. The observer should view the prosthetic side.

Early Stance

➢ Insufficient knee flexion; the floor reaction passes anterior to the knee.

    ¤ Anatomic/physiologic causes include the following:

      » Anterodistal pain—Patient who fears bending the knee may exaggerate knee extension, thus causing excessive pressure on the distal end of the tibia.

      » Poor balance—Patient fears allowing the ipsilateral knee to flex.

      » Extensor synergy, seen in patients who have cerebrovascular accident in addition to amputation.

      » Knee extensor contracture.

      » Knee extensor weakness—Patient compensates by forcing the knee posteriorly.

    ¤ Prosthetic causes include the following:

      » Shoe that has a lower heel or a more resilient heel than that for which the prosthesis had been aligned.

      » Prosthetic foot that has a heel cushion that is too resilient.

      » Prosthetic foot malaligned in plantar flexion. Shank should be perpendicular to the floor in the sagittal and frontal planes.

      » Socket malaligned in insufficient flexion.

      » Socket malaligned posterior in relation to the prosthetic foot.

      » Suspension that interferes with knee flexion.

➢ Excessive knee flexion (*buckling*); the floor reaction passes posterior to the knee.

    ¤ Anatomic/physiologic causes include the following:

      » Knee extensor weakness.

      » Knee flexor contracture.

    ¤ Prosthetic causes include the following:

      » Shoe that has a higher heel or a firmer heel than that for which the prosthesis had been aligned.

      » Prosthetic foot that has too firm a heel cushion.

      » Prosthetic foot malaligned in dorsiflexion.

      » Socket malaligned in excessive flexion.

      » Socket malaligned anterior in relation to the prosthetic foot.

      » Suspension that causes knee flexion.

      » Prosthesis too long.

Late Stance

➢ Early knee flexion (*drop off*); floor reaction passes posterior to the knee.

    ¤ Anatomic, physiologic, and prosthetic causes include the following:

      » Most of the factors identified with excessive knee flexion in early stance cause this late stance deviation. Height of the shoe heel and the resilience of the prosthetic heel cushion, however, are not relevant at late stance.

➢ Delayed knee flexion (*climbing the hill*); the floor reaction passes anterior to the knee.

    ¤ Anatomic, physiologic, and prosthetic causes include the following:

      » Problems associated with insufficient flexion in early stance, except for the shoe heel and prosthetic heel cushion, can also cause this late stance abnormality.

➢ Step length discrepancy; prosthetic step is longer than step with sound foot.

    ¤ Anatomic/physiologic causes include the following:

      » Hip and/or knee flexor contracture.

      » Poor balance.

      » Pain in amputation limb.

    ¤ Prosthetic causes include the following:

      » Prosthesis too long.

Frontal Plane Analysis

Ordinarily, at midstance during single support on the prosthesis, the knee shifts slightly within the prosthesis. Shift is inevitable as the rigid portion of the socket compresses the soft tissues of the amputation limb. Movement of the prosthetic socket brim is known as *thrust*.

Usually, the prosthesis is aligned to position the floor reaction medial to the knee, increasing load on the pressure-tolerant proximomedial aspect of the amputation limb. If the patient walks with a cane, or if the prosthesis has an elastic sleeve, distal pin, or suction suspension, thrust will be less conspicuous.

The observer should stand behind the patient, noting the movement of the knee in relation to the socket during midstance on the prosthesis.

> Excessive lateral thrust; brim shifts laterally to a marked extent. Floor reaction passes medial to the knee. This may cause reddening of the proximomedial aspect of the amputation limb and, possibly, discomfort in this area.
  ⌑ Prosthetic causes include the following:
    » Excessive adduction of the socket.
    » Excessive lateral displacement of the socket (foot inset).
> Medial thrust. Floor reaction passes lateral to the knee. Patient is apt to complain about too much pressure on the fibular head and will probably walk with a wide base.
  ⌑ Prosthetic causes include the following:
    » Socket abduction.
    » Medial displacement of the socket (foot outset).

Frontal plane abnormalities are rarely caused by anatomic or physiologic factors.

TROUBLE-SHOOTING GAIT PROBLEMS

> Gait disorders related to anatomic/physiologic causes:
  ⌑ Anterodistal pain: Insufficient knee flexion, delayed knee flexion.
  ⌑ Poor balance: Insufficient knee flexion, delayed knee flexion, long prosthetic step.
  ⌑ Extensor synergy: Insufficient knee flexion, delayed knee flexion.
  ⌑ Hip flexor contracture: Long prosthetic step.
  ⌑ Knee extensor contracture: Insufficient knee flexion, delayed knee flexion.
  ⌑ Knee extensor weakness: Excessive knee flexion, insufficient knee flexion, early knee flexion.
  ⌑ Knee flexor contracture: Excessive knee flexion, early knee flexion, long prosthetic step.
  ⌑ Pain in amputation limb: Long prosthetic step.
> Gait disorders related to prosthetic causes:
  ⌑ Suspension inferring with knee flexion: Insufficient knee flexion, delayed knee flexion.
  ⌑ Suspension causing knee flexion: Excessive knee flexion, early knee flexion.
  ⌑ Socket malaligned in insufficient flexion: Insufficient knee flexion, delayed knee flexion.
  ⌑ Socket malaligned in excessive flexion: Excessive knee flexion, early knee flexion.

⌑ Socket malaligned posterior to prosthetic foot: Insufficient knee flexion, delayed knee flexion.
⌑ Socket malaligned anterior to prosthetic foot: Excessive knee flexion, early knee flexion.
⌑ Socket malaligned in excessive adduction: Excessive lateral thrust.
⌑ Socket malaligned in abduction: Medial thrust.
⌑ Prosthetic foot heel cushion too resilient: Insufficient knee flexion.
⌑ Prosthetic foot heel cushion too stiff: Excessive knee flexion.
⌑ Prosthetic foot malaligned in plantar flexion: Insufficient knee flexion, delayed knee flexion.
⌑ Prosthetic foot malaligned in dorsiflexion: Excessive knee flexion, early knee flexion.
⌑ Prosthetic foot excessively outset: Medial thrust.
⌑ Prosthetic foot excessively inset: Excessive lateral thrust.
⌑ Shoe heel lower than that for which prosthesis was aligned: Insufficient knee flexion.
⌑ Shoe heel higher than that for which prosthesis was aligned: Excessive knee flexion.
⌑ Prosthesis too long: Excessive knee flexion, long prosthetic step.
⌑ Prosthesis too short: Insufficient knee flexion.

REFERENCES

1. Isakov E, Keren O, Benjuya N. Trans-tibial amputee gait: time-distance parameters and EMG activity. *Prosthet Orthot Int.* 2000;24:216-220.
2. Vrieling AH, van Keeken HG, Schoppen T, et al. Gait initiation in lower limb amputees. *Gait Posture.* 2008;27: 423-430.
3. Winter DA, Sienko SE. Biomechanics of below-knee amputee gait. *J Biomech.* 1988;21:361-367.
4. Grumillier C, Martinet N, Paysant J, et al. Compensatory mechanism involving the hip joint of the intact limb during gait in unilateral trans-tibial amputees. *J Biomech.* 2008; 41:2926-2931.
5. Tesio L, Lanzi D, Detrembleur C. The 3-D motion of the centre of gravity of the human body during level walking. II. Lower limb amputees. *Clin Biomech (Bristol, Avon).* 1998;13:83-90.
6. Vanicek N, Strike S, McNaughton L, Polman R. Gait patterns in transtibial amputee fallers vs non-fallers: biomechanical differences during level walking. *Gait Posture.* 2008;27:415-420.

7. Royer TD, Wasilewski CA. Hip and knee frontal plane moments in persons with unilateral, trans-tibial amputation. *Gait Posture*. 2006;23:303-306.

8. Vickers DR, Palk C, McIntosh AS, Beatty KT. Elderly unilateral transtibial amputee gait on an inclined walkway: a biomechanical analysis. *Gait Posture*. 2008;27: 518-529.

9. Nolan L, Wit A, Dudzinski K, et al. Adjustments in gait symmetry with walking speed in transfemoral and transtibial amputees. *Gait Posture*. 2003;17:142-151.

10. Perry J. Amputee gait. In: Smith D, Michael J, Bowker J, eds. *Atlas of Amputations and Limb Deficiencies*. 3rd ed. Rosemont, IL: American Academy of Orthopedic Surgeons; 2004:367-375.

11. Selles R, Bussmann J, Van Soest AJ, Stam H. The effect of prosthetic mass properties on the gait of transtibial amputees: a mathematical model. *Disabil Rehabil*. 2004;26:694-704.

Chapter 7

Transfemoral Prostheses

Transfemoral prostheses (Figure 7-1) consist of the following 5 major components:

1. Foot-ankle assembly
2. Shank
3. Knee unit
4. Socket
5. Suspension

As with every prosthesis, prescription of each component for a particular patient depends on the physical examination[1] and the person's fiscal assets.

FOOT-ANKLE ASSEMBLY

Any foot-ankle assembly can be used with most transfemoral prostheses. Feet with a shank component, for example, Flex-Foot (Ossur, Aliso Viejo, California), are suitable because there is no restriction on the length of the transfemoral shank. Energy-storing foot-ankle units enabled a small sample of transfemoral prosthesis wearers to walk faster than with nondynamic feet.[2] Walking with an ankle with restricted sagittal mobility is associated with relatively great prosthetic knee flexion.[3] Some knee units, however, must be used with a particular prosthetic foot. These limitations are included in the discussion of knee units.

SHANK

The relatively light weight of the endoskeletal shank presents a distinct advantage for the transfemoral prosthesis. Because the shank is a smaller part of the transtibial prosthesis, the weight difference between endo- and exoskeletal shanks is minimal. In contrast, in a transfemoral prosthesis, the shank is full length and thus heavier. The endoskeletal shank also enables minor changes in alignment of the prosthesis. The same array of vertical and transverse shock absorbers noted in Chapter 3 are applicable to transfemoral prostheses for active wearers. The transverse shock absorber is likely to reduce shear stress between the socket and the thigh.[4]

KNEE UNIT

Virtually all transfemoral prostheses include a knee unit. The rare exception pertains to a prosthesis for a young child with a transfemoral amputation or limb deficiency. The first prosthesis may consist of a socket attached to an elongated shank, with suspension and a foot; the simple prosthesis is easy for the youngster to control.

Knee units are mass-produced in sizes to suit toddlers through adults. The units may have one or more of the following features:

➤ *Axis:* Connection between thigh and shank.
➤ *Friction mechanism:* Controls shank movement during swing phase.
➤ *Extension aid:* Assists shank extension during the latter part of swing phase.
➤ *Stabilizer:* Mechanism that resists knee flexion during stance phase.
➤ *Extension mechanism:* Motor that extends the knee during stance phase.

Although all knee mechanisms connect the thigh section to the shank by means of an axis, they may or may not have other features. Many combinations of features are present in contemporary knee units.

Axis

The more common connection is a single axis (Figure 7-2). The shank swings on a transverse bolt. This axis is relatively simple and is used with many other knee attributes.

Edelstein JE, Muroz A.
Lower-Limb Prosthetics and Orthotics: Clinical Concepts (pp 49-60).
© 2011 Taylor & Francis Group.

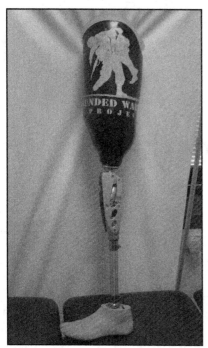

Figure 7-1. Transfemoral prosthesis.

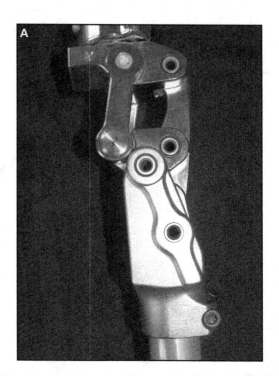

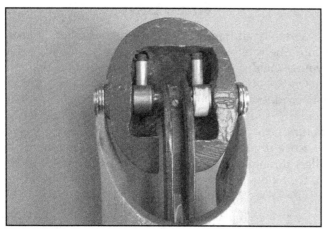

Figure 7-2. Single-axis knee unit.

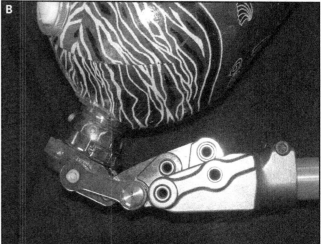

Figure 7-3. Polycentric axis. (A) Extended. (B) Flexed.

The alternate axis is polycentric (Figure 7-3). It consists of 2 or more pairs of bars that pivot proximally and distally. A 4-bar linkage has 2 bars on the medial side of the unit and 2 bars on the lateral side. The top and bottom of each bar pivots on the frame of the knee unit. Unlike the single-axis unit, which has a fixed center of knee rotation, polycentric knee units have a changing axis. As the patient causes the knee to bend, the axis of rotation shifts. The momentary axis is the point of intersection between lines drawn through the proximal and distal pivots of each pair of bars. Other polycentric units have 6 or more pairs of bars.

Two advantages of polycentric units are (1) inherent stability and (2) reduction of shank protrusion when the wearer sits. Stability is achieved by the linkage system.

Through most of the range of knee flexion, the intersection of lines drawn through the pivots is proximal and posterior to the wearer's line of gravity. Consequently, the line of gravity passes anterior to the knee's center of rotation. Proximal location of the intersection is closer to the wearer's hip, facilitating knee unit control.

The knee unit is always distal to the socket. An individual with a long transfemoral amputation limb requires a relatively long socket. Consequently, the additional thickness of the knee unit may cause the socket-knee unit length to exceed the length of the contralateral intact thigh. The asymmetry is most apparent when the wearer sits. The linkage causes the pivoting bars to shift posteriorly, making sitting posture more symmetrical.

Friction

During swing phase, the transfemoral prosthesis behaves like a compound pendulum, with the upper pivot at the anatomic hip and the lower pivot at the knee. If no friction mechanism interferes with the pendular action, the person who walks rapidly will demonstrate movement of the prosthesis that differs from that of the sound leg. During early swing, prosthetic knee flexion is more acute (known as *high heel rise*), and during late swing phase, the prosthetic knee extends abruptly (*terminal impact*). A friction mechanism modifies the pendular action. Constant friction refers to a mechanism that resists shank motion throughout swing phase. The most common design consists of a pair of clamps on the knee bolt (Figure 7-4). The tighter the clamps, the greater the friction. Variable friction occurs when a mechanism resists early and late swing phase more than midswing, mimicking the action of the anatomic knee. In early swing phase, anatomic knee flexion is resisted passively by the viscoelasticity of the quadriceps. In late swing phase, the hamstring muscles actively resist knee extension.

Closely related to the time(s) when friction is applied, whether constant or variable, is the medium that provides friction. A sliding (mechanical) friction mechanism is exemplified by a pair of clamps gripping the knee bolt. The amount of friction does not change if the wearer walks slowly or rapidly. Sliding friction units are relatively simple, inexpensive, and lightweight and suit those at the K1 and K2 levels who are not expected to change walking velocity.

Variable friction (variable damping) is applied by a knee unit that resists the swing of the shank during early and late swing phase. Such knee units are available in both single-axis and polycentric axis models. Variable friction imitates the usual action of the intact knee. Normally, viscoelasticity of the quadriceps muscle resists excessive knee flexion in early swing phase, and active contraction of the hamstring muscles decelerates the swing of the leg during late swing phase. Variable friction units incorporate fluid, air (pneumatic), or oil (hydraulic).

Variable friction fluid units have a cylinder filled with fluid. A piston attached to the axis system moves up and down in the cylinder. During early swing phase, the piston descends. The ease of movement, and hence the amount of resistance, is governed by the type of fluid and the wearer's walking velocity. During late swing phase, the piston ascends. A pneumatic unit uses air as the resistive medium and is less expensive than hydraulic units. Air-filled units provide moderate resistance to the swing of the shank and are most suitable for moderately active wearers, such as K2 or K3. The units may not function optimally in very high altitudes and are not available in very small sizes.

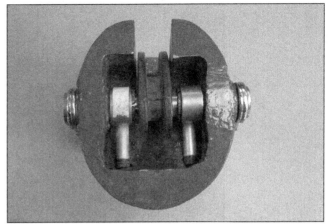

Figure 7-4. Sliding friction showing 2 clamps on the knee bolt.

A hydraulic unit has an oil-filled cylinder. Because oil is denser and more viscous than air, a hydraulic unit provides greater resistance to shank movement and is thus most appropriate for very active individuals, such as K3 or K4. Oil tends to become more viscous in extreme cold environments; however, if the patient flexes and extends the knee a few times, the internal temperature rises, reducing viscosity. Magnetized fluid can also be used as the resistive medium

All fluid units change friction automatically when the wearer changes walking velocity. Thus, fast gait results in greater resistance to the swing of the shank, minimizing the asymmetry between the arcs of the prosthetic and sound legs.

Extension Aid

Many knee units have a mechanism to assist the extension of the shank during the latter part of swing phase. The basic pendular action of the prosthesis would cause the knee to extend; however, some patients like the extra assistance provided by an extension aid so that stance phase on the prosthesis may begin with a fully extended knee. An external extension aid (kick strap) is elastic webbing that is attached to the anterior surface of the socket and the anterior surface of the shank. Knee flexion in early swing phase stretches the elastic. The strap recoils during late swing phase. An internal extension aid consists either of a rod and elastic webbing inside the knee unit (Figure 7-5) or springs (Figure 7-6). Either design resists early swing phase by moving the rod that stretches the webbing or by spring compression. In late swing phase, the webbing or spring recoils, causing the shank to extend.

Although the swing phase action of the external and internal extension aids is the same, action of the aids differs when the wearer sits. With an external extension aid, the prosthetic knee tends to remain extended,

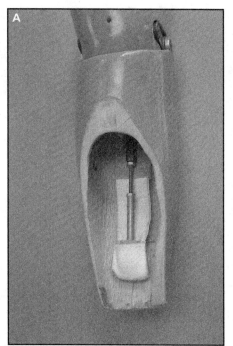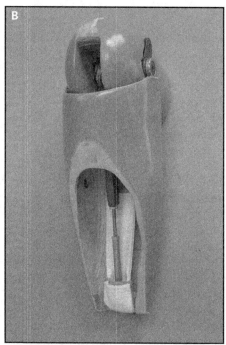

Figure 7-5. Internal extension aid. (A) Extension. (B) Flexion.

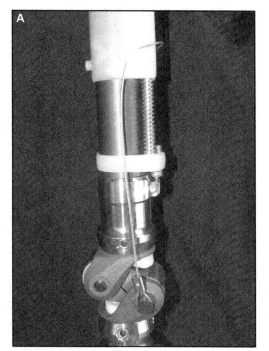

Figure 7-6. Spring extension aid. (A) Extension.
(B) Slight flexion. (C) Full flexion.

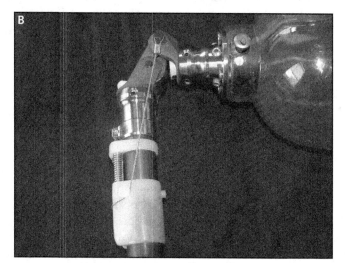

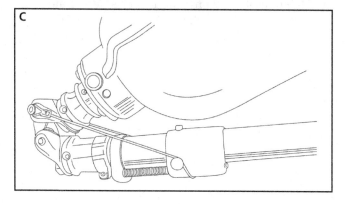

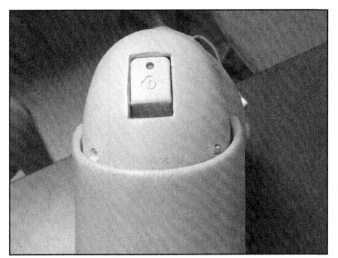

Figure 7-7. Manual lock.

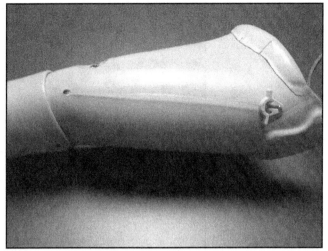

Figure 7-8. Pull cord lock release.

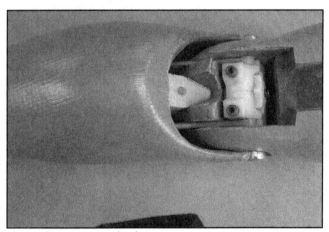

Figure 7-9. Friction brake.

until the individual uses the sound foot to nudge the prosthetic foot posteriorly. With an internal extension aid, when the prosthetic knee is flexed acutely, the aid maintains the knee flexed without any need to move the prosthetic foot. All fluid-controlled knee units incorporate internal extension aid springs. Patients at the K1 and K2 levels should have an extension aid because they tend to walk so slowly that the knee may not be fully extended at the end of swing phase.

Stabilizer

A few models of knee units include a mechanism that resists knee flexion during early and midstance phase. All people who wear transfemoral prostheses should be able to stand without collapse of the knee unit and should be able to bear weight on the prosthesis confidently. Stability can be achieved by aligning the components of the prosthesis so the knee unit is extended or by incorporating a polycentric knee unit. Some people, however, require the additional assistance of a stabilizer. The 2 basic types of stabilizer are a manual lock and a brake.

A manual lock is a spring-loaded knob that fits into a receptacle in the knee unit (Figure 7-7). The patient unlocks the unit by pulling on a lever attached to the knob (Figure 7-8). The manual lock is a simple, inexpensive mechanism that provides stability throughout the gait cycle. Though stability is desirable during early stance phase, the locked unit remains extended throughout the gait cycle. Thus, the individual has to walk with a stiff knee, which is especially conspicuous during swing phase. The wearer must disengage the lock when sitting. The manual lock is indicated for someone at the K1 level or anyone whose occupation requires standing for prolonged periods.

A brake is a mechanism that applies very high friction to resist knee flexion. A friction brake has a wedge that lodges into a curved groove (Figure 7-9). The groove is designed to accommodate the wedge when the wearer initiates stance phase when the prosthetic knee

is either fully extended or flexed through an angle that is no greater than approximately 25 degrees. Without a brake, if the person began stance phase with the prosthetic knee flexed, the prosthesis would be apt to collapse. With a brake, the individual has stability only during early and midstance; during late stance, swing phase, and sitting, the knee unit does not resist flexion. Individuals at the K1 or K2 levels may benefit from a friction brake, although the unit is relatively heavy.

Most hydraulic knee units provide stance control with a braking mechanism, protecting the patient from inadvertent knee flexion and enabling him or her to avoid stumbling. Stance control units also enable the person to select the manual lock mode or deactivate the brake for special activities such as bicycling. Examples of hydraulic units are the Mauch SNS (Swing 'N Stance) unit (Ossur; Figure 7-10) and the Endurance 160 Hydraulic Knee System (Fillauer, Chattanooga, Tennessee). Both of these units enable the user to select (a) swing and stance control, (b) manually locked knee, and (c) swing phase control by changing the position of a lever and applying the appropriate load to the prosthesis.

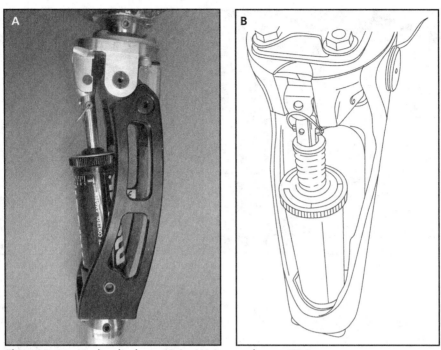

Figure 7-10. Hydraulic knee unit. (A) Lever down. (B) Lever up.

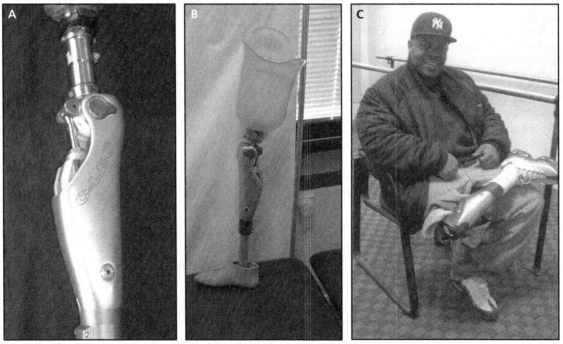

Figure 7-11. C-Leg. (A) Unit. (B) Prothesis. (C) Man sitting with knee rotated.

Electronically controlled knee units include stance control achieved with sensors that detect the tendency of the knee unit to flex and then adjust the braking action accordingly. The knee may have hydraulic control, such as the C-Leg (Otto Bock, Minneapolis, Minnesota; Figure 7-11), which must be worn with the energy-storing C-Walk (Otto Bock). C-Leg's microprocessors gather information from strain gauges in the pylon and knee angle sensors; the data are processed electronically to create a signal to adjust the resistance of the knee, controlling swing phase angle and velocity. The sensors in the pylon determine loading at the heel, toe, and pylon, adjusting stance stability whether the patient is walking on level or uneven terrain, stairs, or slopes. The walker achieves slight prosthetic knee flexion in early stance phase. The individual can change the mode of the knee

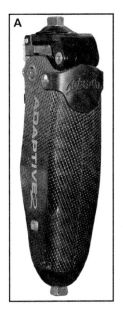
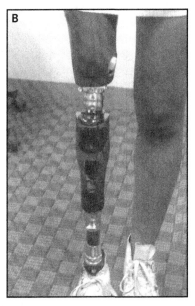
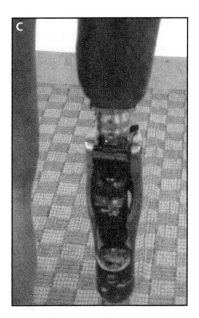
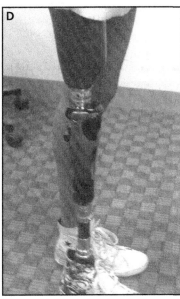
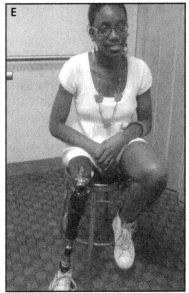

Figure 7-12. Adaptive 2 Knee. (A) Unit. (Reprinted with permission from Endolite.) (B) Anterior view. (C) Posterior view. (D) Lateral view. (E) Woman sitting.

from walking, standing on a locked knee, or freely swinging either by tapping the prosthetic toe while standing or using a handheld remote control. The Plié MPC knee (Freedom Innovations, Irvine, California) is another computerized hydraulic swing and stance control unit that allows the patient to select the amount of knee stiffness to suit the intended activity.

Other electronic knees combine pneumatic swing phase control with hydraulic stance control. The Intelligent Prosthesis and the Adaptive 2 Knee (Endolite, Miamisburg, Ohio; Figure 7-12) both include a pneumatic cylinder for swing phase control. The Self-Learning Knee (DAW, San Diego, California) has 4-bar linkage with pneumatic stance control and magnetized

swing control; the unit determines the walker's slowest and fastest speeds and adjusts accordingly. The Smart IP (Endolite) has mechanical stance control and pneumatic swing control.

A knee unit that utilizes magnetized fluid is the RHEO KNEE (Ossur; Figure 7-13). The magnetized fluid offers the patient proportional resistance to the force applied by the patient. The unit has force and angle sensors that respond to the wearer's gait pattern; the unit also incorporates a stabilizer mechanism.

Electronically controlled knee units are appropriate for active individuals at the K3 or, in some instances, the K4 level. The compact version of the C-Leg is designed for people at the K2 level. Some patients at K2 also

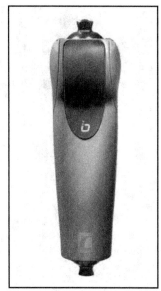

Figure 7-13. RHEO KNEE. (Photo courtesy of Ossur.)

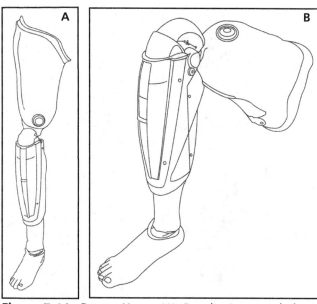

Figure 7-14. Power Knee. (A) Prosthesis extended. (B) Prothesis flexed.

preferred the C-Leg.[5,6] The patient must recharge or replace the batteries periodically. The relative heaviness of electronic units may make stair ascent and other climbing activities more difficult, although optimal weight of the prosthesis remains undetermined.[7] They are not intended for very short people, children, or obese patients. They are more expensive than other knee units, although limited evidence suggests that the units are cost effective.[8]

Comparison of performance demonstrated that the RHEO unit caused the least metabolic rate, followed by C-Leg and then Mauch SNS.[9] Subjects chose faster walking speeds when wearing the C-Leg but did not use less oxygen than when walking with the Mauch SNS.[10] Investigation of oxygen consumption by a small group wearing the Intelligent Prosthesis and then the C-Leg showed slightly better efficiency with C-Leg.[11] Others confirmed minimal improvement with the C-Leg[12] and with the Intelligent Prosthesis.[13] Two subjects, ages 75 and 81, were successfully fitted with the Intelligent Prosthesis, walking faster with less fatigue than with nonmicroprocessor knee units.[14] Others reported no significant difference in energy consumption when subjects walked with microprocessor units.[15,16] Younger adults wearing the Intelligent Prosthesis achieved velocity equal to able-bodied age-mates.[17] Microprocessor units also improved gait kinematics.[18,19]

People were able to descend stairs, climb hills, maneuver over obstacles more easily, and had fewer stumbles with the C-Leg.[6,20-22]

Those wearing microprocessor units also scored high on measures of self-confidence and body image,[22] could walk without as much cognitive attention,[23,24] and had better subjective responses than with older units.[25,26]

Extension Mechanism

The extension mechanism has a motor that extends the knee unit when the wearer ascends stairs or rises from a chair. The unit, Power Knee (Ossur; Figure 7-14), has multiple microprocessors that assess the direction and force of movement. The Power Knee can forcibly extend, aiding the wearer in rising from a chair to standing, as well as in ascending stairs step over step. The unit is bulky, heavy, noisy, and expensive.

Contrary to the generally favorable response to microprocessor knee units is a study that showed that subjects preferred manually locked knees to freely swinging knees.[27]

Locking Rotator

A locking rotator installed above the knee unit (see Figure 7-11C) enables the wearer to sit with crossed legs and to sit on the floor in a tailor fashion.

SOCKET

As is true of all prostheses, the socket is the most important component because the patient inserts the amputation limb into it. Transfemoral sockets are generally made of a combination of a flexible thermoplastic socket lodged in a thermosetting plastic frame[28] (Figure 7-15). Compared with a rigid thermosetting plastic socket, the flexible plastic socket provides several benefits:

> ➤ Greater comfort when the wearer sits because the plastic yields to the contour of the chair.

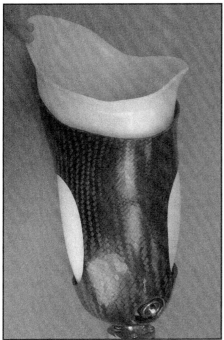

Figure 7-15. Flexible socket in a rigid frame.

➤ Better heat dissipation through the thinner material.

➤ Translucency so that the clinician can see any areas of high pressure or space between the socket and the amputation limb.

➤ Easier modification because the thermoplastic socket shape can be altered by heating the plastic (with the socket off the patient) or by trimming the proximal margin; in contrast, a rigid socket can only be modified by adding material to the socket interior or grinding the plastic in the areas where the socket does not fit comfortably.

The thermoplastic socket, however, may tear if subjected to marked stress.

Many people wear the socket, whether rigid or flexible, next to the skin. Others, however, may interpose socks with or without a liner between the skin and the socket. The same array of liners is available for transfemoral sockets as described for transtibial sockets.

Chapter 8 describes socket designs. The socket is set into the thigh section, which matches the length of the contralateral thigh.

Growing experience with osseous integrated prostheses[29-33] suggests that some patients may achieve greater comfort and function with bony attachment of the prosthesis, eliminating the socket. Most of these individuals have amputations caused by trauma or tumor.

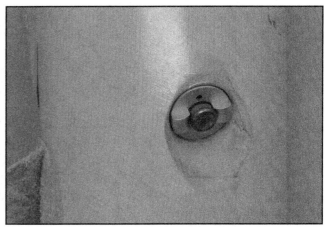

Figure 7-16. Suction valve.

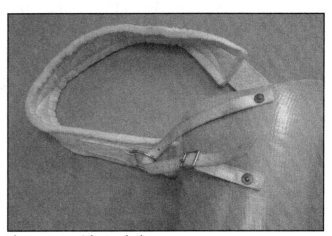

Figure 7-17. Silesian belt.

SUSPENSION

Suction is probably the most popular form of transfemoral suspension. At the proximal margin of the socket, fit must be snug. The socket has a one-way air expulsion valve (Figure 7-16) The patient removes the valve and then inserts the thigh into the socket; the amputation limb displaces air in the socket through the valve hole. Inserting the valve prevents air from reentering the socket. Consequently, atmospheric pressure keeps the socket on the patient's thigh. Suction suspension eliminates reliance on a belt or strap around the torso, giving the wearer maximum control. The patient must maintain stable limb volume so that proximal socket fit remains snug; thus, the most likely candidate has a firm tissue without volume fluctuation.

Partial suction suspension involves use of a suction valve; however, the patient also wears one or more socks to create a snug fit. Because air will enter between the threads of the socks, partial suction suspension requires auxiliary suspension (usually a Silesian belt; Figure 7-17). The belt is attached to the proximal lateral aspect of the socket above and posterior to the greater

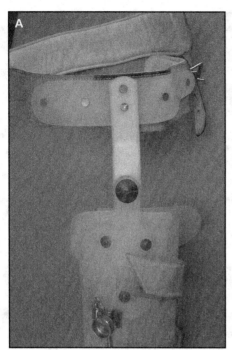
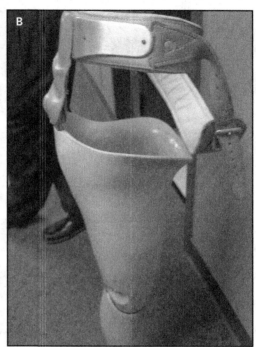

Figure 7-18. Pelvic band. (A) Nylon. (B) Steel.

trochanter. A second attachment is on the anterior midline of the socket at or slightly below the level of the ischial tuberosity. The Silesian belt augments suspension and reduces the tendency of the prosthesis to rotate internally or abduct. Partial suction suspension is indicated for people whose thigh volume varies.

Another suspension option utilizes a lanyard or strap from the distal end of the socket liner. The patient dons the liner, passes the lanyard or strap through a hole or slit in the bottom of the socket up the anterior aspect of the socket, and secures the lanyard or strap to a fixture near the proximal edge of the socket. Donning lanyard or strap suspension is easier than applying suction suspension. The patient can wear a sock over the liner to increase the snugness of the socket. Unlike the lanyard, which may permit the liner to rotate within the socket, the broad strap provides more secure fixation of the thigh and liner in the socket.

Pelvic band suspension (Figure 7-18) includes a rigid metal or nylon single-axis joint and a belt around the torso. The distal end of the joint is attached to the proximolateral aspect of the socket and the proximal end is secured to the belt. The axis should lie proximal and anterior to the greater trochanter. If the pelvic band fits snugly, pelvic band suspension limits hip abduction and adduction, as well as internal and external rotation. Pelvic band suspension may be used to augment suction suspension, enabling the patient to wear 1 or more socks to accommodate limb volume changes. Alternatively, the patient may prefer to eliminate the valve, relying only on the pelvic band for suspension.

Ordinarily, pelvic band suspension is worn with a relatively loose socket, making it comfortable for the person who dislikes socket snugness. It is also easier to don than a prosthesis with suction or partial suction suspension. The drawbacks of pelvic band suspension are less control of socket position, greater bulk around the torso, and greater weight of the prosthesis.

Prosthetic Durability

The longevity of the prosthesis depends, in part, on the age and activity of the user, with younger patients requiring more repairs and replacements of the prosthesis. During a 10-year period, the average requirement was one new prosthesis, 3.3 new sockets, and 25 repairs.[34]

Prescription Guidelines

Patients classified at the K1-2 level may benefit from a prosthesis that includes an energy-storing foot, endoskeletal shank, knee unit with sliding friction and an extension aid, a thermoplastic socket in a rigid frame, and partial suction suspension. A manually locked knee may be necessary for the individual at K1.

Those at K3 may benefit from microprocessor-controlled hydraulic knee unit, and the very active person at K4 will make good use of a hydraulic knee unit, as well as vertical and transverse shock absorbers. The person who frequently sits cross-legged may like a locking rotator unit.

REFERENCES

1. Friel K. Componentry for lower extremity prostheses. *J Am Acad Orthop Surg*. 2005;13:326-335.

2. Graham LE, Datta D, Heller B, et al. A comparative study of conventional and energy-storing prosthetic feet in high-functioning transfemoral amputees. *Arch Phys Med Rehabil*. 2007;88:801-806.

3. Lee S, Hong J. The effect of prosthetic ankle mobility in the sagittal plane on the gait of transfemoral amputees wearing a stance phase controlled knee prosthesis. *Proc Inst Mech Eng H*. 2009;223:263-271.

4. Van der Linden ML, Twiste N, Rithalia SV. The biomechanical effects of the inclusion of a torque absorber on trans-femoral amputee gait: a pilot study. *Prosthet Orthot Int*. 2002;26:35-43.

5. Wetz HH, Hafkemeyer U, Drerup B. The influence of the C-Leg knee-shin system from the Otto Bock Company in the care of above-knee amputees: a clinical-biomechanical study to define indications. *Orthopade*. 2005;34:298-319.

6. Hafner BJ, Smith DG. Differences in function and safety between Medicare Functional Classification Level-2 and -3 transfemoral amputees and influence of prosthetic knee joint control. *J Rehabil Res Dev*. 2009;46:417-433.

7. Cumming JC, Barr S, Howe TE. Prosthetic rehabilitation for older dysvascular people following a unilateral transfemoral amputation [serial on CD-ROM]. *Cochrane Database Syst Rev*. 2006;18:CD005260.

8. Brodtkorb T-H, Henriksson M, Johannesen-Munk, Thidell F. Cost-effectiveness of C-Leg compared with non-microprocessor-controlled knees: a modeling approach. *Arch Phys Med Rehabil*. 2008;89:24-30.

9. Johansson JL, Sherrill DM, Riley PO, et al. A clinical comparison of variable-damping and mechanically passive prosthetic knee devices. *Am J Phys Med Rehabil*. 2005;84:563-575.

10. Orendurff MS, Segal AD, Klute GK, et al. Gait efficiency using the C-Leg. *J Rehabil Res Dev*. 2006;43:239-246.

11. Chin T, Machida K, Sawamura S, et al. Comparison of different microprocessor controlled knee joints on the energy consumption during walking in trans-femoral amputees: Intelligent Knee prosthesis (IP) versus C-Leg. *Prosthet Orthot Int*. 2006;30:73-80.

12. Seymour R, Engbretson B, Kott K, et al. Comparison between the C-Leg microprocessor-controlled prosthetic knee and nonmicroprocessor-controlled prosthetic knees: a preliminary study of energy expenditure, obstacle course performance and quality of life survey. *Prosthet Orthot Int*. 2007;31:51-61.

13. Datta D, Heller B, Howitt J. A comparative evaluation of oxygen consumption and gait pattern in amputees using Intelligent Prostheses and conventionally damped knee swing-phase control. *Clin Rehabil*. 2005;19:398-403.

14. Chin T, Maeda Y, Sawamura S, et al. Successful prosthetic fitting of elderly trans-femoral amputees with Intelligent Prosthesis (IP): a clinical pilot study. *Prosthet Orthot Int*. 2007;31:271-276.

15. Kaufman KR, Levine JA, Brey RH, et al. Energy expenditure and activity of transfemoral amputees using mechanical and microprocessor-controlled prosthetic knees. *Arch Phys Med Rehabil*. 2008;89:1380-1385.

16. Jepson F, Datta D, Harris I, et al. A comparative evaluation of the Adaptive knee and CaTech knee joints: a preliminary study. *Prosthet Orthot Int*. 2008;32:84-92.

17. Chin T, Sawamura S, Shiba R, et al. Effect of an Intelligent Prosthesis (IP) on the walking ability of young transfemoral amputees: comparison of IP users with able-bodied people. *Am J Phys Med Rehabil*. 2003;82:447-451.

18. Kaufman KR, Levine JA, Brey RH, et al. Gait and balance of transfemoral amputees using passive mechanical and microprocessor-controlled prosthetic knees. *Gait Posture*. 2007;26:489-493.

19. Segal AD, Orendurff MS, Klute GK, et al. Kinematic and kinetic comparisons of transfemoral amputee gait using C-Leg and Mauch SNS prosthetic knees. *J Rehabil Res Dev*. 2006;43:857-870.

20. Kahle JT, Highsmith MJ, Hubbard SL. Comparison of nonmicroprocessor knee mechanism versus C-Leg on Prosthesis Evaluation Questionnaire, stumbles, falls, walking tests, stair descent, and knee preference. *J Rehabil Res Dev*. 2008;45:1-14.

21. Hafner BJ, Willingham LL, Buell NC, et al. Evaluation of function, performance, and preference as transfemoral amputees transition from mechanical to microprocessor control of the prosthetic knee. *Arch Phys Med Rehabil*. 2007;88:207-217.

22. Swanson E, Stube J, Edman P. Function and body image levels in individuals with transfemoral amputations using the C-Leg. *J Prosthet Orthot*. 2005;17:80-84.

23. Heller BW, Datta D, Howitt J. A pilot study comparing the cognitive demand of walking for transfemoral amputees using the Intelligent Prosthesis with that using conventionally damped knees. *Clin Rehabil*. 2000;14:518-522.

24. Williams RM, Turner AP, Orendurff M, et al. Does having a computerized prosthetic knee influence cognitive performance during amputee walking? *Arch Phys Med Rehabil*. 2006;87:989-994.

25. Datta D, Howitt J. Conventional versus microchip controlled pneumatic swing phase control for trans-femoral amputees: user's verdict. *Prosthet Orthot Int*. 1998;22:129-135.

26. Stinus H. Biomechanics and evaluation of the microprocessor-controlled C-Leg exoprosthesis knee joint. *Z Orthop Ihre Grenzgeb*. 2000;138:278-282.

27. Devlin M, Sinclair LB, Colman D, et al. Patient preference and gait efficiency in a geriatric population with transfemoral amputation using a free-swinging versus a locked prosthetic knee joint. *Arch Phys Med Rehabil*. 2002;83:246-249.

28. Kapp SL. Transfemoral socket design and suspension options. *Phys Med Rehabil Clin N Am*. 2000;11:569-583.

29. Hagberg K, Brånemark R. One hundred patients treated with osseointegrated transfemoral amputation prostheses: rehabilitation perspective. *J Rehabil Res Dev*. 2009;46:331-344.

30. Hagberg K, Brånemark R, Gunterberg B, Rydevik B. Osseointegrated trans-femoral amputation prostheses: prospective results of general and condition-specific quality of life in 18 patients at 2-year follow-up. *Prosthet Orthot Int.* 2008;32:29-41.

31. Hagberg K, Haggstrom E, Uden M, Brånemark R. Socket versus bone-anchored trans-femoral prostheses: hip range of motion and sitting comfort. *Prosthet Orthot Int.* 2005;29:153-163.

32. Sullivan J, Uden M, Robinson KP, Sooriakumaran S. Rehabilitation of the trans-femoral amputee with an osseointegrated prosthesis: the United Kingdom experience *Arch Phys Med Rehabil.* 2002;83:242-246.

33. Brånemark R, Brånemark P-I, Rydevik B, Myers RR. Osseointegration in skeletal reconstruction and rehabilitation: a review. *J Rehabil Res Dev.* 2001;38:175-181.

34. Nair A, Hanspal RS, Zahedi MS, et al. Analyses of prosthetic episodes in lower limb amputees. *Prosthet Orthot Int.* 2008;32:42-49.

Transfemoral Biomechanics

The goals of transfemoral biomechanics are the same as for all prostheses (ie, to maximize comfort and function). The means of achieving these goals are also similar to that for other prostheses.

SOCKET DESIGNS

The custom-made permanent transfemoral socket is either formed over a plaster model of the patient's thigh or by means of computer-aided design and computer-aided manufacture (CAD-CAM). Regardless of the method, the ideal socket maximizes pressure over socket tissue while minimizing pressure over sensitive areas. Because the thigh has a single, central bone enveloped by soft tissue, the contours of each transfemoral socket vary much more than that of the transtibial socket, which encases a relatively bony amputation limb. Amputation disturbs the balance of hip muscles. If the iliotibial tract is not sutured to the femur, the patient will avoid an abduction contracture but will risk a flexion contracture because the iliopsoas muscle is intact. Abduction contracture is avoided only if the hip adductors are fixed to the femur.[1]

Although every transfemoral socket is unique, the 2 principal designs are quadrilateral and ischial containment and its variants.[2,3] Both of these shapes provide total contact, including touching the distal end of the amputation limb. Measurement of socket interface pressures and electromyography suggest a significant correlation between muscle activity and interface pressure at the biceps femoris and rectus femoris.[4]

Quadrilateral

The older design is quadrilateral. The proximal margin resembles a rectangle (Figure 8-1). The anterior wall features an adductor tendon relief (concavity) in the anteromedial corner. The medial two-thirds of the anterior wall has a buildup (convexity) over the area of the femoral (Scarpa's) triangle to maximize the contact area over the sensitive femoral artery, vein, and nerve. In the anterolateral corner is a gentle relief for the rectus femoris muscle. The posterior wall has a hamstring tendon relief in the posteromedial corner. A gluteus maximus channel (relief) in the posterolateral corner provides room for the bulging muscle as it contracts. The lateral wall has a relief for the greater trochanter. The anteroposterior dimension of the proximal socket is somewhat larger than the mediolateral dimension.

The posterior brim of the quadrilateral socket has a horizontal shelf to enable ischiogluteal weight bearing. The posterior and medial brims are at the level of the ischial tuberosity, which rests on the posterior brim. The anterior and lateral brims are approximately 3 inches higher to increase contact area, thereby reducing pressure (Figure 8-2).

Ischial Containment

The proximal margin of the ischial containment is somewhat oval (Figure 8-3), with the mediolateral dimension smaller than the anteroposterior dimension. The posterior and medial walls are relatively high to encase the ischial tuberosity (Figures 8-4 and 8-5). The anterior wall is slightly lower, and the lateral wall is approximately at the same level as the posterior and medial walls. The relatively high posterior, medial, and lateral walls encase the inferior pelvis. The socket, however, must not impinge on the ischiopubic ascending ramus.

A comparison of the quadrilateral and ischial containment sockets indicates that the ischial containment socket distributes pressure more evenly, especially on the anterior and posterior walls; pressure distribu-

Edelstein JE, Muroz A.
Lower-Limb Prosthetics and Orthotics: Clinical Concepts (pp 61-64).
© 2011 Taylor & Francis Group.

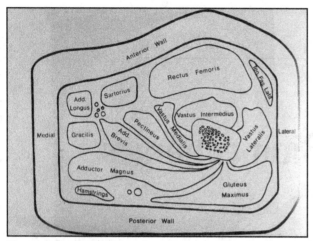

Figure 8-1. Quadrilateral socket, superior view.

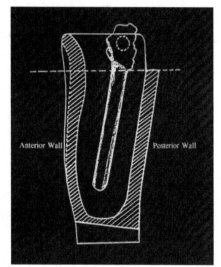

Figure 8-2. Quadrilateral socket, medial view.

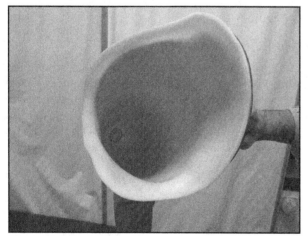

Figure 8-3. Ischial containment socket, superior view.

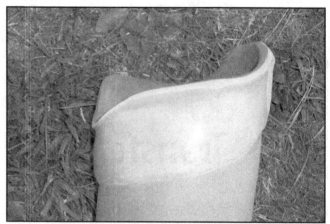

Figure 8-4. Ischial containment socket, posterior view.

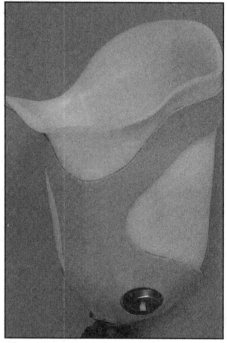

Figure 8-5. Ischial containment socket, medial view.

tion on the lateral and medial walls is similar in both designs.[5] Other investigators[6] reported that subjects rated the ischial containment as more comfortable when they walked and sat. Computerized tomography and radiography both demonstrated that this design kept the femur more adducted.

Variations of the ischial containment design are numerous. Some alter the trim line of the socket to increase lateral stabilization. Others have changed the frame so that it has an anterodistal projection which may foster more active muscular control of the prosthesis (Figure 8-6).

ALIGNMENT

Socket comfort is influenced by the shape of the socket and the alignment of the socket relative to the rest of the prosthesis. Frontal and sagittal alignment contribute to comfort by directing forces on the amputated limb strategically.

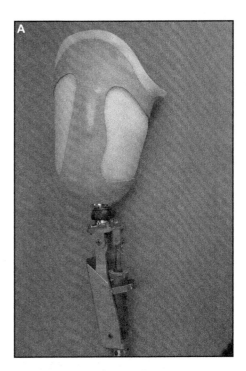

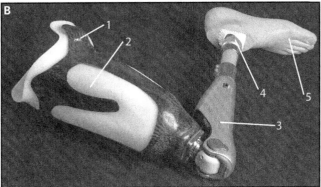

Figure 8-6. Ischial containment socket. (A) Lateral view. (B) Frame with anterodistal projection. (1) Frame. (2) Socket. (3) Knee unit and shank. (4) Foot bolt. (5) Foot. (Courtesy of Hanger Prosthetics & Orthotics, Inc.)

Sagittal Plane

Giving the patient appropriate control of the prosthetic knee is the principal purpose of alignment in the sagittal plane. The individual at the K1 functional level requires a very stable alignment, whereas someone at the K4 level needs a prosthesis in which the knee unit is easy to flex and extend. Sagittal alignment is influenced by the patient's physical ability as well as the type of knee unit.

The socket is flexed approximately 5 degrees (Figure 8-7) in order to:

➤ Facilitate contraction of the hip extensors, especially gluteus maximus.

➤ Prevent excessively lordotic standing posture.

➤ Provide a range through which the hip can hyperextend during mid- and late stance.

➤ Aid in positioning the ischial tuberosity on the posterior brim, for the patient wearing a quadrilateral socket.

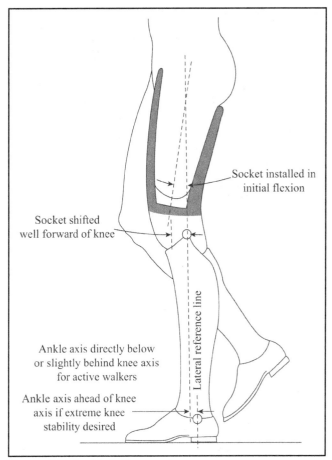

Figure 8-7. Sagittal alignment.

The knee axis is aligned relative to the hip and ankle axes (lateral reference line). Anterior placement of the knee axis increases the ease of flexing the knee; posterior alignment increases the stability of the prosthesis. Consequently, the K1 patient usually has the knee aligned relatively posteriorly, whereas the K4 individual has a more anterior placement. Knee units that have hydraulic stance control are usually placed somewhat anteriorly because the unit has inherent stability.

Foot placement and structure also influence stability. A foot that is aligned relatively anterior to the knee will increase the stability of the prosthesis. A relatively resilient heel cushion also increases stability.

Shoe selection modifies stability. A prosthesis with a high, rigid shoe heel will be less stable than one that has a low, resilient heel.

Other means of increasing sagittal stability include a cane or walker, which places the patient's weight line well in front of the prosthetic knee axis. A polycentric knee axis is also inherently more stable because the instant center of rotation is posterior to the weight line for most of the excursion of the knee. Knee units equipped with stance control increase stability in early stance phase. A manually locked knee offers maximum stability.

Frontal Plane

The socket is slightly adducted to reduce the tendency of the pelvis to lower on the amputated side (Figure 8-8). The shorter the amputation limb, the greater the tendency for pelvic displacement. Outsetting the prosthetic foot also increases frontal plane stability; however, the resulting wide base causes the patient to exaggerate lateral trunk bending. A snugly fit pelvic band contributes to frontal stability because the mechanical hip joint resists frontal plane motion.

A cane or walker aids frontal stability by enabling the patient to obtain upward force from the floor to the hand on the assistive device, thus resisting the downward motion of the pelvis. The device also transfers a variable amount of the load from the pelvis to the hand.

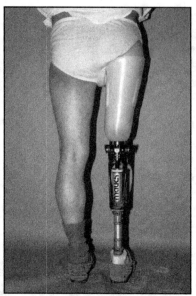

Figure 8-8. Frontal alignment.

REFERENCES

1. Jaegers SM, Arendzen JH, de Jongh HJ. Changes in hip muscles after above-knee amputation. *Clin Orthop.* 1995;319:276-284.

2. Kapp SL. Transfemoral socket design and suspension options. *Phys Med Rehabil Clin N Am.* 2000;11:569-583.

3. Schuch CM, Pritham CH. Current transfemoral sockets. *Clin Orthop Relat Res.* 1999;361:48-54.

4. Hong JH, Mun MS. Relationship between socket pressure and EMG of two muscles in trans-femoral stumps during gait. *Prosthet Orthot Int.* 2005;29:59-72.

5. Lee VS, Solomonidis SE, Spence WD. Stump-socket interface pressure as an aid to socket design in prostheses for trans-femoral amputees—a preliminary study. *Proc Inst Mech Eng H.* 1997;211:167-180.

6. Hachisuka K, Umezu Y, Ogata H, et al. Subjective evaluations and objective measurements of the ischial-ramal containment prosthesis. *J UOEH.* 1999;21:107-118.

Chapter 9

Transfemoral Static Evaluation

Evaluation of socket fit, as well as prosthetic alignment and construction, is a critical phase of rehabilitation. The patient should have the benefit of optimum comfort and stability prior to learning to use the prosthesis; otherwise, the individual will be obliged to compensate for inadequacies in the prosthesis.

Administration of the transfemoral evaluation mirrors that which was described in Chapter 5. The patient and prosthesis should be examined prior to prosthetic training (initial evaluation) and at the completion of basic training (final evaluation).

Equipment for performing the evaluation includes a checklist of items to be evaluated, several pieces of plywood, each approximately 9 × 12 × 0.5-inch, an armless unupholstered chair, parallel bars, and a table.

1. Is the prosthesis as prescribed? Verify that the foot, shank, knee unit, socket, and suspension are the same as in the prescription. Very occasionally, the clinical team determines that the patient would benefit from different component(s); if the change(s) are reflected in an amended prescription, then the prosthesis is satisfactory. If not, the prosthesis must include the prescribed components.

2. Can the patient don the prosthesis easily? Although the patient has not been trained to don the prosthesis, the individual should be able to insert the amputation limb into the socket with minimal difficulty. At the time of the final evaluation, the patient should be able to don the prosthesis accurately, independently, and rapidly. If the patient cannot don the prosthesis easily, the socket may need adjustment.

STANDING

3. Is the patient comfortable when standing with the heel midlines 6 in (15 cm) apart? (Figure 9-1).

The patient should stand in the best obtainable posture with minimal support facing forward. Feet should be on a line parallel with the shoulders. Feet may be separated so that the midlines are approximately 6 inches apart, representing a compromise between the normal walking base of 2 to 4 inches (5 to 10 cm) and a standing at ease position with feet in line with the shoulders. Record the patient's comments about overall comfort.

➢ If the individual complains of discomfort, note specific painful areas. Response to other items in the evaluation will confirm or refute the response to this item.

4. Is any flesh roll above the socket minimal? Check all sides of the brim to determine whether there is any overhanging flesh (Figure 9-2). A medial flesh roll may compel the wearer to widen the walking base. Confirm whether any overhang is excessive when the prosthesis is removed.

➢ Prolonged redness indicates that the socket is too tight and needs adjustment.

5. Is the patient free from vertical pressure in the perineum? Ask the patient to adduct the prosthesis and bear full weight on it (Figure 9-3). Question the individual regarding feelings of comfort or discomfort along the medial brim. Discomfort suggests that the brim is impinging on the adductor nerve. The quadrilateral socket should have a relief for the adductor longus tendon. The medial brim of the ischial containment socket should not press tissue excessively. Confirm whether the pressure is excessive when the prosthesis is removed.

➢ Prolonged redness indicates that the socket needs adjustment.

Edelstein JE, Muroz A.
Lower-Limb Prosthetics and Orthotics: Clinical Concepts (pp 65-70).
© 2011 Taylor & Francis Group.

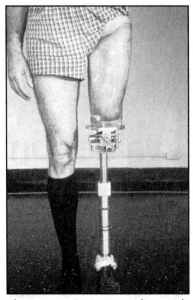

Figure 9-1. Patient standing with heel midlines 6 inches apart, anterior view.

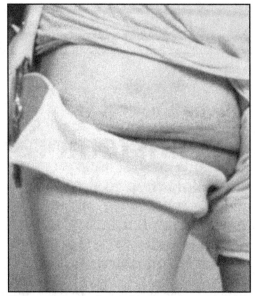

Figure 9-2. Socket brim showing the flesh overhang.

6. Do the contours and color of the prosthesis match the opposite limb? Compare the shape and color of the prosthesis with that of the sound limb and note any marked disparity.

➢ If there is a considerable difference, reserve judgment until item #27, which pertains to the patient's appraisal of the prosthesis.

7. Is the prosthesis the correct length? The patient should stand in the same position as specified for item #3. Ask the individual to bend forward. Assess the symmetry of the torso. If the person does not have a fixed scoliosis, compare the heights of the anterior superior iliac spines, the iliac crests, and the posterior superior iliac spines. If both spines are not parallel with the floor, insert as many pieces of plywood under the shorter leg as needed to place the pelvis in the level position. Measure the height of the plywood. If less than 0.5-inch (1 cm), the prosthesis is most likely the proper height.

➢ If the patient requires more than a 0.5-inch lift under the prosthesis, any of the following aspects of the prosthesis may be deficient:

  ¤ The socket is too loose, causing the amputation limb to bear excessive weight distally. Usually the patient will complain of distal pain. Additional socks may alleviate the problem; otherwise, the socket needs adjustment.

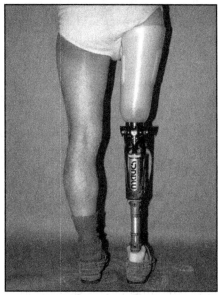

Figure 9-3. Patient standing, posterior view, with prosthesis adducted.

¤ The heel on the prosthetic foot is too soft. The prosthesis will appear too short and the patient will likely shift weight posteriorly. Verify the adequacy of the heel during gait analysis. A soft heel will cause the patient to walk with limited knee flexion.

¤ The shank may be too short. The clinician has no reference points to measure shank length in a cosmetically finished prosthesis. In the absence of other deficiencies, one may infer that the shank is too short.

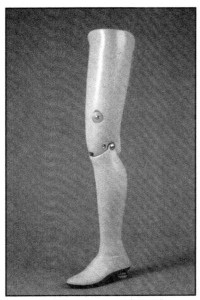

Figure 9-4. Prosthesis, lateral view.

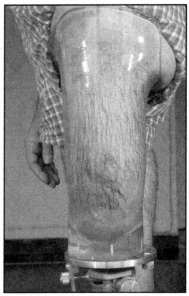

Figure 9-5. Quadrilateral socket, lateral view.

◻ The thigh section may be too short. Reserve judgment until evaluating the seated patient. Any discrepancy between lengths of the thighs and the shanks will be apparent.

➤ If the patient requires more than a 0.5-inch lift under the sound leg:

◻ The socket is too tight, preventing the amputation limb from lodging correctly in the socket. The wearer may complain of circumferential or proximal pain. If adjustment of sock thickness does not correct the problem, the socket will have to be adjusted.

◻ The heel on the prosthetic foot is too firm. The patient may shift weight anteriorly and will tend to walk with excessive knee flexion.

◻ The shank or the thigh section may be too long.

8. Is the knee stable? Have patient stand within parallel bars or other safe environment. Stand perpendicular to the patient to protect the person in the event of an inadvertent knee collapse (Figure 9-4). Punch the back of the prosthetic knee forcefully. Note whether the knee moves in response to the blow and, if so, the extent of movement. A knee unit that has a manual lock, a friction brake, or hydraulic stance control should not move. A unit that does not have a mechanical stabilizer should flex slightly then return to full extension.

➤ If a knee unit with a stabilizer moves, the prosthesis should be returned to the prosthetist for adjustment of the knee unit. If a prosthesis that has a knee unit lacking a stabilizer collapses, the sagittal alignment is unstable and requires adjustment. If the knee unit in the same type of prosthesis fails to flex, the sagittal alignment is excessively stable and requires adjustment.

9. When the socket valve is removed, is the distal tissue firm? Instruct the patient to remain standing and not to start walking. Remove the valve and palpate the flesh at the valve hole. The flesh should have the consistency of the examiner's thenar eminence, indicating that the socket is reasonably snug.

➤ If the flesh is excessively taut, the socket may be too snug and may require adjustment. If flesh does not protrude slightly at the valve hold, the socket may be too loose distally and may require adjustment.

QUADRILATERAL SOCKET

10. Does the ischial tuberosity rest on the posterior brim (Figure 9-5)? Have the patient stand within parallel bars or another safe environment. Stand perpendicular to the patient. Ask the patient to lean forward just enough so that you can palpate the ischial tuberosity. Once you have located the tuberosity, ask the patient to resume upright posture. Determine whether the tuberosity is directly over the posterior brim.

➤ If the tuberosity is posterior to the brim, the socket is too small and should be adjusted. If the tuberosity does not contact the brim, the patient may not have donned the socket completely. Remove the prosthesis and repeat the donning process. If the tuberosity is still too high, the socket is too small.

11. Is the posterior brim approximately parallel to the floor? Observe the alignment of the posterior brim.

➤ If the medial half of the posterior brim is tilted downward, the patient may not be bearing sufficient weight on the lateral portion of the brim. The socket may need adjustment.

12. Is the adductor longus tendon located in the anterior-medial corner? Ask the patient to contract the adductor longus muscle. Palpate the tendon in the anteromedial aspect of the thigh. The tendon should occupy a relief in the socket. In addition, question the patient regarding comfort, particularly in the anteromedial aspect of the socket.

➤ If the tendon is not in its relief or if the patient complains of discomfort, the socket needs adjustment.

ISCHIAL CONTAINMENT SOCKET

13. Does the posterior-medial corner of the socket cover the ischial tuberosity? Stand behind the patient and observe the posterior aspect of the socket to determine whether it covers the ischial tuberosity.

➤ If the tuberosity is not covered, the socket may need adjustment.

14. Can the patient hyperextend the hip on the amputated side comfortably? Ask the patient to hyperextend the hip. Question the individual regarding comfort.

➤ If the patient cannot hyperextend or is uncomfortable, the socket may need adjustment.

15. Can the patient flex the hip 90 degrees comfortably, without socket gapping? Ask the patient to flex the hip. Observe whether the socket remains snug on the amputation limb. Question the patient regarding comfort.

➤ If the patient cannot flex the hip or is uncomfortable, or if the socket gaps, the socket may need adjustment.

16. Can the patient abduct the hip on the amputated side comfortably, without socket gapping? Ask the patient to abduct the hip. Observe whether the socket remains snug on the amputation limb. Question the patient regarding comfort.

➤ If the patient cannot abduct the hip or is uncomfortable, or if the socket gaps, the socket may need adjustment.

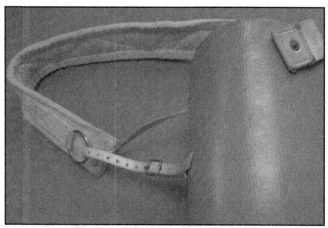

Figure 9-6. Anterior and lateral attachments of a Silesian belt.

SUSPENSION

17. Does the Silesian belt control prosthetic rotation and abduction adequately? Note whether the prosthetic foot is approximately 6 inches lateral to the sound foot and matches the toe-out angle of the sound foot.

➤ If the prosthetic foot does not mirror the position of the sound foot, 1 or both attachments of the Silesian belt may need adjustment. The lateral attachment should be superior and posterior to the greater trochanter for optimum rotational control. The midpoint between the 2 anterior attachments should be slightly below the level of the ischial tuberosity and should be on the midline of the anterior aspect of the socket (Figure 9-6).

18. Does the pelvic band conform to the torso? Note whether the upper and lower borders of the pelvic band contact the posterior trunk.

➤ If only 1 border contacts the trunk, the patient may experience excessive pressure at the point of contact. If neither border contacts the trunk, the pelvic band may be too loose. Reserve judgment about the fit of the pelvic band until the patient sits because pelvic rotation will alter the fit of the pelvic band. The band should fit comfortably during standing and sitting. Otherwise, the band requires adjustment.

SITTING

19. Can the patient sit comfortably with hips and knees flexed 90 degrees? Ask the patient to sit in an adult-sized straight chair. Posture should be symmetrical with both hips and both knees flexed 90 degrees. Feet should be flat on the floor. Record the wearer's comments about sitting comfort.

➢ If the patient complains of discomfort, ask the individual to specify painful area(s). Depending on the patient's comments, the socket or the suspension may need adjustment.

20. Does the socket remain secure on the thigh, without gapping or rotating? Observe whether the brim contacts the anterior thigh without gapping. Determine whether the rotational position of the socket matches the sound thigh.

➢ If the socket does not fit snugly or if it is not symmetrical with the contralateral thigh, socket fit with or without alignment of the prosthesis may need adjustment.

21. Are both thighs approximately the same length and height from the floor? Ordinarily, both thighs should be of equal length, and both shanks should also be equal in height. If, however, the patient has a long amputation limb, the prosthetic thigh may be slightly longer and the shank correspondingly shorter so that standing posture can be symmetrical.

➢ If length discrepancy exists in the absence of a long amputation limb, the thigh or the shank may need adjustment.

22. Can the patient lean forward to touch the shoes? Regardless of socket design, the patient should be able to flex at the waist to reach the shoes.

➢ If the patient cannot reach forward comfortably, the anterior brim may need a broader curvature or the brim may need to be lowered slightly.

WALKING

23. Is the patient's performance in level walking satisfactory? Although the individual who receives his or her first prosthesis will not have had much gait training, the prosthetist will have guided the patient through a few steps to accomplish the alignment procedure. Judgments made at initial evaluation are tentative; however, any gross gait abnormalities should be recorded. Chapter 10 details gait problems encountered by some people who wear transfemoral prostheses.

24. Is the patient's performance on stairs and ramps satisfactory? This item can be omitted at the initial evaluation. If the patient has marginal functional prognosis, such as K1, the item is also irrelevant. Otherwise, the person should demonstrate confidence on stairs and ramps.

➢ The individual at K2-4 who is unable to traverse stairs and ramps safely may require additional training.

25. Does the suspension function properly? Observe the suspension component as the patient walks.

The patient should be able to walk without untoward shifting of the prosthesis. The individual may need to adjust the valve when starting to walk; however, repeated valve adjustment suggests that the valve is not functioning properly.

➢ If the suspension appears inadequate, the component usually requires adjustment.

26. Does the prosthesis operate quietly? Listen to the prosthesis as the patient walks. If the prosthesis includes an articulated foot, listen for metallic noises indicating excessive contact between joint surfaces. Also listen to the knee unit as the patient passes through swing phase.

➢ A prosthesis that is unacceptably noisy usually requires maintenance.

27. Does the patient consider the prosthesis satisfactory as to comfort, function, and appearance? Solicit the person's opinion, noting any favorable and unfavorable comments. The new wearer may be disappointed in the appearance or function of the prosthesis; however, with experience and emotional adjustment to prosthetic use, many complaints resolve spontaneously.

➢ If the individual is dissatisfied, referral to the prosthetic clinical team is indicated. Problems that are identified should be resolved.

PROSTHESIS OFF THE PATIENT

28. Is the skin free of abrasions or other discolorations attributable to this prosthesis? Examine the skin of the amputation limb after prosthetic wear and compare it with the examination conducted prior to donning the prosthesis, looking for any new color changes.

➢ Redness persisting for more than 10 minutes may necessitate adjustment of the socket.

29. Is the socket interior smooth? Touch all portions of the socket to determine whether any roughness exists, particularly if a suspension component has been riveted through the socket.

➢ A socket that has any coarse areas should have those areas smoothed.

30. With the prosthesis fully flexed on a table, can the thigh piece be brought to at least the vertical position? Place the prosthesis in the kneeling position on the table. The thigh section should tilt slightly posteriorly indicating that the patient will be able to assume a stable position when kneeling (Figure 9-7). If the individual has a long amputation limb, however, the thigh section may be vertical.

➢ If the thigh section tilts anteriorly, the posterior aspect of the socket or knee unit may need adjustment to permit a more acute flexion angle.

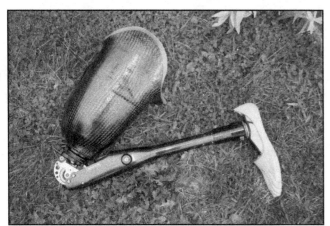

Figure 9-7. Side view of the prosthesis flexed with socket slightly tilted backward.

31. If the socket is totally rigid, is a back pad attached? A back pad made of felt upholstered with leather should be attached to the posterior aspect of the socket (Figure 9-8). The pad muffles noise when the patient sits on an unupholstered chair and reduces abrasion of the wearer's trousers or skirt.

➢ If the rigid socket does not have a back pad, a pad should be installed.

32. Is the construction satisfactory? Determine whether the plastic portions are uniform. If the prosthesis has an articulated foot, look for a thin leather guard surrounding the ankle. Check all rivets and other fasteners for smooth placement. Check for uniformity of stitching. Any construction deficiencies should be rectified.

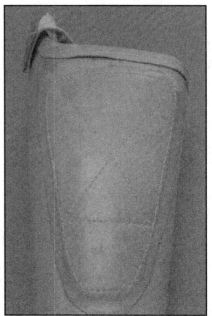

Figure 9-8. Posterior view of socket showing back pad.

33. Do all components function satisfactorily? If the prosthesis has a suction valve, make certain that the air hole is not occluded. Examine any strap fastenings that may be present. If the foot has any adjustment feature, check that it is easy to operate. If any component does not function satisfactorily, the component should be adjusted or replaced.

Chapter 10

Transfemoral Gait Analysis

People who wear transfemoral prostheses walk differently than able-bodied adults. Gait characteristics reflect 2 basic factors. First there are inherent anatomic differences between prosthesis wearers and able-bodied individuals.[1-5] The patient must cope with the absence of knee and foot musculature and the associated sensory input, as well as impaired function of proximal musculature. Most wearers do not have a closed kinematic chain in stance phase because they lack rigid continuity from the amputation limb to the floor. Second, design deficiencies in contemporary prostheses interfere with achieving optimal gait. Complicating anatomic and prosthetic problems are difficulties that can be corrected or reduced, including pain in the amputation limb and the contralateral knee, contracture, weakness, instability, incoordination, and deficits in prosthetic fit and alignment.

TYPICAL TRANSFEMORAL GAIT

Step length is generally asymmetrical, with a longer step on the prosthetic side enabling the walker to remain on the intact, sensate leg for more time.[3,6-8] Absence of the anatomic knee joint deprives the patient of sensory receptors in the knee, as well as normal quadriceps and hamstring muscle power on the amputated side. Consequently, most people begin stance phase on the prosthesis with the knee extended. Knee units that have stance-stabilizing mechanisms, however, permit the individual to achieve heel contact with a slightly flexed knee. Alignment usually is designed to keep the knee unit extended during most of stance phase.

Prosthetic gait is typically slower,[1,9] especially among those with vascular disease.[4] The walking base is wider.[6] Severance of the adductor magnus creates imbalance, favoring hip abduction.[10] Subjects exhibit increased excursion of the center of mass, with lateral trunk bending toward the prosthetic side during stance

on the prosthesis.[2,3,11] The torso shifts toward the prosthesis during stance phase on the prosthesis. Gluteus medius contraction causes the femoral remnant to compress soft tissues on the lateral aspect of the amputation limb. In the absence of a closed kinematic chain, which occurs during normal stance phase, the hip abductors cannot control trunk movement effectively. Amputation renders their distal insertions unstable. During swing phase, patients tend to elevate the pelvis.[12] Those with shorter amputation limbs walk with greater pelvic tilt.[3,13] Patients also exert greater muscle activity[5,14,15] and consume more energy (energy consumption is discussed in Chapter 16).[1] Arm swing is also asymmetrical, with greater excursion on the contralateral upper limb.[16,17]

Patients initiate gait with active contraction of the ankle muscles on the intact leg, regardless of the leg taking the first step.[18,19] Gait is terminated with decreased peak braking ground reaction force in the prosthesis and longer braking force in the intact limb.[20]

Components of the prosthesis also influence the walking pattern. A socket that unloads the pelvis tends to load the soft tissues of the thigh; conversely, a socket with higher margins restrains hip extension. During double support with the prosthesis behind the sound limb, the wearer tilts the pelvis anteriorly and flexes the hip on the intact side, thereby overcoming the socket's interference with hip motion on the amputated side.[21]

The type of knee unit affects the ease of walking. The locking knee unit was preferred by older patients with dysvascular amputation, even though they were accustomed to a freely swinging knee unit. They walked farther and faster with the locked unit.[22] Comparison of gait with mechanically and microprocessor-controlled knee units demonstrates greater velocity with prostheses equipped with microprocessor units[23,24]; subjects walked with a flexed prosthetic knee in early stance[25]

Edelstein JE, Muroz A.
Lower-Limb Prosthetics and Orthotics: Clinical Concepts (pp 71-78).
© 2011 Taylor & Francis Group.

and had fewer stumbles.[26,27] Hip muscular activity decreased when subjects walked with prostheses having a magnetorheological-based knee unit.[28]

Distal components also contribute to the walking pattern. A torque absorber may reduce thigh chafing.[29] Energy-storing feet are associated with faster walking, although they did not reduce the asymmetry of load between the intact and prosthetic limbs.[30] Experimentation with prosthetic ankles having various ranges of sagittal motion suggests that a foot-ankle unit with limited mobility causes greater flexion of the prosthetic knee than does an ankle providing maximum motion.[31] The weight of the prosthesis appears to have no significant effect on gait, although many wearers preferred a somewhat heavier prosthesis.[32]

A few investigations of gait on surfaces other than level floors demonstrate that people wearing transfemoral prostheses exerted more muscular effort on the intact side during stair ascent.[33] When walking on hills, subjects could not increase prosthetic knee flexion but compensated with greater flexion of the intact knee, particularly when ascending the ramp.[34]

Elite runners demonstrated greater asymmetry between the prosthetic and intact limbs when they increased running speed.[35]

ABNORMAL TRANSFEMORAL GAIT

In contrast to the relative simplicity of transtibial gait analysis, transfemoral gait can present many abnormalities. This discussion will thus group abnormalities into 6 categories:

1. Lateral displacements of the prosthesis
2. Trunk shifts
3. Rotations
4. Excessive knee motion
5. Insufficient knee motion
6. Step length discrepancies

For each abnormality, anatomic, physiologic, and prosthetic causes are described. In some instances, the same patient may demonstrate several abnormalities. Corrective intervention directed at the prosthetic fault(s) is usually more expedient than improving the anatomic or physiologic disorders. Inadequacies that often can be eliminated include improper donning, use of an inappropriate shoe, socket misfit or malalignment, malfunctioning components, and improper prosthesis height.

LATERAL DISPLACEMENTS OF THE PROSTHESIS

The prosthesis should move forward with minimal lateral displacement, maintaining a walking base of approximately 2 to 4 inches (5 to 10 cm) between the heel centers.

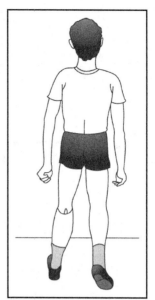

Figure 10-1. Abducted gait.

Abduction

This stance phase abnormality is noted when the walking base is excessively wide (Figure 10-1). Abduction is associated with lateral trunk bending.

➤ Anatomic/physiologic causes include the following:
  ¤ Hip abductor contracture.
  ¤ Weak hip abductors.
  ¤ Laterodistal thigh pain may indicate the need for a socket relief at the site of pain.
  ¤ Adductor tissue roll; soft tissue should be contained within the socket.
  ¤ Balance instability, which may be reduced with the use of a cane.
➤ Prosthetic causes include the following:
  ¤ Prosthesis longer than contralateral lower limb.
  ¤ Abducted hip joint on a pelvic band.
  ¤ Inadequate lateral socket wall adduction.
  ¤ Sharp or high medial socket wall.
  ¤ Foot outset excessively.

Circumduction

During swing phase, the patient brings the prosthesis forward in a semicircle (Figure 10-2). Circumduction may be combined with abduction.

➤ Anatomic/physiologic causes include the following:
  ¤ Hip abductor contracture.
  ¤ Poor control of the knee unit; the patient flings the prosthesis forward in a semicircular motion to avoid or limit flexion of the prosthetic knee.

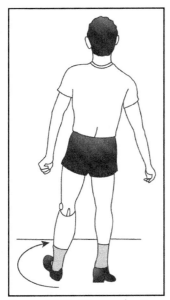

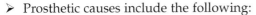

Figure 10-2. Circumduction.

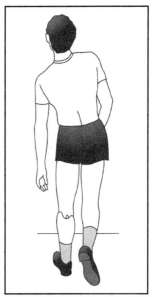

Figure 10-3. Lateral trunk bending.

➢ Prosthetic causes include the following:
  ¤ Prosthesis longer than contralateral lower limb; patient achieves swing phase clearance by circumducting the prosthesis.
  ¤ Locked knee unit; in the presence of a locked knee unit, the prosthesis should be shortened approximately 0.5-inch to permit swing phase clearance.
  ¤ Loose friction mechanism fails to control the swing of the prosthetic knee.
  ¤ Inadequate suspension may cause the prosthesis to lower during swing phase and thus become functionally longer.
  ¤ Small or tight socket does not accommodate the amputation limb; failure to lodge the thigh fully in the socket creates apparent lengthening of the prosthesis.
  ¤ Loose socket will slip downward during swing phase.
  ¤ Foot malaligned in plantar flexion also lengthens the prosthesis.

TRUNK SHIFTS

Ideally, the patient will maintain the trunk erect with the same minimal movement in the frontal, transverse, or sagittal planes as seen in able-bodied gait. Trunk shifts are most obvious during early stance phase on the prosthesis.

Lateral Bending

The patient exaggerates lateral flexion of the trunk toward the amputated side during stance on the prosthesis (Figure 10-3). Regardless of the cause of lateral trunk bending, a cane will eliminate the abnormality because it reestablishes a rigid connection between the torso and the floor. The cane is more effective if used on the side opposite to the prosthesis.

➢ Anatomic/physiologic causes include the following:
  ¤ Hip abductor contracture places the abductors in a slack position, hampering muscle contraction.
  ¤ Weak hip abductors.
  ¤ Hip pain. Normally, hip abductors must exert substantial force to counteract the tendency of the torso to drop to the unsupported, swing side, with the result being relatively great pressure in the hip joint, which may be painful; by shifting the trunk over the hip, the patient reduces the demand on the hip abductors and thus the pressure on the hip.
  ¤ Balance instability.
  ¤ Short amputation limb reduces the weight of the thigh, which contributes to stabilizing the distal insertion of the hip abductors; the short limb also reduces the area over which the socket can apply medially directed force to counteract the tendency for the trunk to shift laterally.

➢ Prosthetic causes include the following:
  ¤ Short prosthesis necessitates shifting the trunk over the prosthesis during stance phase.
  ¤ Inadequate lateral socket wall adduction reduces stabilization of the hip abductor muscles.
  ¤ Sharp or high medial wall is likely to be painful, forcing the patient to move away from the discomfort.
  ¤ Foot outset excessively.

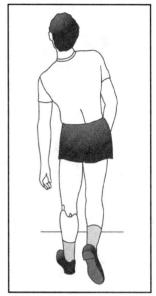

Figure 10-4. Lordosis.

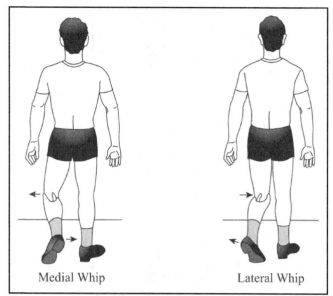

Figure 10-5. Lateral and medial whips.

Forward Bending

The patient leans forward during stance on the prosthesis.
> Anatomic/physiologic causes include the following:
  ¤ Hip flexor contracture.
  ¤ Balance instability.
  ¤ Poor control of the knee unit.
> Prosthetic causes include the following:
  ¤ Unstable knee unit tends to collapse during early stance phase.
  ¤ Short walker or crutches compels the patient to lean forward.

Lordosis

The pelvis tilts forward to an abnormal extent (Figure 10-4).
> Anatomic causes include the following:
  ¤ Hip flexor contracture tilts the pelvis posteriorly.
  ¤ Weak hip extensors and abdominal muscles fail to stabilize the trunk during early stance phase on the prosthesis.

The prosthetic cause is inadequate socket flexion. Slight socket flexion facilitates contraction of the hip extensors and restores the normally flexed alignment of the proximal femur.

ROTATIONS

The prosthesis should move forward in a relatively straight line as the patient makes the transition from stance to swing phase and from swing back to stance phase.

Whips (Figure 10-5) occur during the transition from stance to swing phase of the prosthesis and are observed from the rear of the patient. The shank should swing forward with minimal transverse plane movement. A medial whip is seen when the heel of the shoe on the prosthesis rotates medially during late stance and early swing phase and then rotates laterally during late swing. Lateral whip designates the opposite movement.
> Physiologic causes include the following:
  ¤ Prosthesis donned in malrotation; contraction of muscles located improperly in the socket forces the socket, and thus the entire prosthesis, into exaggerated rotation.
> Prosthetic causes include the following:
  ¤ Faulty socket contour that does not accommodate thigh muscles properly.
  ¤ Knee bolt malrotated. External rotation of the knee bolt may lead to medial whip. Internal rotation has the opposite effect.
  ¤ Foot malrotation can also disturb the transition from stance to swing phase.

Foot rotation at heel contact is forefoot pivoting on the heel (Figure 10-6). This abnormality can cause the patient to fall because the prosthesis is not stable when the individual transfers weight to it. There is no anatomic or physiologic cause for this disorder.
> Prosthetic causes include the following:
  ¤ Prosthetic foot heel cushion is too stiff to absorb the shock of heel contact sufficiently.
  ¤ Malrotated foot does not accept the patient's weight adequately.

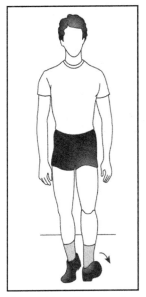
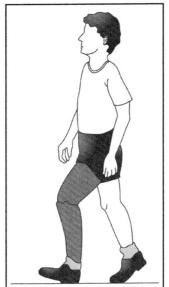
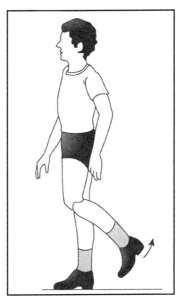
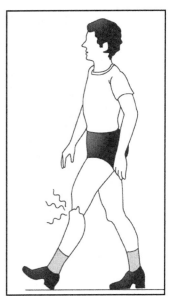

Figure 10-6. Foot rotation at heel contact. **Figure 10-7.** Knee collapse. **Figure 10-8.** High heel rise. **Figure 10-9.** Terminal impact.

EXCESSIVE KNEE MOTION

The prosthetic shank should mirror the motion of the contralateral leg with regard to its range of motion and direction of movement.

Knee collapse occurs during stance phase on the prosthesis (Figure 10-7).

➢ Anatomic/physiologic causes include the following:

  ✄ Weak hip extensors.

  ✄ Hip flexor contracture.

➢ Prosthetic causes include the following:

  ✄ Inadequate socket flexion.

  ✄ Knee axis too far anterior.

  ✄ Shoe heel higher than that for which prosthesis was designed.

  ✄ Prosthetic foot aligned in dorsiflexion.

  ✄ Prosthetic foot heel cushion too stiff.

High heel rise occurs during early swing phase (Figure 10-8). The heel on the prosthesis rises higher than the contralateral heel because the prosthetic knee is flexed excessively. Although the shoe is observed, the problem concerns knee control.

Physiologic cause is forceful hip flexion. Patients with poor control of the knee unit may intentionally fling the prosthesis forward to insure that the knee will be extended at the end of swing phase and the beginning of the next stance phase. The initial hip flexion causes the knee to flex excessively. Forceful hip motion can produce a noise that signals the patient that the prosthetic knee is safely extended. This maneuver is usually seen only with knee units that have sliding friction mechanisms. In contrast, fluid-controlled knee units, whether hydraulic or pneumatic, will automatically increase friction in response to forceful hip motion.

➢ Prosthetic causes include the following:

  ✄ Inadequate friction, particularly in units with sliding friction mechanisms.

  ✄ The knee unit does not resist the force exerted by forceful hip flexion.

  ✄ Slack extension aid fails to restrain upward motion of the shank.

Terminal impact occurs at the end of swing phase (Figure 10-9). The shank accelerates forward and may produce an audible signal if the knee unit does not have an adequate damper.

Physiologic cause is forceful hip flexion exhibited by patients who are fearful that the prosthetic knee will not be stable at the end of stance phase.

➢ Prosthetic causes include the following:

  ✄ Inadequate friction, particularly in units with sliding friction mechanisms.

  ✄ Taut extension aid hastens forward motion of the shank.

  ✄ If the patient exhibits both high heel rise and terminal impact, most likely the friction is insufficient. If high heel rise occurs in the absence of terminal impact, the extension aid is too loose. If terminal impact occurs without high heel rise, the extension is too taut. These abnormalities are less common with prostheses having fluid-controlled knee units.

INSUFFICIENT KNEE MOTION

During swing phase the prosthesis must clear the floor by approximately 0.5-inch. Otherwise, the patient risks tripping. Because the prosthetic ankle usually remains stationary during swing phase, the patient usually flexes the knee unit to obtain swing phase clearance.

Vaulting is exaggerated plantar flexion of the sound ankle during swing phase of the prosthesis (Figure 10-10). Contraction of the triceps surae is usually sufficient to lift the body at least 0.5-inch, enabling the prosthesis to swing through easily. Vaulting is a common compensation among children and young adults because it enables advancing the prosthesis rapidly without having to use forceful hip motion on the amputated side.

The physiologic cause is poor control of the knee unit; rather than using hip flexors on the amputated side to flex the prosthetic knee, the patient relies on the plantar flexors on the intact side to obtain swing phase clearance.

> Prosthetic causes include the following:
  - ¤ Prosthesis longer than contralateral lower limb.
  - ¤ Locked knee unit. In the presence of a locked knee unit, the prosthesis should be shortened approximately 0.5-inch to permit swing phase clearance.
  - ¤ Loose friction mechanism fails to control the swing of the prosthetic knee.
  - ¤ Inadequate suspension may cause the prosthesis to lower during swing phase and thus become functionally longer.
  - ¤ Small or tight socket does not accommodate the amputation limb; failure to lodge it fully in the socket creates apparent lengthening of the prosthesis.
  - ¤ Loose socket will slip downward during swing phase.
  - ¤ Foot malaligned in plantar flexion also lengthens the prosthesis.

Hip hiking is an alternate method for clearing the prosthetic foot during swing phase. On the amputated side, the patient contracts the quadratus lumborum and other related pelvic musculature to elevate the pelvis and thus the entire prosthesis. This compensation is easier to perform than vaulting and thus is more common among older adults.

Physiologic and prosthetic causes are the same as for vaulting.

STEP LENGTH DISCREPANCY

Longer step on the prosthetic side. Step length discrepancy also tends to alter the rhythm of walking with excessive time spent on the sound leg.

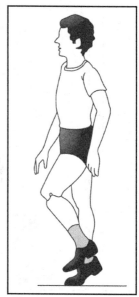

Figure 10-10. Vaulting.

> Anatomic/physiologic causes include the following:
  - ¤ Hip flexor contracture usually shortens the affected leg, thus making steps unequal in length.
  - ¤ Balance instability may make the patient reluctant to bear weight on the prosthesis; a long prosthetic step increases the time spent on the sound leg.

The prosthetic cause is usually an uncomfortable socket that interferes with placing much weight on the prosthesis and contributes to a long prosthetic step.

TROUBLE-SHOOTING GAIT PROBLEMS

> Gait disorders related to anatomic/physiologic causes:
  - ¤ Hip abductor contracture: Abduction, circumduction, lateral bending.
  - ¤ Hip flexor contracture: Lordosis, forward bending, step length discrepancy, knee collapse.
  - ¤ Weak hip abductors: Abduction, lateral bending.
  - ¤ Weak hip extensors and abdominals: Lordosis, knee collapse.
  - ¤ Laterodistal thigh pain: Abduction.
  - ¤ Hip pain: Lateral bending.
  - ¤ Adductor tissue roll: Abduction.
  - ¤ Balance instability: Abduction, lateral bending, forward bending, step length discrepancy.
  - ¤ Poor knee control: Circumduction, vaulting, hip hiking.

¤ Prosthesis donned in rotation: Whip.

¤ Forceful hip flexion: High heel rise, terminal impact.

¤ Short amputation limb: Lateral bending.

¤ Walker or crutches too short: Forward bending.

➤ Gait disorders related to prosthetic causes:

¤ Prosthesis longer than contralateral lower limb: Abduction, circumduction, vaulting, hip hiking.

¤ Short prosthesis: Lateral bending.

¤ Abducted hip joint on a pelvic band: Abduction.

¤ Inadequate lateral socket wall adduction: Abduction, lateral bending.

¤ Uncomfortable socket: Step length discrepancy.

¤ Inadequate socket flexion: Lordosis, knee collapse.

¤ Sharp or high medial socket wall: Abduction, lateral bending.

¤ Socket does not accommodate thigh muscle contraction: Whip.

¤ Tight socket: Circumduction, vaulting, hip hiking.

¤ Loose socket: Circumduction, vaulting, hip hiking.

¤ Knee axis too far anterior: Knee collapse.

¤ Knee axis malrotated: Whip.

¤ Locked knee unit: Circumduction, vaulting, hip hiking.

¤ Unstable knee unit: Forward bending.

¤ Insufficient friction: Circumduction, high heel rise, terminal impact, vaulting, hip hiking.

¤ Slack extension aid: High heel rise.

¤ Taut extension aid: Terminal impact.

¤ Foot plantar flexed: Circumduction, vaulting, hip hiking.

¤ Foot outset: Abduction, lateral bending.

¤ Foot malrotated: Whip, rotation on heel contact.

¤ Foot aligned in dorsiflexion: Knee collapse.

¤ Foot heel cushion too stiff: Rotation on heel contact, knee collapse.

¤ Shoe heel higher than that for which prosthesis was designed: Knee collapse.

¤ Inadequate suspension: Circumduction, vaulting, hip hiking.

REFERENCES

1. Boonstra AM, Schrama J, Fidler V, Eisma WH. The gait of unilateral transfemoral amputees. *Scand J Rehabil Med.* 1994;26:217-223.

2. Skinner HB, Effeney DJ. Gait analysis in amputees. *Am J Phys Med.* 1995;64:82-89.

3. Jaegers SM, Arendzen JH, de Jongh JH. Prosthetic gait of unilateral transfemoral amputees: a kinematic study. *Arch Phys Med Rehabil.* 1995;76:736-743.

4. Perry J. Amputee gait. In: Smith D, Michael J, Bowker J, eds. *Atlas of Amputations and Limb Deficiencies.* 3rd ed. Rosemont, IL: American Academy of Orthopedic Surgeons; 2004:375-384.

5. Bae TS, Choi K, Hong D, Mun M. Dynamic analysis of above-knee amputee gait. *Clin Biomech (Bristol, Avon).* 2007;22:557-566.

6. Hof AL, van Bockel RM, Schoppen T, Postema K. Control of lateral balance in walking: experimental findings in normal subjects and above-knee amputees. *Gait Posture.* 2007;25:250-258.

7. Tesio L, Lanzi D, Detrembleur C. The 3-D motion of the centre of gravity of the human body during level walking. II. Lower limb amputees. *Clin Biomech (Bristol, Avon).* 1998;13:83-90.

8. Schmid M, Beltami G, Zambarbieri D, Verni G. Centre of pressure displacements in trans-femoral amputees during gait. *Gait Posture.* 2005;21:255-262.

9. Hagberg K, Haggstrom E, Brånemark R. Physiological cost index (PCI) and walking performance in individuals with transfemoral prostheses compared to healthy controls. *Disabil Rehabil.* 2007;29:643-649.

10. Gottschalk FA, Stills M. The biomechanics of trans-femoral amputation. *Prosthet Orthot Int.* 1994;18:12-17.

11. Buckley JG, O'Driscoll D, Bennett SJ. Postural sway and active balance performance in highly active lower-limb amputees *Am J Phys Med Rehabil.* 2002;81:13-20.

12. Michaud SB, Gard SA, Childress DS. A preliminary investigation of pelvic obliquity patterns during gait in persons with transtibial and transfemoral amputation. *J Rehabil Res Dev.* 2000;37:1-10.

13. Baum BS, Schnall BL, Tis JE, Lipton JS. Correlation of residual limb length and gait parameters in amputees. *Injury.* 2008;39:728-733.

14. Nolan L, Wit A, Dudzinski K, et al. Adjustments in gait symmetry with walking speed in transfemoral and transtibial amputees. *Gait Posture.* 2003;17:142-151.

15. Nolan L, Lees A. The functional demands on the intact limb during walking for active trans-femoral and transtibial amputees. *Prosthet Orthot Int.* 2000;24:117-125.

16. Donker SF, Beek PJ. Interlimb coordination in prosthetic walking: effects of asymmetry and walking velocity. *Acta Psychol (Amst).* 2002;110:265-288.

17. Goujon-Pillet H, Sapin E, Fodé P, Lavaste F. Three-dimensional motions of trunk and pelvis during trans-femoral amputee gait. *Arch Phys Med Rehabil.* 2008;89: 87-94.

18. van Keeken HG, Vrieling AH, Hof AL, et al. Controlling propulsive forces in gait initiation in transfemoral amputees. *J Biomech Eng.* 2008;130:011002.

19. Vrieling AH, van Keeken HG, Schoppen T, et al. Gait initiation in lower limb amputees. *Gait Posture.* 2008;27: 423-430.

20. Vrieling AH, van Keeken HG, Schoppen T, et al. Gait termination in lower limb amputees. *Gait Posture.* 2008;27: 82-90.

21. Rabuffetti M, Recalcati Ferrarin M. Transfemoral amputee gait: socket-pelvis constraints and compensation strategies. *Prosthet Orthot Int.* 2005;29:183-192.

22. Devlin M, Sinclair LB, Colman D, et al. Patient preference and gait efficiency in a geriatric population with transfemoral amputation using a free-swinging versus a locked prosthetic knee joint. *Arch Phys Med Rehabil.* 2002;83:246-249.

23. Segal AD, Orendurff MS, Klute GK, et al. Kinematic and kinetic comparisons of transfemoral amputee gait using C-Leg and Mauch SNS prosthetic knees. *J Rehabil Res Dev.* 2006;43:857-870.

24. Orendurff MS, Segal AD, Klute GK, et al. Gait efficiency using the C-Leg. *J Rehabil Res Dev.* 2006;43:239-246.

25. Kaufman KR, Levine JA, Brey RH, et al. Gait and balance of transfemoral amputees using passive mechanical and microprocessor-controlled prosthetic knees. *Gait Posture.* 2007;26:489-493.

26. Hafner BJ, Smith DG. Differences in function and safety between Medicare Functional Classification Level-2 and -3 transfemoral amputees and influence of prosthetic knee joint control. *J Rehabil Res Dev.* 2009;46:417-433.

27. Kahle JT, Highsmith MJ, Hubbard SL. Comparison of nonmicroprocessor knee mechanism versus C-Leg on Prosthesis Evaluation Questionnaire, stumbles, falls, walking tests, stair descent, and knee preference. *J Rehabil Res Dev.* 2008;45:1-14.

28. Johansson JL, Sherrill DM, Riley PO, et al. A clinical comparison of variable-damping and mechanically passive prosthetic knee devices. *Am J Phys Med Rehabil.* 2005;84:563-575.

29. Van der Linden ML, Twiste N, Rithalia SV. The biomechanical effects of the inclusion of a torque absorber on trans-femoral amputee gait: a pilot study. *Prosthet Orthot Int.* 2002;26:35-43.

30. Graham LE, Datta D, Heller B, et al. A comparative study of conventional and energy-storing prosthetic feet in high-functioning transfemoral amputees. *Arch Phys Med Rehabil.* 2007;88:801-806.

31. Lee S, Hong J. The effect of prosthetic ankle mobility in the sagittal plane on the gait of transfemoral amputees wearing a stance phase controlled knee prosthesis. *Proc Inst Mech Eng H.* 2009;223:263-271.

32. Meikle B, Boulias C, Pauley T, Devlin M. Does increased prosthetic weight affect gait speed and patient preference in dysvascular transfemoral amputees? *Arch Phys Med Rehabil.* 2003;84:1657-1661.

33. Bae TS, Choi K, Mun M. Level walking and stair climbing gait in above-knee amputees. *J Med Eng Technol.* 2009;33:130-135.

34. Vrieling AH, van Keeken HG, Schoppen T, et al. Uphill and downhill walking in unilateral lower limb amputees. *Gait Posture.* 2008;28:235-242.

35. Burkett B, Smeathers J, Barker T. Walking and running inter-limb asymmetry for Paralympic trans-femoral amputees, a biomechanical analysis. *Prosthet Orthot Int.* 2003;27:36-47.

Chapter 11

Partial Foot Amputations and Prostheses

Absence of part of the foot is usually less disabling than transtibial amputation. Distal amputation, however, does disturb the individual's standing balance and gait. Amputation necessitated by vascular disease also should be viewed as a harbinger of possible future limb loss, with appropriate vigilance directed by avoiding the further loss of both lower limbs.

In most instances, when the patient stands, weight is likely to shift posteriorly. Partial foot amputations and disarticulations are *end-bearing* (ie, the patient can support full weight through the lower limb) and thus usually more comfortable than *peripheral bearing* amputations (ie, weight borne around the periphery of the amputation limb). If the other foot is intact, the individual is likely to bear disproportionate weight on it. When the patient walks, swing phase may pose difficulty retaining the shoe on the foot, unless the shoe fastens high on the dorsum. In late stance phase, loss of 1 or more toes compromises propulsion normally augmented by the intrinsic flexors. If the amputation involves the proximal part of the foot, another problem is added; namely, control of early stance with avoidance of foot slap.

Ordinarily the patient will manage better with a shoe with a closed upper, rather than a sandal. The more proximal the amputation, the more important it is that the shoe fastens high on the dorsum of the foot. Management often combines prosthetic and orthotic designs.[1,2]

PHALANGEAL AMPUTATION

Loss of 1 or more distal phalanges (Figures 11-1 and 11-2) has minimal effect on standing and walking; however, running may be hampered because propulsion in late stance is slightly lessened. Absence of any of the middle phalanges further limits action of the intrinsic muscles. The most serious phalangeal amputation involves the proximal phalanges, the site of insertion of the plantar aponeurosis (fascia). Weakening of this tough undergirding of the foot causes the longitudinal arch to lower, thus impairing comfortable standing, especially for extended durations. Compared with amputation of the lesser toes, there is a greater compromise on late stance propulsion and standing balance from the removal of both phalanges of the first (great) toe. The 2 sesamoids at the hallux head may be sources of irritation unless they are also removed. Removal of the second toe is associated with hallux valgus.

Although some people function without any shoe modification, optimum management includes an orthosis to aid stability while supporting and protecting the foot.[3] The device should support the longitudinal arch support to compensate for the weakening of the plantar aponeurosis, particularly if several toes are missing; a resilient cover for the orthosis reduces pressure concentration. Many patients walk more easily with a shoe having a rigid sole.[4] A toe filler in the shoe will restore the normal appearance of the upper portion of the shoe; the proximal margin of the filler should have a silicone pad under the metatarsal heads.[5] Some people opt for a more cosmetic prosthesis that includes a toe filler and arch support and covers the entire foot (Figures 11-3 and 11-4). Although a rocker bar on the shoe sole will aid propulsion, many patients are reluctant to have their shoes modified.[6] If a rocker bar is used, its apex should lie immediately posterior to the metatarsal heads.

RAY AMPUTATION

Absence of the phalanges and the associated metatarsal of a single toe create an abnormally narrow foot, which may interfere with comfortable standing. If the first or fifth ray is missing, the patient will shift weight to the lateral or medial border of the foot, respectively. Gait

Edelstein JE, Muroz A.
Lower-Limb Prosthetics and Orthotics: Clinical Concepts (pp 79-86).
© 2011 Taylor & Francis Group.

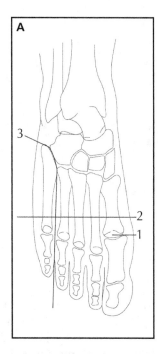

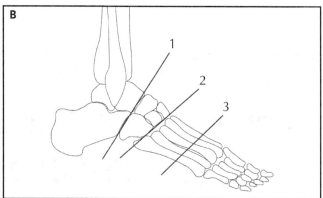

Figure 11-1. Superior and lateral views of a foot skeleton. A: (1) Metatarsophalangeal disarticulation. (2) Transmetatarsal amputation. (3) Ray resection. B: (1) Chopart disarticulation. (2) Lisfranc disarticulation. (3) Transmetatarsal amputation. (Reprinted with permission from Carroll K, Edelstein JE. *Prosthetics and Patient Management: A Comprehensive Clinical Approach.* Thorofare, NJ: SLACK Incorporated; 2006.)

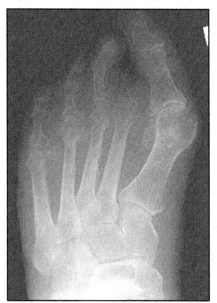

Figure 11-2. Digit amputation. (Reprinted with permission from Carroll K, Edelstein JE. *Prosthetics and Patient Management: A Comprehensive Clinical Approach.* Thorofare, NJ: SLACK Incorporated; 2006.)

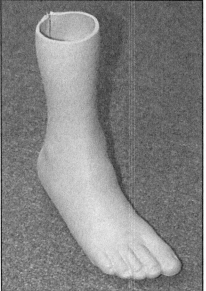

Figure 11-3. Foot prosthesis. (Reprinted with permission from Carroll K, Edelstein JE. *Prosthetics and Patient Management: A Comprehensive Clinical Approach.* Thorofare, NJ: SLACK Incorporated; 2006.)

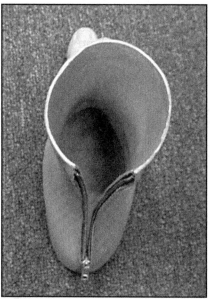

Figure 11-4. Foot prosthesis, rear entry. (Reprinted with permission from Carroll K, Edelstein JE. *Prosthetics and Patient Management: A Comprehensive Clinical Approach.* Thorofare, NJ: SLACK Incorporated; 2006.)

is minimally disturbed,[7] although the vigorous walker may notice diminished propulsive force in late stance.

The shoe on the amputated side should include a longitudinal filler to equalize left and right foot widths. A rocker sole bar may also be helpful.

TRANSMETATARSAL AMPUTATION

Amputation through the metatarsal shafts (Figures 11-5 and 11-6) exaggerates the problems already cited.

Healing is apt to be prolonged because the thin dorsal skin is relatively fragile with scant blood supply.[8] When the patient resumes walking, each step tends to shift the amputation limb forward against the dorsal surgical scar. During standing, posterior weight shift[5] and flattening of the longitudinal arch occur. Propulsion may be diminished because all intrinsic flexors are lost, necessitating increased power generation across the hip joints.[9,10] During swing phase the patient may have difficulty retaining the shoe on the shortened foot.

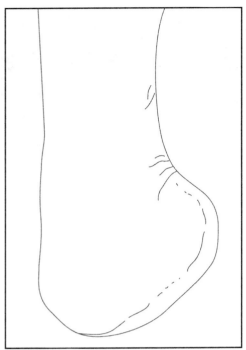

Figure 11-5. Transmetatarsal amputations.

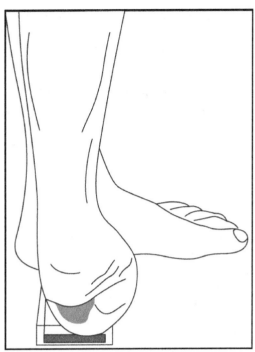

Figure 11-6. Chopart disarticulation.

Although some people manage with only a toe filler in the shoe,[5] comprehensive care includes a custom-made socket to protect the amputation scar. A toe filler can be secured to the socket so that ordinary shoes can be worn. Nevertheless, lacing or a strap on the proximal dorsum of the foot is desirable to prevent shoe slippage during swing phase. A longitudinal arch support[11] is useful. If wound healing is markedly delayed, the patient may benefit from an ankle-foot orthosis with a proximal weight-bearing cuff and a solid ankle; the orthosis transfers stress from the foot to the proximal leg. A shoe with a resilient heel will enable slight plantar flexion during early stance, compensating for the solid orthotic ankle. A rocker bar will facilitate late stance.

LISFRANC DISARTICULATION

Division of the foot at the tarsometatarsal joints (see Figure 11-1B) is rarely performed today, although it is less traumatic than transmetatarsal amputation and is sometimes used as a limb salvage procedure.[12] Devised by Jacques Lisfranc (1790-1847), the disarticulation involves removal of all metatarsals and phalanges, removing the entire forefoot. Prior to the introduction of anesthesia in the mid-19th century, the relatively rapid disarticulation was generally safer than amputation through the bones. Because the insertions of the extrinsic toe extensors are lost, the foot tends to plantar flex. Consequently, the standing base may be further reduced. Posterior weight shift also interferes with comfortable standing. Late stance propulsion is reduced.

The shorter foot is apt to slip from the shoe during swing phase.

To minimize pes equinus, the patient should keep the Achilles tendon stretched. Although one can function with just a toe filler in the shoe, the amputation limb is usually fitted in a custom-made socket with attached toe filler.[5] A longitudinal arch support is beneficial. The shoe should fasten on the proximal dorsum and should have a rocker bar.

CHOPART DISARTICULATION

Chopart disarticulation is rare in contemporary practice. The difficulties created by Chopart disarticulation and the management are similar to that recommended for Lisfranc disarticulation. Francis Chopart (1743-1795) described removal of the mid- and forefoot, leaving only the talus and calcaneus (see Figures 11-1B, 11-6, and 11-7). The muscular balance of the foot is severely disrupted because the patient has lost all extensor insertions, including the most proximal attachment of the anterior tibialis on the base of the first cuneiform, as well as the metatarsals. Concurrently, the powerful triceps surae remains undisturbed. The resulting equinus deformity can make standing uncomfortable and can create a leg length discrepancy. Additionally, the patient may develop genu recurvatum when attempting to stand on the altered foot. Surgical stabilization of the ankle can alleviate this problem. Early stance is altered because the patient strikes the distal margin of the talus if the equinus deformity has not been corrected. As with the other partial foot losses, weight shifts posteriorly and late stance propulsion is weak. Retaining the shoe during swing phase is difficult. Nevertheless, young healthy adults may function well.[13]

Several prosthetic approaches are available. The simplest measure is strapping the shortened foot to an ankle-foot orthosis (Figure 11-8). The posterior upright of the orthosis will prevent the foot from slipping from the shoe during swing phase and may counteract the tendency of the knee to hyperextend. Although the orthosis may have a toe filler, the upper portion of the shoe will tend to develop an unnatural transverse crease. More comprehensive management involves fitting the patient with a socket to which a shoe filler is attached. The socket enables the individual to wear a low shoe without any proximal componentry. A rocker bar can assist propulsion. For those who experience foot pain, the socket can be attached to side bars and a calf band, creating a modified ankle-foot orthosis; the superstructure stabilizes the foot.[14] A patellar tendon bone (PTB) weight-relieving ankle-foot orthosis reduces stress on the amputation limb; the device includes a synthetic forefoot replacement.[5] To counteract genu recurvatum, the device may include posterior uprights.[15] Another approach involved a silicone prosthesis that enabled subjects to walk faster with less trunk inclination toward the amputated side.[16]

CALCANEAL AMPUTATIONS

In the presence of foot trauma, the calcaneus may be sectioned or removed. In 1854, Nicolai Pirogoff sectioned the calcaneus vertically and then fused the posterior portion to the tibia, thereby minimizing loss of leg length. In 1939, H. B. Boyd described transverse sectioning of the calcaneus, shifting the bone forward and then fusing it to the tibia, thereby preserving the heel fat pad. Both procedures preserve nearly the entire length of the leg and provide an end-bearing amputation limb without the need for a prosthesis.[17,18] Neither is common in current practice because gait is awkward and appearance is abnormal inasmuch as the patient cannot wear an ordinary prosthetic foot. Recent reports of calcanectomy report qualified success with patients wearing shoes with resilient insoles and walking with the aid of assistive devices.[19,20] Figure 11-9 illustrates a Boyd prosthesis.

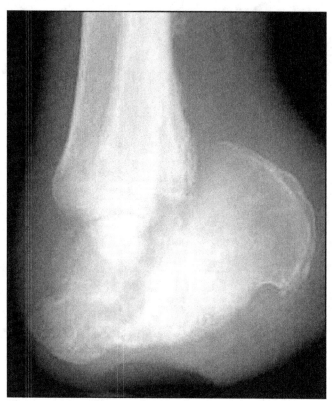

Figure 11-7. Chopart disarticulation with Achilles tendon contracture. (Reprinted with permission from Carroll K, Edelstein JE. *Prosthetics and Patient Management: A Comprehensive Clinical Approach*. Thorofare, NJ: SLACK Incorporated; 2006.)

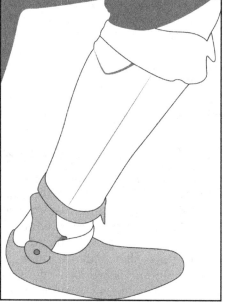

Figure 11-8. Chopart disarticulation prosthesis.

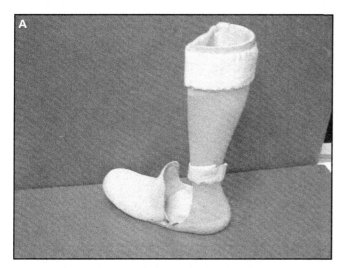

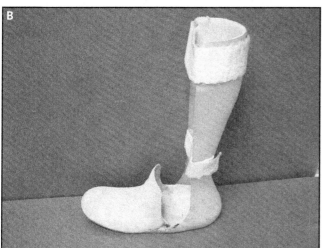

Figure 11-9. Boyd prosthesis. (A) Posterolateral view. (B) Lateral view.

ANKLE DISARTICULATION AND SYME'S AMPUTATION

Ankle disarticulation, more common than Lisfranc and Chopart disarticulations, involves removal of the entire foot, leaving the tibial and fibular malleoli intact. Syme's amputation is an alternative procedure. In 1843, James Syme discussed ablation of the foot of a patient who had osteomyelitis. The leg is amputated through the distal cortical bone of the tibia and fibula (Figure 11-10). Although all tarsals are removed, the calcaneal fat pad is preserved. The overlying skin is sutured to the anterior aspect of the leg, producing a distal cushion.[21,22] Ideally, the limb is end-bearing. The patient retains almost the full length of the leg to control a prosthesis.

Removal of the entire foot, whether by disarticulation or Syme's amputation, creates a slight leg length discrepancy. The patient can walk short distances without any prosthesis, although the individual will lean the trunk toward the amputated side. The length discrepancy allows room for a prosthetic foot specifically designed for this amputation level; with the prosthesis, the legs will be equal in length and symmetrical posture is restored. Some patients with Syme's amputation dislike the bulbous contour at the ankle. Paradoxically, patients who wear a Syme's prosthesis performed better than those with midfoot amputation. With a Syme's prosthesis, subjects concentrated load during the early stance phase in the center of the anatomic heel, transferring weight along the midline of the foot. Those with midfoot amputation loaded the posterolateral aspect of the heel and then transferred weight diagonally across the foot, achieving less propulsive force.[10]

The Syme's prosthesis consists of a Syme's prosthetic foot and a socket. Versions of the SACH (Otto Bock, Minneapolis, Minnesota), SAFE (Campbell-Child, White City, Oregon), Carbon Copy 2 (Ohio Willow Wood, Mount Sterling, Ohio), Flex-Foot (Ossur, Aliso Viejo, California), and Seattle foot (Trulife, Poulsbo, Washington) are manufactured to suit the Syme's prosthesis (Figures 11-11 through 11-13). These feet have a smaller clearance between the proximal margin of the foot and the end of the socket, compared with feet designed for transtibial prostheses.

Two basic socket designs are in current use. Patients who retain the full width of the distal leg usually have a bulbous distal end of the amputation limb. In order to lodge the distal end of the amputation limb in the bottom of the socket, the socket requires either an opening or an elastic liner. If the socket has an opening, the wearer maneuvers the amputation limb into the socket. Once the limb is fully seated, the individual straps a plastic panel over the socket opening. The socket that does not have a side opening requires an elastic liner to enable the bulbous limb to pass to the end of the socket. Compared to a socket with a side opening, the socket that does not have a side opening is more streamlined; however, if the amputation limb is markedly bulbous, it may be very difficult to don the streamlined socket. Patients who have an amputation limb that is not very bulbous can be accommodated with a streamlined socket.

Compared with individuals of comparable age and overall physical condition, those with Syme's amputation enjoy better function, walking more rapidly with less energy expenditure. Athletes perform very well if the prosthesis includes an energy-storing foot.

PARTIAL FOOT AMPUTATION IN PATIENTS WITH DIABETES

Diabetes is the leading cause of foot amputation. Recent chart reviews of patients with diabetes concur that interphalangeal amputations predominate, with

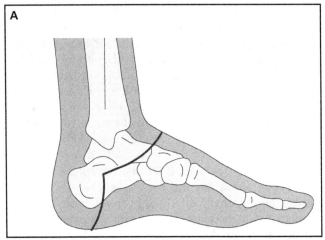 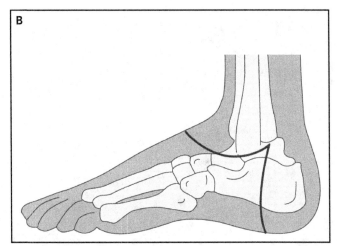

Figure 11-10. Syme's incisions. (A) Medial view. (B) Lateral view.

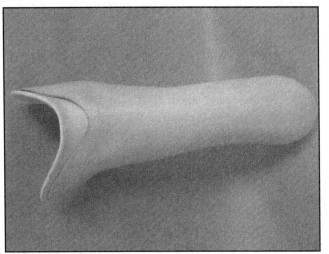 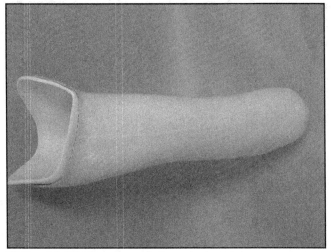

Figure 11-11. Syme's carbon fiber/epoxy laminate socket with DAW Everflex insert; Syme's socket, anterior view.

Figure 11-12. Syme's socket, posterior view.

limb salvage greater than 80% at 5 years.[23] At 5 years, more than 60% of patients with toe amputation required revision, whereas fewer than half had revision of midfoot amputation.[24] An earlier series demonstrated that diabetic patients with toe osteomyelitis, but good circulation, achieved successful rehabilitation.[25] Of 89 patients with ray amputation, at the 1-year follow-up, 12% had developed new ulcerations on the amputated side. Patients were provided with shoes with a rocker bottom sole and custom-molded insoles and had intensive ambulatory check-ups.[26] Protecting the insensate foot from excessive pressure is imperative.[27] Among those with transmetatarsal amputation, healing occurred in 57%, but postsurgical complications developed in 87% of patients.[28] A review of 26 diabetic patients noted that at the 1-year follow-up, half had healed at the Syme level with nearly all functioning well with the Syme's prosthesis; the others had died or had more proximal amputation.[29] Other clinicians note the trend toward amputation within the foot, rather than at more proximal site.[30]

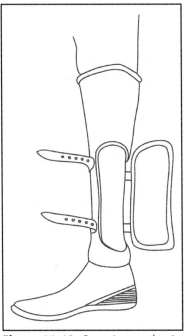

Figure 11-13. Syme's prosthesis.

REFERENCES

1. Berke GM, Rheinstein J, Michael JW, Stark GE. Biomechanics of ambulation following partial foot amputation: a prosthetic perspective. *J Prosthet Orthot.* 2007;19:85-88.

2. Yonclas PP, O'Donnell CJ. Prosthetic management of the partial foot amputee. *Clin Podiatr Med Surg.* 2005;22:485-502.

3. Philbin TM, Leyes M, Sferra JJ, Donley BG. Orthotic and prosthetic devices in partial foot amputations. *Foot Ankle Clin.* 2001;6:215-228.

4. Rommers GM, Diepstraten HJ, Bakker E, Lindeman E. Shoe adaptation after amputation of the II-V phalangeal bones of the foot. *Prosthet Orthot Int.* 2006;30:324-329.

5. Dillon MP, Barker TM. Comparison of gait of persons with partial foot amputation wearing prosthesis to matched control group: observational study. *J Rehabil Res Dev.* 2008;45:1317-1334.

6. Sobel E, Japour CJ, Giorgini RJ, et al. Use of prostheses and footwear in 110 inner-city partial-foot amputees. *J Am Podiatr Med Assoc.* 2001;91:34-49.

7. Ramseler LE, Jacob HA, Exner GU. Foot function after ray resection for malignant tumors of the phalanges and metatarsals. *Foot Ankle Int.* 2004;25:53-58.

8. Thomas SR, Perkins JM, Magee TR, Galland RB. Transmetatarsal amputation: an 8-year experience. *Ann R Coll Surg Engl.* 2001;83:164-166.

9. Dillon MP, Barker TM. Preservation of residual foot length in partial foot amputation: a biomechanical analysis. *Foot Ankle Int.* 2006;27:110-116.

10. Pinzur MS, Wolf B, Havey RM. Walking pattern of midfoot and ankle disarticulation amputees. *Foot Ankle Int.* 1997;18:635-638.

11. Tang SF, Chen CP, Chen MJ, et al. Transmetatarsal amputation prosthesis with carbon-fiber plate: enhanced gait function. *Am J Phys Med Rehabil.* 2004;83:124-130.

12. DeCotis MA. Lisfranc and Chopart amputations. *Clin Podiatr Med Surg.* 2005;22:385-393.

13. Zinger W, Holtslag HR, Verleisdonk EJ. Serious foot injury: consider partial amputation designed to preserve leg-length and a weight-bearing stump. *Ned Tijdschr Geneeskd.* 2007;151:789-794.

14. Hirsch G, McBride ME, Murray DD, et al. Chopart prosthesis and semirigid foot orthosis in traumatic forefoot amputation: comparative gait analysis. *Am J Phys Med Rehabil.* 1996;75:283-291.

15. Baima J, Trovato M, Hopkins M, Delateur B. Achieving functional ambulation in a patient with Chopart amputation. *Am J Phys Med Rehabil.* 2008;87:510-513.

16. Burger H, Erzar D, Maver T, et al. Biomechanics of walking with silicone prosthesis after midtarsal (Chopart) disarticulation. *Clin Biomech (Bristol, Avon).* 2009;24:510-516.

17. Grady JF, Winters CL. The Boyd amputation as a treatment for osteomyelitis of the foot. *J Am Podiatr Med Assoc.* 2000;90:234-239.

18. Taniguchi A, Tanaka Y, Kadono K, et al. Pirogoff ankle disarticulation as an option for ankle disarticulation. *Clin Orthop Relat Res.* 2003;414:322-328.

19. Geertzen JH, Jutte P, Rompen C, Salvans M. Calcanectomy, an alternative amputation? Two case reports. *Prosthet Orthot Int.* 2009;33:78-81.

20. Bollinger M, Thordarson DB. Partial calcanectomy: an alternative to below knee amputation. *Foot Ankle Int.* 2002;23:927-932.

21. Hudson JR, Yu GV, Marzano R, Vincent AL. Syme's amputation: surgical technique, prosthetic considerations, and case reports. *J Am Podiatr Med Assoc.* 2002;92:232-246.

22. Yu GV, Schinke TL, Meszaros A. Syme's amputation: a retrospective review of 10 cases. *Clin Podiatr Med Surg.* 2005;22:395-427.

23. Sheahan MG, Hamdan AD, Veraldi JR, et al. Lower extremity minor amputations: the roles of diabetes mellitus and timing of revascularization. *J Vasc Surg.* 2005;42:476-480.

24. Izumi Y, Satterfield K, Lee S, Harkless LB. Risk of reamputation in diabetic patients stratified by limb and level of amputation: a 10-year observation. *Diabetes Care.* 2006;29:566-570.

25. Kerstein MD, Welter V, Gahtan V, Roberts AB. Toe amputation in the diabetic patient. *Surgery.* 1997;122:546-547.

26. Dalla Paola L, Faglia E, Caminiti M, et al. Ulcer recurrence following first ray amputation in diabetic patients: a cohort prospective study. *Diabetes Care.* 2003;26:1874-1878.

27. Sage RA. Biomechanics of ambulation after partial foot amputation: prevention and management of reulceration. *J Prosthet Orthot.* 2007;19:P77-P79.

28. Pollard J, Hamilton GA, Rush SM, Ford LA. Mortality and morbidity after transmetatarsal amputation: retrospective review of 101 cases. *J Foot Ankle Surg.* 2006;45:91-97.

29. Frykberg RG, Abraham S, Tierney E, Hall J. Syme amputation for limb salvage: early experience with 26 cases. *J Foot Ankle Surg.* 2007;46:93-100.

30. Dupre JC, Dechamps E, Pillu M, Despeyroux L. The fitting of amputated and nonamputated diabetic feet: a French experience at the Villiers-Saint-Denis Hospital. *J Am Podiatr Med Assoc.* 2003;93:221-228.

Chapter 12

Knee and Hip Disarticulations and Prostheses

Knee and hip disarticulations are uncommon in contemporary practice. Consequently, few clinicians acquire substantial experience in managing patients who have these disarticulations. Whether it is a knee or hip disarticulation, patients tend to be somewhat younger and thus in better physical condition to withstand the rigors of prosthetic rehabilitation. The individual's overall health and disease prognosis will determine whether management should include fitting a prosthesis.

KNEE DISARTICULATION

Amputation through the cortical bone of the distal femur and disarticulation of the tibiofemoral joint are both classified as *knee disarticulation*. Etiologies of knee disarticulation include tumor,[1] trauma, vascular disease,[2-7] and severe knee and hip contractures.[8] The distal end of the amputation limb varies, with some retaining the patella, often fused to the femur.[9] A few have the femoral condyles trimmed to reduce distal bulbousness. In most instances, the amputation limb presents a broad end-bearing surface that enhances comfort and avoids the need for ischial weight bearing and provides a long lever arm with strong musculature with which the patient can control the prosthesis.

KNEE DISARTICULATION PROSTHESIS

The knee disarticulation prosthesis consists of a foot, shank, knee unit, and socket (Figure 12-1). Ordinarily, the socket provides sufficient suspension. Any type of foot is suitable for this prosthesis. Ordinarily, the shank is endoskeletal, although an exoskeletal shank would suffice.

Compared with wearers of transfemoral prostheses, individuals wearing knee disarticulation prostheses generally enjoy greater function. Consequently, the disarticulation prosthesis should probably have a fluid-controlled knee unit made specifically for this type of

prosthesis. These units have a thinner proximal attachment compared with knee units intended for transfemoral prostheses.

A problem peculiar to the knee disarticulation level pertains to the height of the shank. Because the thigh is usually full length, the shank is often shortened slightly to compensate for the length of the thigh with the knee unit. When the patient stands and walks, the disparity between shank length on the prosthetic side and on the sound side is not noticeable. When the individual sits, however, the thigh on the prosthetic side is apt to project farther forward than the sound thigh.

One approach to this problem is to substitute a pair of side bars with single-axis joints. The proximal bar is riveted to the socket. The distal bar ordinarily is secured to an exoskeletal shank. The mechanical knee joints are in line with the anatomic knee joint, enabling a nearly symmetrical seating posture. The serious drawback of side bars and single-axis joints is that the joints do not have a friction mechanism. When the user walks rapidly, the shank tends to swing through an abnormally larger arc.

The other approach involves installation of a knee disarticulation unit that has a friction mechanism, ideally fluid controlled. The slightly asymmetrical sitting posture is usually of less importance than the better, swing-phase control.

Two principal socket designs are available, depending on the shape of the distal end of the thigh. If the end is bulbous, a socket with an anterior opening will be easier for the patient to don. The individual secures the opening using straps with hook and pile closures or laces. If, however, the thigh has relatively straight sides, a socket without an anterior opening is preferable because of its streamlined contour and greater durability. This socket is donned by inserting the thigh into the top of the socket. Whether or not the socket has an anterior opening, it generally terminates at the proximal

Edelstein JE, Muroz A.
Lower-Limb Prosthetics and Orthotics: Clinical Concepts (pp 87-92).
© 2011 Taylor & Francis Group.

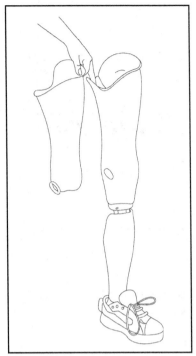

Figure 12-1. Knee disarticulation prosthesis.

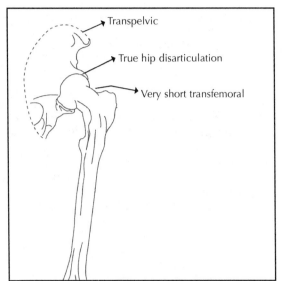

Figure 12-2. Amputation levels: transpelvic, true hip disarticulation, very short transfemoral.

thigh, below the pelvis. The socket is intended to be end bearing through the cortical bone at the distal end of the femur. If the patient cannot tolerate full weight bearing through the femur, the proximal margin of the socket may extend to the pelvis in a manner similar to that of a transfemoral socket. A socket variant has a slit that creates a flexible flap that the wearer can tighten or loosen to accommodate volume changes in the amputation limb.[10]

The knee disarticulation prosthesis ordinarily is aligned with minimal socket flexion because the patient has the full length of the thigh with which to control the prosthesis. Fitting the patient with a temporary prosthesis enabled full weight bearing in 4 weeks.[11]

The functional outcome for patients with knee disarticulation usually exceeds that of people wearing transfemoral prostheses. Knee disarticulation provides end bearing and a long femoral lever arm, unlike midthigh amputation. Some investigators reported that most patients who could walk before surgery were able to walk with a prosthesis.[2] Others had good healing rates but less success with a prosthesis.[7,12]

HIP DISARTICULATION

Several anatomic sites are classified within the general category of *hip disarticulation* because prosthetic fitting and functional outcome are quite similar (Figure 12-2). *True disarticulation* involves removal of the femoral head from the pelvic acetabulum; the

amputation limb usually has much soft tissue over the operative site. Amputation proximal to the greater trochanter, known as *very short transfemoral amputation*, deprives the patient of the natural insertion of the gluteus medius and minimus; however, the bony remnant helps to stabilize the amputation limb in the socket of a modified hip disarticulation prosthesis. Removal of any portion of the pelvis, *transpelvic amputation*, may eliminate the ipsilateral iliac crest and the ischial tuberosity or either bony prominence; consequently, alternate weight-bearing sites must be utilized. Additional problems relate to possible diversion of the urethra and the creation of an ileostomy. Etiologies of hip disarticulation and related amputations include tumors,[13-22] infection,[23] vascular disease,[24] and trauma.[25,26]

If the amputation is part of tumor management, the patient may be undergoing radiation, chemotherapy, or both; radiation may compromise the skin overlying the amputation site, whereas chemotherapy may make the patient unable to engage in a vigorous rehabilitation program.

HIP DISARTICULATION PROSTHESES

Prostheses for high-level amputations include a socket, hip joint, thigh section, knee unit, shank, and foot (Figures 12-3 through 12-7). Contemporary prostheses are based on the Canadian design introduced in 1954.[27] The socket protects the amputation site and provides sufficient area for weight bearing. Individuals with very short transfemoral amputation and those with true hip disarticulation generally rely on the ipsilateral ischial tuberosity, and both iliac crests to support most of their weight. Those with transpelvic amputation may have

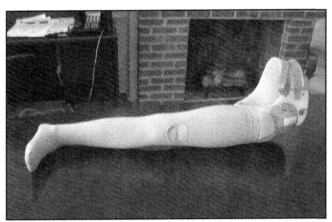

Figure 12-3. Hip disarticulation prosthesis.

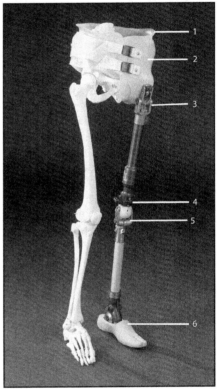

Figure 12-4. Hip disarticulation prosthesis on a skeleton. (1) Iliac crest ridge. (2) Socket. (3) Hip joint. (4) Knee unit. (5) Knee axis. (6) Foot. (Courtesy of Hanger Prosthetics & Orthotics, Inc.)

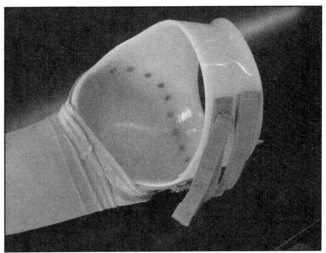

Figure 12-5. Hip disarticulation prosthesis, medial view.

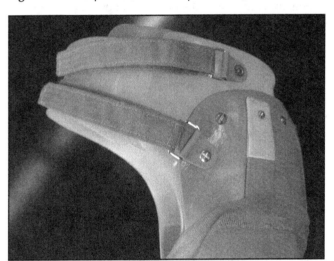

Figure 12-6. Hip disarticulation prosthesis, anterior view.

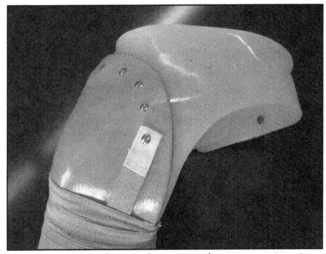

Figure 12-7. Hip disarticulation prosthesis, posterior view.

to depend on abdominal compression with or without impingement on the lower ribs to support weight. A recent variation is a total contact suction design.[28]

Regardless of socket design, it will be attached to the thigh section with a mechanical hip joint. Some joints resemble a ball-and-socket joint; however, transverse and frontal plane motion is markedly limited. Other joints are hinges that provide sufficient flexion for walking and sitting. An extension strap prevents the hip joint from undue flexion when the wearer stands and walks.

The knee unit may feature stance control by means of a hydraulic unit or a manual lock. If the unit does not have a lock, it should include an extension aid. A polycentric knee axis contributes to knee stability.

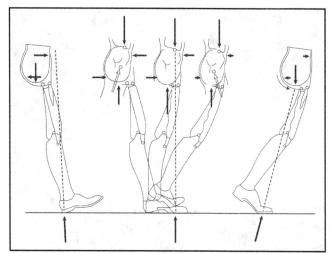

Figure 12-8. Hip and knee extension aids are taut in early stance. In midstance, alignment (rather than extension aids) provides stability. In late stance, extension aids are slack to permit hip and knee flexion.

The shank and thigh sections are usually endoskeletal to minimize prosthetic weight. Often shank length is slightly shorter than the contralateral limb to facilitate swing-phase clearance of the prosthesis. Any type of foot-ankle assembly may be used.

Prosthetic stability is provided by componentry, particularly hip and knee extension aids, and by alignment that positions the hip joint and the knee axis relatively posterior.

At heel contact, the prosthesis is stable because of the alignment of the prosthetic hip and knee joints and tension in the extension aids at both joints (Figure 12-8). Proceeding from stance phase to swing phase is often accomplished by the wearer's deliberate tilting of the pelvis posteriorly to enable the mechanical hip joint to flex. Transferring from standing to sitting requires that the individual intentionally flex the mechanical hip and knee, overriding the extension aids at these joints.

Function with a prosthesis may be limited by difficulty adjusting to the socket and problems related to walking with a rather cumbersome prosthesis.[15-18,20,24,29] Those who forego daily wear may rely on crutches or a walker for household and community ambulation.

Nevertheless, many reports[19,21,25,26,28,30] of successful use of a prosthesis suggest that attempts at rehabilitation are worthwhile, particularly for patients whose amputation was necessitated by tumor or trauma.[23] A wheelchair is important for nearly all people with high amputations, regardless of whether a prosthesis is provided.

REFERENCES

1. Havlícek V, Janícek P, Berka I. Disarticulation of the knee joint. *Acta Chir Orthop Traumatol Cech*. 2003;70:95-99.

2. Bowker JH, San Giovanni TP, Pinzur MS. North American experience with knee disarticulation with use of a posterior myofasciocutaneous flap: healing rate and functional results in seventy-seven patients. *J Bone Joint Surg Am*. 2000;82A:1571-1574.

3. Cull DL, Taylor SM, Hamontree SE, et al. A reappraisal of a modified through-knee amputation in patients with peripheral vascular disease. *Am J Surg*. 2001;182:44-48.

4. Lambregts SA, Hitters WM. Knee disarticulation after total-knee replacement. *Prosthet Orthot Int*. 2002;26: 251-252.

5. Kock HJ, Friederichs J, Ouchmaev A, et al. Long-term results of through-knee amputation with dorsal musculocutaneous flap in patients with end-stage arterial occlusive disease. *World J Surg*. 2004;28:801-806.

6. Morse BC, Cull DL, Kalbaugh C, et al. Through-knee amputation in patients with peripheral arterial disease: a review of 50 cases. *J Vasc Surg*. 2008;48:638-643.

7. Ten Duis K, Bosmans JC, Voesten HG, et al. Knee disarticulation: survival, wound healing, and ambulation: a historic cohort study. *Prosthet Orthot Int*. 2009;33:52-60.

8. Cipriano C, Keenan MA. Knee disarticulation and hip release for severe lower extremity contractures. *Clin Orthop Relat Res*. 2007;462:150-155.

9. Nellis N, Van De Water JM. Through-the-knee amputation: an improved technique. *Am Surg*. 2002;68:466-469.

10. Tingleff H, Jensen L. A newly developed socket design for a knee disarticulation amputee who is an active athlete. *Prosthet Orthot Int*. 2002;26:72-75.

11. Jones ME, Bashford GM, Munro BJ. Development of prosthetic weight bearing in a knee disarticulation amputee. *Aust J Physiother*. 1999;45:309-317.

12. Siev-Ner I, Heim M, Wershavski M, et al. Why knee disarticulation (through-knee amputation) is appropriate for nonambulatory patients. *Disabil Rehabil*. 2000;22:862-864.

13. Renard AJ, Veth RP, Schreuder HW, et al. Function and complications after ablative and limb-salvage therapy in lower extremity sarcoma of bone. *J Surg Oncol*. 2000;73:198-205.

14. Pring ME, Weber KL, Unni KK, Sim FH. Chondrosarcoma of the pelvis: a review of 64 cases. *J Bone Joint Surg Am*. 2001;83:1630-1642.

15. Refaat Y, Gunnoe J, Hornicek FJ, Mankin HJ. Comparison of quality of life after reamputation or limb salvage. *Clin Orthop Relat Res*. 2002;397:298-305.

16. Ferrapie AL, Brunel P, Besse W, et al. Lower limb proximal amputations for a tumor: a retrospective study of 12 patients. *Prosthet Orthot Int*. 2003;27:179-185.

17. Jain R, Grimer RJ, Carter SR, et al. Outcome after disarticulation of the hip for sarcomas. *Eur J Surg Oncol*. 2005;31:1025-1028.

18. Kauzlarić N, Kauzlarić KS, Kolundzić R. Prosthetic rehabilitation of persons with lower limb amputations due to tumour. *Eur J Cancer Care (Engl)*. 2007;16:238-243.

19. Jeon DG, Kim MS, Cho WH, et al. Clinical outcome of osteosarcoma with primary total femoral resection. *Clin Orthop Relat Res*. 2007;457:176-182.

20. Yari P, Dijkstra PU, Geertzen JH. Functional outcome of hip disarticulation and hemipelvectomy: a cross-sectional national descriptive study in the Netherlands. *Clin Rehabil.* 2008;22:1127-1133.

21. Daigeler A, Lehnhardt M, Khadra A, et al. Proximal major limb amputations: a retrospective analysis of 45 oncological cases. *World J Surg Oncol.* 2009;7:15.

22. Zalavras CG, Rigopoulos N, Ahlmann E, Patzakis MJ. Hip disarticulation for severe lower extremity infections. *Clin Orthop Relat Res.* 2009;467:1721-1726.

23. Dénes Z, Till A. Rehabilitation of patients after hip disarticulation. *Arch Orthop Trauma Surg.* 1997;116:498-499.

24. Merimsky O, Kollender Y, Inbar M, et al. Palliative major amputation and quality of life in cancer patients. *Acta Oncol.* 1997;36:151-157.

25. Shin JC, Park CI, Kim YC, et al. Rehabilitation of a triple amputee including a hip disarticulation. *Prosthet Orthot Int.* 1998;22:251-253.

26. Schnall BL, Baum BS, Andrews AM. Gait characteristics of a soldier with a traumatic hip disarticulation. *Phys Ther.* 2008;88:1568-1577.

27. Stark G. Overview of hip disarticulation prostheses. *J Prosthet Orthot.* 2001;13:50-53.

28. Zaffer SM, Braddom RL, Conti A, et al. Total hip disarticulation prosthesis with suction socket: report of two cases. *Am J Phys Med Rehabil.* 1999;78:160-162.

29. Fernández A, Formigo J. Are Canadian prostheses used? A long-term experience. *Prosthet Orthot Int.* 2005;29:177-181.

30. McAnelly RD, Refaeian M, O'Connell DG, et al. Successful prosthetic fitting of a 73-year-old hip disarticulation amputee patient with cardiopulmonary disease. *Arch Phys Med Rehabil.* 1998;79:585-588.

Chapter 13

Bilateral Amputations and Prostheses

People who sustain bilateral lower-limb amputation present formidable challenges to the rehabilitation team. Much depends on the etiology of the amputations, the prior performance of the patient, and the individual's current medical condition. Although Medicare K levels are not applicable to adults with bilateral amputations, the guidelines are helpful in designing rational rehabilitation.

ETIOLOGIES

Bilateral amputation may occur simultaneously, as in the case of trauma (eg, trauma sustained from some land mine explosions).[1] Rarely, bilateral or quadrimembral amputation results from massive infection[2] or as a means of improving the quality of life of a person with spinal cord injury who has had severe lower-limb spasticity, pressure ulcers, and contractures.[3] Another unusual etiology is alcoholism, which creates a management problem beyond consideration of prostheses.[4] A few infants are born with bilateral limb anomaly. These children usually have intact proximal musculature and thus progress very well. Most patients with simultaneous bilateral amputations are generally healthy, although concomitant injuries and emotional issues can compromise rehabilitation.

If bilateral amputation occurs sequentially, the patient generally has peripheral vascular disease. In a few instances, people sustained traumatic amputation and completed prosthetic rehabilitation; years later, they developed vascular disease, which resulted in the contralateral amputation. Several critical issues need to be addressed before the patient with sequential amputations can be considered as a candidate for prostheses. First, was the person fitted with a unilateral prosthesis? How well did the individual use it? It is most unlikely that a dysvascular patient who never wore a single prosthesis will be able to manage a pair of prostheses. The second issue relates to the patient's current medical status. If the person has diabetes, how well is the disease controlled? Diabetes reduces the interval between amputations, compared with patients with bilateral amputation who do not have diabetes. The diabetic patient's cardiac, renal, and visual status bears directly on the ability to benefit from prostheses. Quality of the amputation limbs is paramount; flexion contractures markedly limit the opportunity to benefit from prostheses, as does advanced age and pain.[5]

If it is evident that the patient is not a prosthetic candidate, then rehabilitation should focus on wheelchair mobility. Cosmetic prostheses may be attached to the wheelchair so that the person presents a more normal appearance.

For those deemed suitable for prostheses, several issues unique to bilateral prosthetic fitting demand attention.

FEET SELECTION

Although any type of prosthetic foot may be suitable, both prostheses must have the same foot design from the same manufacturer. Patients are likely to notice subtle differences among feet, particularly the solid ankle, cushion (SACH; Otto Bock, Minneapolis, Minnesota; Kingsley, Costa Mesa, California) feet. The individual's function will be enhanced by a pair of feet that are shorter and wider than the preamputation foot size.

Shorter feet facilitate weight transition from midstance to late stance. Wider feet increase mediolateral stability. Changing foot size entails changing shoe size, which may pose economic difficulties for people who have a large shoe wardrobe.

Edelstein JE, Muroz A.
Lower-Limb Prosthetics and Orthotics: Clinical Concepts (pp 93-96).
© 2011 Taylor & Francis Group.

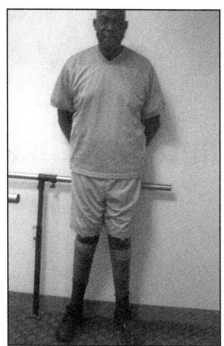

Figure 13-1. Man wearing bilateral transtibial prostheses.

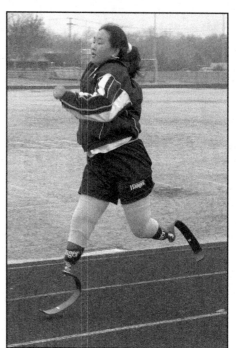

Figure 13-2. Woman running while wearing bilateral transtibial prostheses with Flex-Run Feet. (Reprinted with permission from Carroll K, Edelstein JE. *Prosthetics and Patient Management: A Comprehensive Clinical Approach.* Thorofare, NJ: SLACK Incorporated; 2006.)

BILATERAL TRANSTIBIAL PROSTHESES

Other than a matched pair of prosthetic feet, the other components of bilateral transtibial prostheses need not be the same (Figure 13-1). Endoskeletal shanks are particularly appropriate because slight changes in alignment can have a major effect on the patient's comfort and function. As always, sockets are custom-made for each amputation limb. Suspensions can be selected according to the length of the specific amputation limb and the patient's probable activity level. A pair of thigh corsets should be avoided because patients tend to walk with a wide base to avoid having the medial side bars contact one another; a slightly wider base, however, is common among those wearing bilateral prostheses in order to improve stability. Etiology of amputations does not have a marked effect on gait.[6] Compared with nondisabled adults, those who wore bilateral transtibial prostheses walked slower, had shorter and wider steps, and elevated the pelvis during swing phase. Ankle dorsiflexion and knee flexion in stance phase are reduced.[7] Pelvic elevation on the stance limb is common.[8] Functional performance of some patients who wear bilateral transtibial prostheses is excellent (Figure 13-2).

TRANSTIBIAL/ TRANSFEMORAL PROSTHESES

The components of each prosthesis, with the exception of a matched pair of feet, will depend on the length and condition of each amputation limb.

Patients may prefer foot-ankle units, which provide substantial plantar and dorsiflexion.[9] Any type of prosthetic knee unit can be included in the transfemoral prosthesis. The patient will walk and climb stairs in a manner similar to that of someone wearing a unilateral transfemoral prosthesis.

BILATERAL TRANSFEMORAL PROSTHESES

Fitting a pair of transfemoral prostheses, particularly to a patient with vascular disease, is very difficult. Selection of each of the 5 components of the transfemoral prosthesis (ie, foot, shank, knee unit, socket, and suspension) will be influenced by the person's need for 2 prostheses.

In addition to matching foot design and manufacturer, the clinical team must consider the adjustment of the feet. The resilience of the heel cushions, or plantar flexion bumpers, should enable the wearer to stand with very slight dorsiflexion. This posture reduces the risk of a backward fall, for which the individual would have virtually no protection. Most people who wear a pair of transfemoral prostheses use some type of assistive device, typically a walker. Thus, the minimal forward lean would pose much less risk.

With bilateral prostheses, the most controversial component is the shank, specifically its length. With a unilateral prosthesis, shank length matches the length of the sound leg. Because of formidable stability problems, particularly for the individual who is coping with his or her first pair of prostheses, the shanks typically are shorter than the preamputation leg length. The extreme shortening is seen with a pair of *stubbies* (Figure 13-3). These are short, nonarticulated bilateral transfemoral prostheses. The closer the individual's center of gravity is to the floor, the more stable the person will be. Additionally, stubbies are lighter in weight and easier to control than full-length prostheses. As the patient progresses in rehabilitation, the shanks of the stubbies can be lengthened by substituting longer pylons. By starting with short stature, then gradually lengthening, the wearer is able to determine the optimal height, which usually represents a compromise between function and appearance. Rotator units in the shanks improve gait velocity and reduce the perceived exertion of walking.[10]

Stubbies, however, present several difficulties. The most obvious is the appearance of the patient, who now may be 4 or more inches shorter than prior to the amputations. Trousers need to be shortened. Some people are so distressed by this alteration of body image that they refuse to wear stubbies. Gait is marked by exaggerated pelvic elevation and transverse rotation as well as more hip abduction to obtain limb clearance during swing phase. Transferring into an ordinary, adult-sized chair is more difficult, as is climbing regular 8-inch-high stairs.

Many combinations of knee units have been used successfully. It is not necessary to match knee units. The clinic team should be influenced by Medicare guidelines for the unilateral transfemoral prosthesis. Some units, however, are more appropriate, particularly those with hydraulic stance control. Lacking quadriceps, the typical patient needs an alternate means of stabilizing the knee. Although hydraulic stance control units also have swing phase control, most people who wear bilateral transfemoral prostheses do not walk rapidly and thus do not take much advantage of swing phase accommodation to changes in velocity. One subject achieved better gait, walking farther and faster at lower oxygen consumption when wearing C-Leg (Otto Bock) prostheses.[11] Knee units with sliding friction brakes also aid stance stability. Another option includes 1 knee unit with a manual lock and the other with stance control. Gait will not be as smooth as with a pair of stance control units, but the greater stability afforded by one manual lock may be more important. One should avoid using a pair of manually locked knees for patients who have any potential for climbing stairs. Though this feat is possible with great effort, if neither knee bends, the patient would be limited to staircases wide enough to allow circumducting each prosthesis.

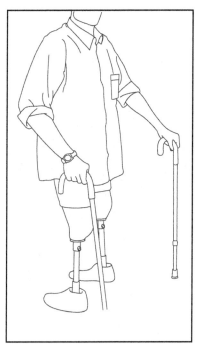

Figure 13-3. Stubby prostheses. Note the posteriorly directed shoes which reduce the wearer's risk of falling backwards.

Sockets, as always, are custom-made and each is unique to the particular amputation limb. Some wearers succeed with a pair of quadrilateral sockets. Nevertheless, more streamlined prostheses include a pair of ischial containment sockets, each of which has a narrower mediolateral dimension, thus reducing the tendency of one socket to collide with the other and minimizing the walking base.

A variety of suspensions are suitable. Patients can learn to don suction-suspended prostheses while sitting. Agile users can manage with bilateral suction suspension; however, most people require additional suspension, such as a Silesian belt designed for bilateral prostheses or an elastic belt.

The functional prospects of patients fitted with bilateral transfemoral prostheses are limited; gait is relatively slow and awkward with high energy consumption, as described in Chapter 14. Young, highly motivated patients, however, are reasonably active when wearing prostheses (Figures 13-4 and 13-5). Nevertheless, most patients rely on a wheelchair for travel in the community.

BILATERAL HIP DISARTICULATION PROSTHESES

Very few people sustain bilateral hip disarticulation; most are not fitted with prostheses and rely on the wheelchair for mobility. Some individuals sit in a socket for

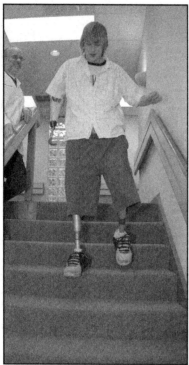

Figure 13-4. Man descending stairs while wearing bilateral transfemoral prostheses and upper-limb prothesis. (Reprinted with permission from Carroll K, Edelstein JE. *Prosthetics and Patient Management: A Comprehensive Clinical Approach.* Thorofare, NJ: SLACK Incorporated; 2006. Courtesy of Hanger Prosthetics & Orthotics, Inc.)

improved trunk control. A novel approach involves adapting the reciprocating gait orthosis so that the patient can achieve upright gait.[12]

REFERENCES

1. Atesalp AS, Erler K, Gür E, et al. Bilateral lower limb amputations as a result of landmine injuries. *Prosthet Orthot Int.* 1999;23:50-54.
2. Hacking HG, Lo-a-Njoe BA, Visser-Meily JM. Multiple amputations due to sepsis: however, functional rehabilitation is possible. *Ned Tijdschr Geneeskd.* 1999;22:1073-1077.
3. Jaffe MS. Elective bilateral above the knee amputation in T4-complete spinal cord injury: a case report. *Spinal Cord.* 2008;46:585-587.
4. Davidson JH, Jones LE, Cornet J, Cittarelli T. Management of the multiple limb amputee. *Disabil Rehabil.* 2002;24:688-699.
5. Traballesi M, Porcacchia P, Averna T, et al. Prognostic factors in prosthetic rehabilitation of bilateral dysvascular above-knee amputee: is the stump condition an influencing factor? *Eura Medicophys.* 2007;43:1-6.

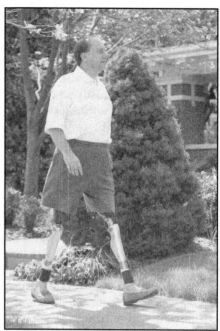

Figure 13-5. Man wearing bilateral prostheses with C-Legs walking in the community. (Reprinted with permission from Carroll K, Edelstein JE. *Prosthetics and Patient Management: A Comprehensive Clinical Approach.* Thorofare, NJ: SLACK Incorporated; 2006.

6. Su P-F, Gard SA, Lipschutz RD, Kuiken TA. Differences in gait characteristics between persons with bilateral transtibial amputations, due to peripheral vascular disease and trauma, and able-bodied ambulators. *Arch Phys Med Rehabil.* 2008;89:1386-1394.
7. Su P-F, Gard SA, Lipschutz RD, Kuiken TA. Gait characteristics of persons with bilateral transtibial amputations. *J Rehabil Res Dev.* 2007;44:491-502.
8. Michaud SB, Gard SA, Childress DS. A preliminary investigation of pelvic obliquity patterns during gait in persons with transtibial and transfemoral amputation. *J Rehabil Res Dev.* 2000;37:1-10.
9. McNealy LL, Gard SA. Effect of prosthetic ankle units on the gait of persons with bilateral trans-femoral amputations. *Prosthet Orthot Int.* 2008;32:111-126.
10. Gitter A, Paynter K, Walden G, Darm T. Influence of rotators on the kinematic adaptations in stubby prosthetic gait. *Am J Phys Med Rehab.* 2002;81:310-314.
11. Perry J, Burnfield JM, Newsam CJ, Conley P. Energy expenditure and gait characteristics of a bilateral amputee walking with C-Leg prostheses compared with stubby and conventional articulating prostheses. *Arch Phys Med Rehabil.* 2004;85:1711-1717.
12. Spence WD, Fowler NK, Nicol AC, Murray SJ. Reciprocating gait prosthesis for the bilateral hip disarticulation amputee. *Proc Inst Mech Eng H.* 2001;215:309-314.

Chapter 14

Prosthetic Gait and Activities Training

Most people who receive their first prosthesis require structured instruction in order to use it with maximum success.[1,2] Prior to training, the clinic team should ascertain whether the patient has a well-healed amputation wound and is in reasonably positive physical and emotional condition. The prosthesis should fit properly, have optimal alignment, and be well constructed.

For all patients, minimum training includes learning to don the prosthesis and being able to transfer from various chairs. Without these skills, the individual is very unlikely to wear the prosthesis or walk in a functional manner.

DONNING PROSTHESES AND DRESSING

Although donning instruction need not begin on the first day of gait training, early in rehabilitation the patient should be taught a method that enables accurate, independent, and rapid donning. Otherwise, the person will have to depend on a family member or friend to assist in the process; in spite of the best intentions, after a while, most people who cannot don the prosthesis independently find it less bothersome simply to avoid coping with the prosthesis. Being able to dress in street clothes is a related, basic activity.

Transtibial Prosthesis

Most transtibial prostheses can be donned while the individual sits. The basic method is the same for prostheses that have cuff suspension with or without a waist belt and fork strap, elastic sleeve suspension, supracondylar brim, or supracondylar-suprapatellar brim suspension. First, the patient dons the required number of amputation limb socks. If the patient has a silicone or urethane liner, this is put on the amputation limb. Second, after removing the resilient liner from the socket, the liner is donned. Securing nylon fabric to the outside of the socket reduces friction between the liner and the socket, thus facilitating donning. Third, the

individual inserts the amputation limb (covered by the socks and/or liner) into the socket. Finally, the person secures the cuff, waist belt, or elastic sleeve if any of these are worn.

The prosthesis with distal pin suspension can also be donned while sitting (Figure 14-1). First, the patient dons the silicone liner, which has a distal pin. Second, the person puts on any socks needed to ensure snug socket fit. The socks will have a distal hole through which the pin is placed. Third, the amputation limb with its liner and socks is inserted into the socket in a manner that permits the pin to engage the locking mechanism in the bottom of the socket. Some patients use a simple device to aid donning.[3]

If thigh corset suspension is used, then the donning procedure has both sitting and standing steps. While seated, first, the patient puts on the amputation limb socks and the socket liner. Second, the amputation limb covered with socks and liner enters the socket. Third, the patient fastens the thigh corset *loosely*. Then the person stands and bears enough weight on the prosthesis in order to lodge the amputation limb fully into the socket. Afterward, the patient fastens the thigh corset *snugly*. If the corset were fully fastened while the patient sat, the amputation limb would tend to be lifted from the socket, creating a space between the bottom of the limb and the bottom of the socket; the limb would tend to develop distal edema.

Transfemoral Prosthesis

Prior to donning a transfemoral prosthesis, the patient should remove the suction valve and place it on a nearby table. Although one can don a transfemoral prosthesis while sitting, it is much easier to accomplish this task while standing. The beginner should stand near a stable support, such as a sturdy chair or parallel bars.

The traditional method involves pulling the thigh into the socket. This requires having a pull sock, a length of tubular cotton stockinet equal to at least twice

Edelstein JE, Muroz A.
Lower-Limb Prosthetics and Orthotics: Clinical Concepts (pp 97-106).
© 2011 Taylor & Francis Group.

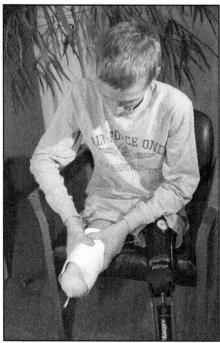

Figure 14-1. Donning liner with pin. (Courtesy of Hanger Prosthetics & Orthotics, Inc.)

the length of the amputation limb. First, the patient dons the pull sock, making certain that the proximal end terminates at the groin. If the sock ends more distally, then the upper thigh will not be lodged within the socket. If the sock ends above the inguinal ligament, it will be very difficult to complete the donning process. Second, insert the thigh with its pull sock into the socket in such a manner that the distal end of the pull sock can be drawn through the valve hole in the socket. Third, pull the end of the pull sock through the valve hole. Fourth, tug on the pull sock while flexing the contralateral hip and knee; this maneuver will shift the skin and underlying soft tissue distally in the socket. Fifth, extend the contralateral hip and knee while relaxing the grip on the pull sock. Repeat the fourth and fifth steps until the thigh settles into the socket. If the suspension is total suction, remove the pull sock and install the valve. If the suspension is partial suction, stuff the end of the pull sock back into the valve hole, then install the valve. Fasten the Silesian belt or pelvic band.

The push method generally is easier. First, the patient applies lotion to the entire thigh. Second, slide the thigh into the socket. Finally, insert the valve and fasten auxiliary suspension, if present. The push method is intended for those who rely on total suction, without wearing a sock over the amputation limb.

Dressing

Although patients in the rehabilitation department may appear in various states of undress, many people shy away from wearing a prosthesis without conventional outer garments.

Donning a skirt, dress, or shorts is relatively simple. The individual should put the sock and shoe on the prosthesis prior to donning it.

The easiest sequence for wearing slacks/trousers/pants/leggings/panty hose involves these steps:

1. Place prosthesis nearby with the amputation limb socks, liners, valve, and any other accessories within reach.
2. While sitting, remove the shoe from the prosthesis. A shoe horn is helpful.
3. Don undergarments.
4. Dress the prosthesis with its sock/legging/panty hose.
5. Insert the prosthesis into the slack/trouser/pant leg.
6. Apply the shoe to the prosthesis.
7. Put the sock/legging/panty hose on the intact foot.
8. Don the shoe on the intact foot.
9. Don the prosthesis with whatever amputation limb socks and/or liners that are needed.
10. Stand; then fasten any closures on the prosthesis.
11. Pull up slacks/trousers/pants to the waist and fasten its closures.

TRANSFERRING TO AND FROM VARIOUS SEATS

On the first day of training, the clinician may assist the individual in rising from the wheelchair. The most stable wheelchair has its rear wheels offset posteriorly to compensate for the posterior shift of the occupant's center of gravity; this placement is particularly important when ascending ramps. Seat, backrest, and armrests should be well fitting. Individuals with trunk and upper-limb weakness benefit from motorized wheelchairs. These chairs are heavier than manually operated wheelchairs; thus, offsetting the rear wheels is unnecessary for stability.

For patients who wear a pair of prostheses, the wheelchair leg rests should swing out to facilitate transfers to other chairs. Footrests with heel guards are essential to prevent the shoes from slipping and to reduce stress on the thighs. Individuals who do not wear prostheses should have a wheelchair that does not have leg rests; in this situation, transferring will be easier. If the wheelchair is positioned near a locked door, the patient can pull on the doorknob to assist in rising. Eventually, the patient must be able to transfer with minimal or no assistance. Otherwise, the likelihood of independent ambulation is dim. Unless training includes getting to and from various chairs, both those that have or those that lack armrests, the person will be limited in daily activities.

In general, the techniques are applicable for individuals wearing either a transtibial or a transfemoral prosthesis. For purposes of transferring, the easiest chair is a heavy armchair or a wheelchair with its brakes locked and the leg rests swung to the side.[4] To rise, the patient maneuvers the buttocks toward the front edge of the chair and places both feet on the floor. The sound foot should be slightly behind the prosthetic foot. The hands may rest on the armrests. Finally, the individual extends both hips and knees and pushes on the armrests to rise. Sitting in the armchair involves approaching the chair obliquely with the sound leg closer to the chair or backing toward the chair so that the sound calf contacts it. The prosthesis is slightly ahead of the sound leg. The patient lowers the buttocks into the chair by means of controlled hip and knee flexion and pushing on the armrests.

Managing a chair that does not have armrests, such as a side chair, toilet seat, or bench, requires the same foot placement. The intact foot is closer to the chair, both on the rising and on the sitting maneuver. Depending on the height of the bench, the patient may be able to control the sit and rising movements with hand pressure on the seating surface.

The individual who wears bilateral prostheses will place the prosthesis encasing the longer, stronger amputation limb closer to the chair.

Transferring into and out of an automobile is relatively easy because the vehicle is stable and offers a rigid frame for grasping. These instructions assume that the car has left-hand drive, as used in North America, and that the car door is swung open. The side of amputation influences the method.

The person who wears a right prosthesis can enter the front passenger seat most easily by reaching into the car with the intact left leg, then sitting, and finally lifting the prosthetic leg into the vehicle. With a left prosthesis, the individual should sit on the side of the seat with both legs outside the car, then lift the prosthesis with or without the aid of the hands to rotate the amputated limb into the car, and finally swing the sound limb into the automobile.

The patient who has a left prosthesis exits from the car by placing the sound right leg obliquely out of the car onto the sidewalk, then lifting the prosthesis so that the prosthetic foot is on the sidewalk. The final step is to extend both hips to rise from the vehicle.

Entering and leaving the car on the driver's side requires reversal of these procedures. The person wearing a left prosthesis reaches that leg into the car and then lifts the prosthesis inside. With a right prosthesis, the driver sits on the side of the left seat with both feet outside the car. The next step requires lifting the prosthesis into the car, following through with the intact left leg. Exiting from the car while wearing a right prosthesis requires swinging the intact leg out of the car, then following through with the prosthesis; the individual

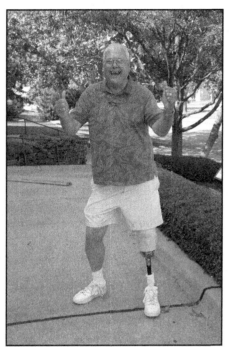

Figure 14-2. Standing balance. (Courtesy of Hanger Prosthetics & Orthotics, Inc.)

should leave sufficient space on the sidewalk for the prosthetic foot. Exiting with a left prosthesis is easiest if the driver rotates the buttocks on the seat so that both feet are outside the car and then steps on the sidewalk with the sound right leg and extends that leg, following with the prosthesis.

EXERCISE

Amputation severs muscles and alters muscular balance. Dysvascular patients, who tend to be older, typically present age-related weakness. Optimum use of a prosthesis depends on restoring strength and coordination throughout the body.[5-7] Exercise for individuals with transtibial amputation should emphasize vastus medialis and hamstring strengthening.[8,9] All patients benefit from increasing strength of the hip abductors.[10,11]

BALANCE AND GAIT TRAINING

A wide range of treatment strategies can be used to enable patients to use their prostheses effectively.[12-15]

Customarily, balance training begins with the patient standing (Figure 14-2) in the parallel bars. The individual may progress more rapidly, however, without using this equipment because detrimental habits can be avoided. Parallel bars encourage the patient to grab the bars and pull upward; this maneuver will not be beneficial when using a cane or walker. Surrounding the patient with metal can create a false sense of security, not available when the person walks in an open area. Finally, very few people own parallel bars, thus obviating transfer of some skills learned in the rehabilitation department to the home.

For the timid individual or one who has major difficulty balancing, body-weight support apparatus is a useful option in the clinic. The user is strapped into a snugly fitting corset that is attached to a steel frame. The device ensures that the patient cannot fall. The clinician can adjust the amount of weight borne through the user's legs, usually starting with 30% of body weight and progressing to full weight borne through both feet. Unweighting the leg facilitates moving it. Some models of the apparatus can be used with a treadmill or on the floor. Gait training is hastened with body-weight support. The apparatus is more expensive than parallel bars and is unlikely to be found in the home.

Weight bearing on the prosthesis is a major goal of balance training.[16,17] Initial balance training, regardless of environment, involves accustoming the patient to transferring weight to and from the prosthesis.[18,19] Continuing strengthening exercises, particularly the hip abductors, is essential for fostering effective balance. Proprioceptive neuromuscular facilitation can improve balance and gait.[12] The clinician should encourage the wearer to shift weight side to side and forward and backward symmetrically. The maneuver is easiest when the sound foot is slightly ahead of the prosthetic foot, placing the line of gravity in front of the knee on the amputated side, thus stabilizing it. Posture should be erect. A full-length mirror, or a face mirror held by the therapist, guides head position. Rhythmic motion is the goal, aided by a metronome, music of appropriate tempo, or asking the patient to sing or count in a uniform beat. Weight shifting enables the patient to perceive the interior contours of the socket as well as the excursions permitted by the prosthetic foot. One-leg balance is an important predictor of eventual prosthetic use. Similarly, static weight bearing through the prosthesis is correlated with walking velocity. Balance confidence is a persistent problem among those with amputation.[20-22] Teaching the patient to shift weight to the intact limb in response to perturbations can help the person to avoid falling.[23]

Weight shifting should include standing with feet on a line and then one foot ahead of the other. The patient should move the torso forward and backward, as well as side to side, always maintaining erect posture.

Training continues with use of a low stool (Figure 14-3). The patient should alternate feet stepping on the stool. The greater challenge occurs when stepping with the sound foot, compelling balance on the prosthesis.

Walking is a natural progression, advancing one foot and then the other.[24] Training should emphasize efficient pelvic motion and symmetrical upper-body movement. Particular elements of gait training that should be stressed are walking velocity and symmetry[25] and short-duration bouts of activity.[26]

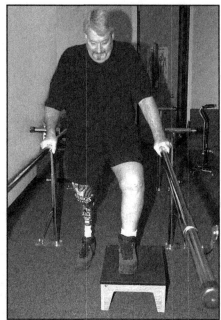

Figure 14-3. Stool step exercise. (Reprinted with permission from Carroll K, Edelstein JE. *Prosthetics and Patient Management: A Comprehensive Clinical Approach*. Thorofare, NJ: SLACK Incorporated; 2006.)

The clinician should consider whether an assistive device is needed. If so, the cane or walker must be measured so that the patient maintains optimal posture.[27,28]

More demanding balance skills emphasize rapid, forceful hip extension, an ability particularly important for those wearing transfemoral prostheses.

OTHER AMBULATORY SKILLS

In addition to walking forward, the individual needs to be able to move sideways, as when in a movie theater aisle, and backward, needed when maneuvering in crowded places. Walking in circles and side-stepping are other useful skills. Dancing is particularly useful, integrating movement in various directions with rhythmic music.

Terrain

People who expect to walk outside the home often encounter asphalt, grass, ramps, and curbs. Within the home, obstacles such as children's toys on the floor and electric cords are often found. Stairs may be present in public places and in many homes. The method that is most useful is to lead with the intact (or stronger) leg. Those wearing unilateral or bilateral transtibial prostheses usually ascend and descend stairs and curbs step-over-step.[29-31] Some people feel safer ascending and descending stairs in the seated position.[32] With transtibial prostheses, patients also traverse ramps[33,34] and obstacles[35,36] leading with either leg.

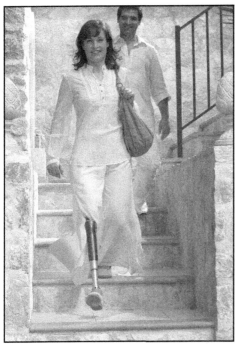

Figure 14-4. Descending stairs. (Reprinted with permission from Otto Bock HealthCare.)

The individual wearing a transfemoral prosthesis ordinarily will ascend stairs and curbs leading with the sound limb and will start stair and curb descent leading with the prosthesis. Depending on the knee unit, the patient may be able to progress to step-over-step descent (Figure 14-4). This method requires flexing the knee unit while bearing weight on the prosthesis. To do so, the patient creates a knee flexion moment by placing the prosthetic forefoot over the edge of the stair and then flexing the ipsilateral hip, enabling the sound leg to lower to the next step. An alternate approach to descending stairs rapidly is to vault down the staircase with the sound lower limb.

Maneuvering up and down stairs is extremely difficult for individuals who wear a pair of transfemoral prostheses. The staircase should be wide and, ideally, be equipped with handrails on both sides. To ascend, the patient circumducts the stronger leg up to the next step and then raises the body onto it. Descent requires controlled lowering of one leg and then the other.

Ascending steep ramps is less difficult if the person proceeds sideways, with the intact (or stronger) leg upwards. Descent is accomplished with the intact (or stronger) leg upward.

Escalators pose a special challenge. In general, the patient will lead with the sound limb when going up and going down. Alternatively, the individual should use stairs or an elevator.

WEARING SCHEDULE

The person who is adjusting to a first prosthesis needs to take special care of the amputation limb.

Frequent skin inspection is essential to detect incipient irritation.[37-39] The clinician should establish a wearing schedule with designated rest periods to avoid skin disorders. The patient should also be instructed in identifying blisters, folliculitis, rashes, and surface wounds. The importance of frequent washing and treating minor blemishes cannot be overemphasized. When the patient is not wearing the prosthesis, the amputation limb should be protected in an elastic shrinker or similar encasement to avoid dependent edema. As the patient becomes accustomed to wearing the prosthesis, the schedule should be altered, with the goal of full-time wear by the time of discharge from rehabilitation.

Wearing clean socks and liners is imperative.[40] The patient should bathe in the evening so that the amputation limb has plenty of time to dry thoroughly.

PROSTHETIC CARE

Caring for the prosthesis is the patient's responsibility. The individual should keep shoes in good repair, replacing the heels and soles as needed. Plastic sockets should be wiped with a damp cloth every evening and left to dry completely. Socks should be washed carefully, with plenty of time for drying. Valves, hinges, and other moving parts should be examined to detect malfunction; abnormalities should be reported to the prosthetist immediately. Straps and other fabric components should also be kept in good repair and replaced when frayed or otherwise imperfect.

ADVANCED ACTIVITIES

People with lower-limb amputations participate in a wide gamut of sports and other advanced ambulatory activities. Sometimes, the individual wears a special prosthesis or adapts the sports equipment. On other occasions, the task is accomplished by modifying the customary technique. In a few instances, the person dispenses with the prosthesis when engaging in a particular activity. The athlete may wish to join a specialized sports organization to exchange ideas and challenge kindred participants. Camping is popular for children and adolescents with amputations and limb deficiencies.

Household Activities

Housework and yard maintenance often involve pushing and pulling. In general, the sound (or stronger) leg should be positioned under the individual's midtorso. This position is also recommended when lowering oneself to the floor. Rising from the floor demands strong bilateral hip extension. Carrying heavy objects is less difficult if the load is handled on the intact side. Climbing ladders is relatively easy, because one can hold both sides of the ladder to maintain balance.

Driving

As with transferring into the car, the side of amputation influences the method of operating the vehicle. The

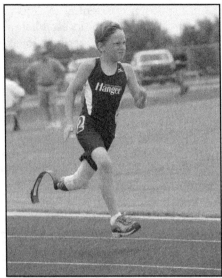

Figure 14-5. Running. (Reprinted with permission from Carroll K, Edelstein JE. *Prosthetics and Patient Management: A Comprehensive Clinical Approach.* Thorofare, NJ: SLACK Incorporated; 2006.)

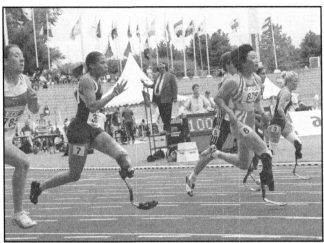

Figure 14-6. Competitive running. (Reprinted with permission from Carroll K, Edelstein JE. *Prosthetics and Patient Management: A Comprehensive Clinical Approach.* Thorofare, NJ: SLACK Incorporated; 2006.)

individual wearing a left prosthesis will drive a car with automatic transmission in the ordinary manner. People who use a right prosthesis may cross the sound, left leg over the prosthesis to operate the pedals. One can install an extension to the accelerator so it can be pushed with the left foot. Hand controls are recommended for those who wear bilateral transfemoral prostheses. Before the patient resumes driving, it is essential to confirm that the emergency light and brake are accessible; if not, either the car needs to be modified or the person's driving technique altered. The same approach applies to operating other vehicles, including airplanes and helicopters. Most adults return to driving,[41,42] although those with right amputation are more likely to have automobile modifications. Individuals wearing a right transtibial prosthesis had faster reaction time when using the intact foot on a left-sided accelerator pedal. Piloting airplanes and helicopters is also pursued by some people who wear prostheses.

Running

Determined runners will benefit from an energy-storing prosthetic foot designed for running[43-45] (Figures 14-5 and 14-6). The special prosthesis is worn when the person runs; the individual also requires a separate prosthesis for walking. Usually, there is no heel component and the prothesis is worn without a shoe. The major impulse will be delivered by the sound leg. This is particularly true for people with transfemoral amputations who run. Disproportionately more propulsion is delivered by the sound leg. World-class runners approach speed records of able-bodied champions. Triathlon competition is possible for those with the physical ability and determination to commit to the systematic practice of swimming, cycling, and running.[46]

Jumping

The patient uses sound leg propulsive force for the upward movement and lands on the sound leg to avoid potentially painful impact between the amputation limb and the prosthetic socket.[47-49] The prosthetic shank should have a vertical shock absorber. Specialized training is indicated for athletes who wish to compete in the long or high jump.

Bicycling

Because prostheses are better able to pull on a pedal than push it, the cyclist should install a toe clip on the pedal so that the prosthesis can pull up on the pedal (Figure 14-7). Some cyclists ride without a prosthesis.

Skiing

One of the most popular sports for athletes with disabilities is skiing. Instructional programs are held throughout the country. Most people with a unilateral amputation prefer not to wear a prosthesis and use equipment modified with the addition of short rudders on the ski poles, known as *three track skiing*. Those with bilateral amputations may enjoy snow sports by sitting in a toboggan or sled; some have ski prostheses that feature marked ankle dorsiflexion and knee flexion.

Swimming

Most people with amputations swim without a prosthesis. To get from the dressing room to the water's edge, they generally hop if the distance is short or use a forearm crutch for longer distances. Custom-made waterproof swim prostheses are available; these should have a drainage channel so that water can flow from the prosthesis. Some people like to swim with a swim fin fitted to a socket or to a pylon. Water skiing and surfing are other sports available to people with amputations.

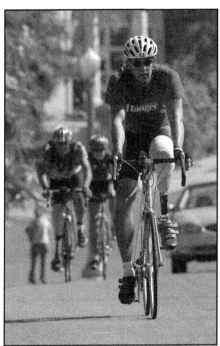

Figure 14-7. Bicycling. (Courtesy of Hanger Prosthetics & Orthotics, Inc.)

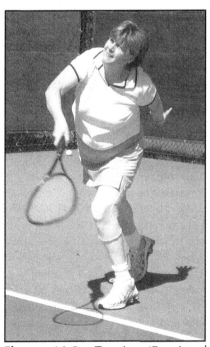

Figure 14-8. Tennis. (Reprinted with permission from Carroll K, Edelstein JE. *Prosthetics and Patient Management: A Comprehensive Clinical Approach.* Thorofare, NJ: SLACK Incorporated; 2006.)

Golf and Other Sports

Skillful performance of golfing,[50] tennis (Figure 14-8), racquet ball, squash, and similar activities involves rotating the torso and leg. Consequently, a transverse

rotator in the shank is desirable to protect the skin of the amputation limb. Soccer[51] can be played with the athlete wearing a prosthesis, with or without crutches. Some agile players depend only on crutches. Amputation does not eliminate the opportunity to play football, baseball, and basketball.

References

1. Wolff-Burke M, Cole ES, Witt M. Basic lower-limb prosthetic training. In: Carroll K, Edelstein JE, eds. *Prosthetics and Patient Management.* Thorofare, NJ: SLACK Incorporated; 2006:109-137.

2. Gailey RS, Clark CR. Physical therapy. In: Smith DG, Michael JW, Bowker JH, eds. *Atlas of Amputations and Limb Deficiencies.* Rosemont, IL: American Academy of Orthopaedic Surgeons; 2004:589-619.

3. Tamir E, Heim M, Oppenheim U, Siev-Ner I. An assistive device designed to convey independent donning of a shuttle lock trans-tibial prosthesis for a multiple limb amputee. *Prosthet Orthot Int.* 2003;27:74-75.

4. Burger H, Kuzelicki J, Marincek C. Transition from sitting to standing after trans-femoral amputation. *Prosthet Orthot Int.* 2005;29:139-151.

5. Deans SA, McFadyen K, Rowe PJ. Physical activity and quality of life: a study of a lower-limb amputee population. *Prosthet Orthot Int.* 2008;32:186-200.

6. Nolan L, Lees A. The functional demands on the intact limb during walking for active trans-femoral and transtibial amputees. *Prosthet Orthot Int.* 2000;24:117-125.

7. Rau B, Bonvin F, de Bie R. Short-term effect of physiotherapy rehabilitation on functional performance of lower limb amputees. *Prosthet Orthot Int.* 2007;31:258-270.

8. Fraisse N, Martinet N, Kpadonou TJ, et al. Muscles of the below-knee amputee. *Ann Readapt Med Phys.* 2008;51: 218-227.

9. Isakov E, Burger H, Krajnik J, et al. Knee muscle activity during ambulation of trans-tibial amputees. *J Rehabil Med.* 2001;33:196-199.

10. Nadollek H, Brauer S, Isles R. Outcomes after transtibial amputation: the relationship between quiet stance ability, strength of hip abductor muscles and gait. *Physiother Res Int.* 2002;7:203-214.

11. Hof AL, van Bockel RM, Schoppen T, Postema K. Control of lateral balance in walking: experimental findings in normal subjects and above-knee amputees. *Gait Posture.* 2007;25:250-258.

12. Yigiter K, Sener G, Erbahceci F, et al. A comparison of traditional prosthetic training versus proprioceptive neuromuscular facilitation resistive gait training with transfemoral amputees. *Prosthet Orthot Int.* 2002;26:213-217.

13. Sjödahl C, Jarnio GB, Persson BM. Gait improvement in unilateral transfemoral amputees by a combined psychological and physiotherapeutic treatment. *J Rehabil Med.* 2001;33:114-118.

14. Sjödahl C, Jarnlo G-B, Söderberg B, Persson BM. Kinematic and kinetic gait analysis in the sagittal plane of trans-femoral amputees before and after special gait re-education. *Prosthet Orthot Int.* 2002;26:101-112.

15. Sjödahl C, Jarnio GB, Söderberg B, Persson BM. Pelvic motion in trans-femoral amputees in the frontal and transverse plane before and after special gait re-education. *Prosthet Orthot Int.* 2003;27:227-237.

16. Jones ME, Bashford GM, Mann JM. Weight bearing and velocity in trans-tibial and trans-femoral amputees. *Prosthet Orthot Int.* 1997;21:183-186.

17. Jones ME, Bashford GM, Munro BJ. Developing prosthetic weight bearing in a knee disarticulation amputee. *Aust J Physiother.* 1999;45:309-317.

18. Matjačić Z, Burger H. Dynamic balance training during standing in people with trans-tibial amputation: a pilot study. *Prosthet Orthot Int.* 2003;27:214-220.

19. Viton JM, Mouchnino L, Mille ML, et al. Equilibrium and movement control strategies in trans-tibial amputees. *Prosthet Orthot Int.* 2000;24:108-116.

20. Miller WC, Speechley M, Deathe AB. Balance confidence among people with lower-limb amputations. *Phys Ther.* 2002;82:856-859.

21. Miller WC, Deathe AB. A prospective study examining balance confidence among individuals with lower limb amputation. *Disabil Rehabil.* 2004;26:875-881.

22. Miller WC, Deathe AB, Speechley M, Koval J. The influence of falling, fear of falling, and balance confidence on prosthetic mobility and social activity among individuals with a lower extremity amputation. *Arch Phys Med Rehabil.* 2001;82:1738-1744.

23. Vanicek N, Strike S, McNaughton L, Polman R. Postural responses to dynamic perturbations in amputee fallers versus nonfallers: a comparative study with able-bodied subjects. *Arch Phys Med Rehabil.* 2009;90:1018-1025.

24. Vrieling AH, van Keeken HG, Schoppen T, et al. Gait initiation in lower limb amputees. *Gait Posture.* 2008;27:423-430.

25. van Velzen JM, van Bennekom CA, Polomski W, Slootman JR. Physical capacity and walking ability after lower limb amputation: a systematic review. *Clin Rehabil.* 2006;20:999-1016.

26. Klute GK, Berge JS, Orendurff MS, et al. Prosthetic intervention effects on activity of lower-extremity amputees. *Arch Phys Med Rehabil.* 2006;87:717-722.

27. Moseley AM, Stark A, Cameron ID, et al. Talk the walk: the importance of teaching patients how to use their walking stick effectively and safely. *Musculoskeletal Care.* 2008;6:150-154.

28. Bateni H, Maki BE. Assistive devices for balance and mobility: benefits, demands, and adverse consequences. *Arch Phys Med Rehabil.* 2005;86:134-145.

29. Jones SF, Twigg PC, Scally AJ, Buckley JG. The gait initiation process in unilateral lower-limb amputees when stepping up and stepping down to a new level. *Clin Biomech (Bristol, Avon).* 2005;20:405-413.

30. Schmalz T, Blumentritt S, Marx B. Biomechanical analysis of stair ambulation in lower limb amputees. *Gait Posture.* 2007;25:267-278.

31. Bae TS, Choi K, Mun M. Level walking and stair climbing gait in above-knee amputees. *J Med Eng Technol.* 2009;33:130-135.

32. Kirby RL, Brown BA, Connolly CM, et al. Handling stairs in the seated position for people with unilateral lower-limb amputations. *Arch Phys Med Rehabil.* 2009;90:1250-1253.

33. Vrieling AH, van Keeken HG, Schoppen T, et al. Uphill and downhill walking in unilateral lower limb amputees. *Gait Posture.* 2008;28:235-242.

34. Vickers DR, Palk C, McIntosh AS, Beatty KT. Elderly unilateral transtibial amputee gait on an inclined walkway: a biomechanical analysis. *Gait Posture.* 2008;27:518-529.

35. Vrieling AH, van Keeken HG, Schoppen T, et al. Obstacle crossing in lower limb amputees. *Gait Posture.* 2007;26:587-594.

36. Hofstad CJ, Weerdesteyn V, van der Linde H, et al. Evidence for bilaterally delayed and decreased obstacle avoidance responses while walking with a lower limb prosthesis. *Clin Neurophysiol.* 2009;120:1009-1015.

37. Meulenbelt HE, Geertzen JH, Jonkman MF, Dijkstra PU. Determinants of skin problems of the stump in lower-limb amputees. *Arch Phys Med Rehabil.* 2009;90:74-81.

38. Baars ECT, Dijkstra PU, Geertzen JH. Skin problems of the stump and hand function in lower limb amputees: a historic cohort study. *Prosthet Orthot Int.* 2008;32:179-185.

39. Dudek NL, Marks MB, Marshall SC. Skin problems in an amputee clinic. *Am J Phys Med Rehabil.* 2006;85:424-429.

40. Hachisuka K, Nakamura T, Ohmine S, et al. Hygiene problems of residual limb and silicone liners in transtibial amputees wearing the total surface bearing socket. *Arch Phys Med Rehabil.* 2001;82:1286-1290.

41. Boulias C, Meikle B, Pauley T, Devlin M. Return to driving after lower-extremity amputation. *Arch Phys Med Rehabil.* 2006;87:1183-1188.

42. Meikle B, Devlin M, Pauley T. Driving pedal reaction times after right transtibial amputations. *Arch Phys Med Rehabil.* 2006;87:390-394.

43. Pailler D, Sautreuil P, Piera JB, et al. Evolution in prostheses for sprinters with lower-limb amputation. *Ann Readapt Med Phys.* 2004;47:374-381.

44. Brown MB, Millard-Stafford ML, Allison AR. Running-specific prostheses permit energy cost similar to nonamputees. *Med Sci Sports Exerc.* 2009;41:1080-1087.

45. Weyand PG, Bundle MW, McGowan CP, et al. The fastest runner on artificial legs: different limbs, similar function? *J Appl Physiol.* 2009;107:903-911.

46. Gailey R, Harsch P. Introduction to triathlon for the lower limb amputee triathlete. *Prosthet Orthot Int.* 2009;33:242-255.

47. Nolan L, Lees A. The influence of lower limb amputation level on the approach in the amputee long jump. *J Sports Sci.* 2007;25:393-401.

48. Nolan L, Patritti BL, Simpson KJ. A biomechanical analysis of the long-jump technique of elite female amputee athletes. *Med Sci Sports Exerc.* 2006;38:1829-1835.

49. Nolan L, Patritti BL. The take-off phase in transtibial amputee high jump. *Prosthet Orthot Int.* 2008;32:160-171.

50. Yazicioglu K, Taskaynatan MA, Guzelkucuk U, Tugcu I. Effect of playing football (soccer) on balance, strength, and quality of life in unilateral below-knee amputees. *Am J Phys Med Rehabil.* 2007;86:800-805.

51. Rogers JP, Strike SC, Wallace ES. The effect of prosthetic torsional stiffness on the golf swing kinematics of a left and a right-sided transtibial amputee. *Prosthet Orthot Int.* 2004;28:121-131.

ORGANIZATIONS

ActiveAmp.org
PO Box 9315
Wilmington, DE 19809
www.activeamp.org

Adaptive Adventures
27888 Meadow Drive
Evergreen, CO 80419
www.adaptiveadventures.org

American Amputee Hockey Association
PO Box 5660
Kalamazoo, MI 49003
www.usahockey.com/aaha

American Amputee Soccer Association
www.ampsoccer.org

Amputee Coalition of America
900 East Hill Avenue
Knoxville, TN 37915
www.amputee-coalition.org

American Ski-Bike Association
PO Box 40
Lake George, CO 80828
www.ski-bike.org

British Limbless Ex-Service Men's Association
185-187 High Road
Chadwell Heath
Romford, Essex RM6 6NA
Great Britain
www.blesma.org

Canadian Amputee Hockey Association
www.canadianamputeehockey.ca

Canadian Association for Disabled Skiing
91 Nelson Street
Barrie, ON L4M 4K4
Canada
www.disabledskiing.ca

Challenged Athletes Foundation
PO Box 910769
San Diego, CA 92191
www.challengedathletes.org

Disabled Sports USA
451 Hungerford Drive, Suite 100
Rockville, MD 20850
www.dsusa.org

Fishing Has No Boundaries, Inc
PO Box 175
Hayward, WI 54843
www.fhnbinc.org

Handicapped Hunting Resource Guide
4008 West Michigan Avenue
Jackson, MI 49202
www.disabledhunting.net

International Paralympic Committee
Adenauerallee 212-214
53113 Bonn, Germany
www.paralympic.org

National Ability Center
PO Box 682799
Park City, UT 84068
www.nac1985.org

National Amputee Golf Association
11 Walnut Hill Road
Amherst, NH 03031
www.nagagolf.org

National Sports Center for the Disabled
PO Box 1290
Winter Park, CO 80482
www.nscd.org

Spokes 'n Motion
2226 South Jason Street
Denver, CO 80223
www.spokesnmotion.com

USA Swimming—Adapted Swimming Committee
One Olympic Plaza
Colorado Springs, CO 80909
www.usaswimming.org

USA Water Ski
1251 Holy Cow Road
Polk City, FL 33868
www.usawaterski.org

US Adaptive Recreation Center
PO Box 2897
Big Bear Lake, CA 92315
www.usarc.org

US Hand Cycling Federation
PO Box 3538
Evergreen, CO 80437
www.ushf.org

US Paralympic—US Olympic Committee
One Olympic Plaza
Colorado Springs, CO 80909
www.usparalympics.org

US Sled Hockey Association
1775 Bob Johnson Drive
Colorado Springs, CO 80906
www.usahockey.com

War Amputations of Canada
1 Maybrook Drive
Scarborough, ON M1V 5K9
Canada
www.waramps.ca

Chapter 15

Lifelong Management of Older Patients

Richard A. Frieden, MD

Many factors differentiate the care of the younger person with limb loss from the management of the older adult. These differences are relevant regardless of whether the person had a lower-limb amputation as a youth and is now aging with the condition or has had the amputation after age-related and acquired comorbidities began to take their toll.

AGING AND THE ETIOLOGY OF AMPUTATION

As the population ages, peripheral arterial disease (PAD) due to atherosclerosis is becoming one of the most common and possibly most undertreated chronic illnesses in the United States. The rate of dysvascular amputations continues to increase, whereas the number of traumatic and cancer-related amputations has declined.[1] Atherosclerosis is accelerated by diabetes mellitus; currently, these 2 conditions account for over 90% of the major lower-limb amputations performed annually in the United States, most involving patients over the age of 60.

Other risk factors and comorbidities associated with PAD are related to aging, including smoking, hypertension, hyperlipidemia, obesity, inactive lifestyle, and a family history of vascular or heart disease.

Juvenile obesity combined with an earlier diagnosis of type 2 (adult-onset) diabetes significantly increases the possibility of limb loss in early adulthood.[2] These young people then need to confront aging with an amputation. The rate of reamputation at a more proximal level is higher for people with amputation due to diabetes.[3] The risk of further ipsilateral surgery is greatest within the first 6 months after initial amputation.[4]

Screening and preventive measures take place earlier and are more widespread. Revascularization techniques (including endovascular methods)[5] are advancing. Nevertheless, the rate of lower-limb amputation has not decreased significantly, partly because many comorbidities in the aging population can lead to injury and the need for amputation. As longevity extends, the pool of potential amputees keeps increasing.[6,7] Although there was a transient decrease in amputations when improved revascularization methods were introduced, the rate of amputations rose again when hospitals and surgeons reached maximal capacity for performing these procedures.[6]

REVASCULARIZATION AND LIMB SALVAGE

Prevention of amputation by revascularization is a complex topic.[7-16] The procedure should not be used as a means of obtaining a more distal amputation level, such as when attempting to save a knee joint.[13] The financial and temporal costs of revascularization must be weighed against those of primary amputation and prosthetic rehabilitation.[14] Primary amputation is associated with fewer postoperative complications than a secondary, more proximal, amputation after attempted revascularization.[7] Delaying an amputation that occurs while waiting to see whether the bypass is successful allows more time for systemic complications to arise.[17] Limb ischemia is a harbinger of systemic vasculopathy; thus, a high index of suspicion is needed to prevent significant morbidity and mortality.[18]

AMPUTATION SURGERY AND PERIOPERATIVE CARE

Medical stability, including the ability to withstand metabolic stress due to sepsis, anesthesia, and the surgery itself, is the primary concern in the older patient.

Edelstein JE, Muroz A.
Lower-Limb Prosthetics and Orthotics: Clinical Concepts (pp 107-112).
© 2011 Taylor & Francis Group.

Assessing both the individual's level of functioning prior to the onset of leg ischemia and the need for amputation is critical in determining postoperative expectations.[19]

The energy expenditure required to ambulate with and without a prosthesis should be considered before surgery. With advancing age, exercise tolerance decreases and the likelihood of more proximal amputation increases. Because the metabolic demand of walking with crutches without a prosthesis is greater than with a prosthesis, crutch walking is considered to be a good predictor of the ability of young people to use a prosthesis.[20] As adults age and balance declines, testing ambulation with a walker without a prosthesis enables a more accurate assessment.[21] Cardiac and pulmonary function testing should be conducted in patients with known risk factors who face amputation.

Another concern is the need to proceed with prosthetic fitting and training quickly. Early ambulation may not increase the risk to the contralateral limb and can reduce the debilitating effects of prolonged inactivity due to months of conservative treatment, reduce dependency, and improve the quality and possibly length of life for the person with limb loss.[20] Delays in fitting and training, whether due to insurance or healing, could mean the onset of comorbidities that may adversely affect ambulation. Interruptions to the rehabilitation process need to be resolved rapidly so they do not jeopardize the functional outcome.[22] Survival following lower-limb amputation is impaired by advanced age, cardiovascular and renal disease, and a more proximal amputation level.[23]

AGE-ASSOCIATED RISK FACTORS THAT INTERFERE WITH PROSTHETIC TRAINING

The risk of injurious falls is greater for the elderly.[24,25] This can jeopardize both the contralateral limb as well as the residual limb; either injury can impede ambulation with a prosthesis.[26]

The person with severe arthritis in the shoulders or hands will have difficulty using a walker or crutches. Arthritic changes in the back or hips hamper shifting weight from side to side.[26]

Systemic disabling diseases and their sequelae (eg, diabetic retinopathy and neuropathy) are more likely among the elderly. Diminished sensation combined with poor nutrition and circulatory insufficiency can lead to skin breakdown, with a decreased ability to heal.[19,26-28] Difficulty donning a prosthesis properly due to hand impairment can cause skin problems.[29]

Other losses that may occur with aging affect lean body mass, bone density, and vision; neurological diseases are more likely to occur.[28] Nevertheless, these conditions do not necessarily contraindicate prosthetic fitting. Adaptations to assist in donning the prosthesis are available; family members can aid the patient to apply the prosthesis, stand, and start walking. Use of a prosthesis solely for ease of transfers is worthwhile.

DIAGNOSTIC ASSESSMENT

Assessment scales and treatment protocols designed for younger adults are not always applicable to the elderly because the scales do not take into account the older person's altered physiology and life circumstances.

Gait analysis of persons with limb loss[30] indicates that older people walk differently than do younger adults.[26,31] Elderly patients increase the use of the intact leg for push-off[32]; the gait is slower and is correlated with overall diminished functional status.[33]

Predicting functional outcomes in the elderly is difficult. Assessments of balance, cognition, and the number and type of comorbidities are important. At one time, being older than 55 years was itself considered a negative factor predicting against optimal functioning.[34] Though age, per se, is no longer considered to be an obstacle to prosthetic use, the comorbidities that arise with aging cannot be ignored. More physical activity and greater social participation are expected of the younger person. Negative perceptions of the elderly that may adversely influence decision making include the assumptions that all older adults have decreased motivation and adaptability, increased psychological distress, increased physical limitations, and impaired judgment.[35] In addition to age, factors that influence quality of life after amputation include depression, perceived prosthetic mobility, social support, comorbidities, prosthetic problems, and social activity.[36]

PROSTHETIC PRESCRIPTION

A wide range of componentry is available for the prostheses of older people. The prosthetic prescription should take into account the specific needs and capacities of the individual, rather than applying a template prescription based on age or diagnosis alone. The universal goal is to improve the quality of life and the degree of independence. Effective communication between the patient, prosthetist, and other members of the rehabilitation team is part of this process.[37]

Less has been published concerning specific component selection for the elderly, partly because more resources are allotted to the care of younger people and more research has been conducted using younger subjects.[38] As with other aspects of care of the aging population, stereotyping older people as frail and unable to benefit from newer technologies still persists. The logic then follows that relatively sedentary people need lightweight, uncomplicated devices that do not require much maintenance, whereas more active people benefit from sophisticated devices such as microprocessor knee units and energy-storing feet. Paradoxically, though newer safety features that might benefit the elderly are available, increased expense means that reimbursement policies limit access.[38]

PREVENTION OF FUTURE LIMB LOSS

After unilateral amputation, the remaining leg needs even closer scrutiny. The ability of a person to walk will be compromised if the intact limb is threatened. The principles already described are applicable, including general screening; foot inspection, hygiene, shoe selection and fitting; and systemic disease modification, incorporating diet and smoking cessation.

Guiding patients and families in the prevention of future limb loss by implementation of risk factor detection and modification is important in light of the continuing risk of amputation despite therapeutic interventions.[39] The specifics of these processes are described in earlier chapters.

As with many conditions associated with aging, one needs to be aware that the pain of PAD may be mistaken for—or dismissed as—"arthritis" or "getting old." This false impression must be corrected. Symptoms can range from exercise-induced pain, such as intermittent claudication through numbness and rest pain; infection and tissue damage may be evident. The experience of pain influences using a prosthesis. Consequently, elucidating the cause of discomfort and instituting measures to reduce it, including educating the patient and support system, are important.[40]

The details of prescribing prostheses and training patients to use them are described elsewhere in this book.

AGING WITH AN AMPUTATION

The aging person with limb loss needs regular follow-up as the manifestations of growing older become increasingly more evident, including fragile skin and restricted joint motion, aggravated by poor nutrition. As the mechanisms used to maintain balance and correct for perturbations start to fail, falls tend to increase. A 2-pronged approach encompassing balance training and environmental modification is important.

Programs for older adults need to accommodate for the older person's decreased physical and (occasionally) mental capacity, as well as consider the increased risk to the ischemic remaining leg and greater need to control comorbidities, and recognize altered socioeconomic realities.

Resumption of employment and high-level activities are appropriate goals for young people. In contrast,

increased comfort, improvement in self-care and walking skills, and decreased reliance on caregivers are more usual goals for the elderly. Factors such as age, physical condition, psychological and cognitive status, and social resources influence functional goals and quality of life.[41] The tempo of rehabilitation needs to accommodate the patient.[42,43] Older individuals often require longer hospital stays and lengthier rehabilitation, are more likely to go to a nursing home after the acute hospital stay,[44] and are less likely to use a prosthesis on a long-term basis.[45]

Some elderly patients set aside their prostheses shortly after training is concluded[46]; perhaps half do so within 6 months after discharge.[47] Decreased use of a prosthesis is correlated with advanced age, female gender, possession of a wheelchair, cognitive impairment, a higher level of disability, presence of cerebrovascular disease, the need for reamputation or contralateral amputation, and dissatisfaction with the prosthesis.[48,49] In contrast, successful prosthetic fitting is associated with younger age, marriage, fewer comorbidities, a more distal amputation level, and the ability to be discharged home.[50] With advancing age, function after transfemoral amputation declines more rapidly than it does after transtibial amputation.[51] Furthermore, because the likelihood of bilateral surgery increases with age, more discussion is needed regarding amputation levels and prosthetic components.[52,53]

Although a wheelchair is provided to nearly all persons with limb loss, many prefer an alternative, such as walking with crutches or crawling.[54] Mobility solely at the wheelchair level may be necessary in the presence of bilateral amputation. Powered mobility should be considered if there is decreased ability to self-propel a manual wheelchair. Lower cardiopulmonary endurance and the loss of mobility within the home due to arthritis and stroke, among other conditions, makes wheeled mobility a rational option.

MUSCULOSKELETAL COMPLICATIONS

Osteoarthritis (OA) in the hip and knee of the contralateral side often arises in persons with unilateral limb loss,[55] probably due to a combination of increased stress during stance phase and greater load on the intact side, unequal leg lengths, and similar biomechanical changes. More proximal amputation levels have a greater tendency to demonstrate arthritic disease. The presence of OA and the need for joint replacement influence prosthetic mobility.[56]

Tendonopathy or bursitis may result from disturbed body mechanics and posture during gait. Altered tendon pull and abnormal joint motions create inflammation at and over muscle-bone attachments.

The lower back is a frequent site of pain in patients with lower-limb amputations. Lower back pain occurs more often in those using transfemoral prostheses than transtibial prostheses, and more commonly than in the general population.[57,58] Pain may be caused by disturbed body mechanics over time with or without degenerative changes in the spine of the older person.

Osteoporosis has been demonstrated radiographically in the bones of the amputated limb.[59] This may be related to a combination of disuse muscle atrophy, lack of weight bearing through the skeleton,[60] abnormal biochemical processes, and atherosclerosis.

Heterotopic ossification has been reported in cases of posttraumatic amputation.[61] This may relate to the nearby muscle and nerve injuries, similar to the mechanism in other traumatic injuries. Prevention includes the use of nonsteroidal antiinflammatory drugs and local radiation. Prosthetic modification is a more common intervention than surgical excision.

People who undergo amputation due to tumor face musculoskeletal problems secondary to their pathology and treatment. Neuropathy, bone loss, muscle atrophy, fibrosis, fractures, and limb length discrepancy are not uncommon.[62] All of these difficulties worsen with advancing age.

SUMMARY

Older adults who undergo amputation are significantly impacted by comorbidities, general deconditioning, loss of mobility, and lack of social support. These problems are compounded by a lack of knowledge about caring for the residual limb and prosthesis as well as the need to maintain general health.

People who sustained limb loss at an early age and who became successful ambulators may find increasing difficulties as they age. In addition to musculoskeletal complications,[63] acquired chronic diseases, which occur more frequently as people age, can adversely affect function after amputation. Prosthetic designs may need modification and different components may be needed to accommodate the changing requirements of the older patient.

REFERENCES

1. Dillingham TR, Pezzin LE, MacKenzie EJ. Limb amputation and limb deficiency: epidemiology and recent trends in the United States. *South Med J.* 2002;95:875-883.

2. Vinicor F. Diabetes: preventing lower-extremity amputations. *inMotion.* 2001;11:15-16.

3. Dillingham TR, Pezzin LE, Shore AD. Reamputation, mortality and health care costs among persons with dysvascular lower-limb amputations. *Arch Phys Med Rehabil.* 2005;86:480-486.

4. Izumi Y, Satterfield K, Lee S, Harkless LB. Risk of reamputation in diabetic patients stratified by limb and level of amputation. *Diabetes Care.* 2006;29:566-570.

5. Rowe VL, Lee W, Weaver FA, Etzioni D. Patterns of treatment for peripheral arterial disease in the United States: 1996-2005. *J Vasc Surg.* 2009;49:910-917.

6. Feinglass J, Brown JL, LoSasso A, et al. Rates of lower-extremity amputation and arterial reconstruction in the United States, 1979 to 1996. *Am J Public Health.* 1999;89:1222-1227.

7. Van Niekerk LJA, Stewart CPU, Jain ASA. Major lower limb amputation following failed infrainguinal vascular bypass surgery: a prospective study on amputation levels and stump complications. *Prosthet Orthot Int.* 2001;25:29-33.

8. Newman AB. Peripheral arterial disease: insights from population studies of older adults. *J Am Geriatr Soc.* 2000;48:1157-1162.

9. Fletcher DD, Andrews KL, Hallett JW Jr, et al. Trends in rehabilitation after amputation for geriatric patients with vascular disease: implications for future health resource allocation. *Arch Phys Med Rehabil.* 2002;83:1389-1393.

10. Pomposelli FB Jr, Arora S, Gibbons GW, et al. Lower extremity arterial reconstruction in the very elderly: successful outcome preserves not only the limb but also residential status and ambulatory function. *J Vasc Surg.* 1998;28:215-225.

11. Kistner RL. Management of severe leg ischemia in the elderly patient. *Geriatrics.* 1968;23:93-96.

12. Skversky N, Zislis JM. Peripheral-vascular disorders and the aged amputee. *Geriatrics.* 1970;25:142-149.

13. Callow AD, Mackey WC. Costs and benefits of prosthetic vascular surgery. *Int Surg.* 1988;73:237-240.

14. Robinson KP. Long posterior flap amputation in geriatric patients with ischaemic disease. *Ann R Coll Surg Engl.* 1976;58:440-451.

15. O'Brien TS, Lamont PM, Crow A, et al. Lower limb ischaemia in the octogenarian: is limb salvage surgery worthwhile? *Ann R Coll Surg Engl.* 1993;75:445-447.

16. Persson B. Lower limb amputation part 1: amputation methods—a 10-year literature review. *Prosthet Orthot Int.* 2001;25:7-13.

17. Weiss GN, Gorton A, Read RC, Neal LA. Outcomes of lower extremity amputations. *J Am Geriatr Soc.* 1990;38:877-883.

18. Henke PK. Contemporary management of acute limb ischemia: factors associated with amputation and in-hospital mortality. *Semin Vasc Surg.* 2009;22:34-40.

19. Dacher JE. Rehabilitation and the geriatric patient. *Nurs Clin North Am* 1989;24:225-237.

20. Wilson, AB. Limb prosthetics today. *Artif Limbs.* 1963;7:1-42.

21. Steinberg FU, Sunwoo IS, Roettger RF. Prosthetic rehabilitation of geriatric amputee patients: a follow-up study. *Arch Phys Med Rehabil.* 1985;66:742-745.

22. Meikle B, Devlin M, Garland M. Interruptions to amputee rehabilitation. *Arch Phys Med Rehabil.* 2002;83:1222-1228.

23. Mayfield JA, Reiber GE, Maynard C, et al. Survival following lower-limb amputation in a veteran population. *J Rehabil Res Dev.* 2001;38:341-345.

24. Miller WC, Speechley M, Deathe B. The prevalence and risk factors of falling and fear of falling among lower extremity amputees. *Arch Phys Med Rehabil.* 2001;82:1042-1047.

25. Miller WC, Deathe B, Speechley M, Kovac J. The influence of falling, fear of falling, and balance confidence on prosthetic mobility and social activity among individuals with a lower extremity amputation. *Arch Phys Med Rehabil.* 2001;82:1238-1244.

26. Leonard JA Jr. The elderly amputee. In: Felsenthal G, Garrison SJ, Steinberg FU, eds. *Rehabilitation of the Aging and Elderly Patient.* Baltimore, MD: Williams & Wilkins; 1994:397-406.

27. Dunlop DD, Manheim LM, Sohn M-W, et al. Incidence of functional limitation in older adults: the impact of gender, race, and chronic conditions. *Arch Phys Med Rehabil.* 2002;83:964-971.

28. Andrews KL. Rehabilitation in limb deficiency. 3. The geriatric amputee. *Arch Phys Med Rehabil.* 1996;77:S14-S17.

29. Baars ECT, Dijkstra PU, Geertzen JHB. Skin problems of the stump and hand function in lower limb amputees: a historic cohort study. *Prosthet Orthot Int.* 2008;32:179-185.

30. Perry J. Amputee gait. In: Smith DG, Michael JW, Bowker JH, eds. *Atlas of Amputation and Limb Deficiencies: Surgical, Prosthetic, and Rehabilitation Principles.* 3rd ed. Rosemont, IL: American Academy of Orthopaedic Surgeons; 2004:367-384.

31. Kerrigan DC, Todd MK, Della Croce U, et al. Biomechanical gait alterations independent of speed in the healthy elderly: evidence for specific limiting impairments. *Arch Phys Med Rehabil.* 1998;79:317-322.

32. Lemaire ED, Fisher FR, Robertson DGE. Gait patterns of elderly men with trans-tibial amputation. *Prosthet Orthot Int.* 1993;17:27-37.

33. Hubbard WA, McElroy GK. Benchmark data for elderly, vascular trans-tibial amputees after rehabilitation. *Prosthet Orthot Int.* 1994;18:142-149.

34. Russek AS. Management of amputees in the older age group. *Int J Phys Med.* 1960;4:51-56.

35. Kurichi JE, Kwong PL, Reker DM, et al. Clinical factors associated with prescription of a prosthetic limb in elderly veterans. *J Am Geriatr Soc.* 2007;55:900-906.

36. Asano M, Rushton P, Miller WC et al. Predictors of quality of life among individuals who have a lower limb amputation. *Prosthet Orthot Int.* 2008;32:231-243.

37. Pezzin LE, Dillingham TR, Mackenzie EJ, et al. Use and satisfaction with prosthetic limb devices and related services. *Arch Phys Med Rehabil.* 2004;85:723-729.

38. Highsmith MJ. Barriers to the provision of prosthetic services in the geriatric population. *Top Geriatr Rehabil.* 2008;24:325-331.

39. Wrobel JS, Charns MP, Diehr P, et al. The relationship between provider coordination and diabetes-related foot outcomes. *Diabetes Care.* 2003;26:3042-3047.

40. Desmond D, Gallagher P, Henderson-Slater D, Chatfield R. Pain and psychosocial adjustment to lower limb amputation amongst prosthesis users. *Prosthet Orthot Int.* 2008;32:244-252.

41. Deans SA, McFadyen AK, Rowe PJ. Physical activity and quality of life: a study of a lower-limb amputee population. *Prosthet Orthot Int.* 2008;32:186-200.

42. Hamilton EA, Nichols PJR. Rehabilitation of the elderly lower-limb amputee. *Br Med J.* 1972;2:95-99.

43. Hutchins PM. The outcome of severe tibial injury. *Injury.* 1981;13:216-219.

44. Dillingham TR, Pezzin LE, Mackenzie EJ. Discharge destination after dysvascular lower-limb amputation. *Arch Phys Med Rehabil.* 2003;84:1662-1668.

45. Kerstein MD, Zimmer H, Dugdale FE, Lerner E. What influence does age have on rehabilitation of amputees? *Geriatrics.* 1975;30:67-71.

46. Cutson TM, Bongiorni D, Michael JW, Kochersberger G. Early management of elderly dysvascular below-knee amputees. *J Prosthet Orthot.* 1994;6:62-66.

47. Mazet R Jr. The geriatric amputee. *Artif Limbs.* 1967;11:33-41.

48. Cumming JC, Barr S, Howe TE. Prosthetic rehabilitation for older dysvascular people following a unilateral transfemoral amputation [serial on CD-ROM]. *Cochrane Database Syst Rev.* 2006;CD005260.

49. Bilodeau S, Hebert R, Desrosiers J. Lower limb prosthesis utilization by elderly amputees. *Prosthet Orthot Int.* 2000;24:126-132.

50. Fletcher DD, Andrews KL, Butters MA, et al. Rehabilitation of the geriatric vascular amputee patient: a population-based study. *Arch Phys Med Rehabil.* 2001;28:776-779.

51. Goldberg RT. New trends in the rehabilitation of lower extremity amputees. *Orthot Prosthet.* 1985;39:29-40.

52. Pinzur MS, Smith D, Tornow D, et al. Gait analysis of dysvascular below-knee and contralateral through-knee bilateral amputees: a preliminary report. *Orthopedics.* 1993;16:875-879.

53. Brodza WK, Thornhill HL, Zarapkar SE, et al. Long-term function of persons with atherosclerotic bilateral below-knee amputation living in the inner city. *Arch Phys Med Rehabil.* 1990;71:895-900.

54. Stokes D, Curzio J, Berry A, et al. Pre prosthetic mobility: the amputees' perspectives. *Disabil Rehabil.* 2009;31:138-143.

55. Burke MJ, Roman V, Wright V. Bone and joint changes in lower limb amputees. *Ann Rheum Dis.* 1978;37:252-254.

56. Mak J, Solomon M, Faux S. Ipsilateral total hip arthroplasty in a dysvascular below-knee amputee for advanced hip osteoarthritis: a case report and review of the literature. *Prosthet Orthot Int.* 2008;32:155-159.

57. Ehde DM, Smith DG, Czerniecki JM, et al. Back pain as a secondary disability in persons with lower limb amputations. *Arch Phys Med Rehabil.* 2001;82:731-734.

58. Ephraim PL, Wegener ST, MacKenzie EJ, et al. Phantom pain, residual limb pain, and back pain in amputees: results of a national survey. *Arch Phys Med Rehabil.* 2005;86:1910-1919.

59. Rush PJ, Wong JS, Kirsh J, Devlin M. Osteopenia in patients with above knee amputation. *Arch Phys Med Rehabil.* 1994;75:112-115.

60. Yazicioglu K, Tugcu I, Yilmaz B, et al. Osteoporosis: a factor on residual limb pain in traumatic trans-tibial amputations. *Prosthet Orthot Int.* 2008;32:172-178.

61. Potter BK, Burns TC, Lacap AP, et al. Heterotopic ossification following traumatic and combat-related amputations: prevalence, risk factors, and preliminary results of excision. *J Bone Joint Surg Am.* 2007;89:476-486.

62. Aksnes LH, Bruland ØS. Some musculo-skeletal sequelae in cancer survivors. *Acta Oncol.* 2007;46:490-496.

63. Murnaghan JJ, Bowker JH. Musculoskeletal complications. In: Smith DG, Michael JW, Bowker JH, eds. *Atlas of Amputation and Limb Deficiencies: Surgical, Prosthetic, and Rehabilitation Principles.* 3rd ed. Rosemont, IL: American Academy of Orthopaedic Surgeons; 2004:683-700.

Chapter 16

Prosthetic Functional Outcomes

A major goal of prosthetic training is maximizing the patient's functional capacity. Function can be measured by energy expenditure and subjective responses, as well as the activities that patients pursue (as described in Chapter 14).

ENERGY EXPENDITURE

Physical activity requires the expenditure of energy, most commonly measured as *oxygen consumption*. People who have lower-limb amputation and walk at a self-selected walking speed typically use about as much oxygen as able-bodied adults who walk at their comfortable walking speed. The distinction between the 2 groups is that able-bodied adults select a faster pace. The person with an amputation compensates by walking slower and thus covering less distance in a given time period; an alternate means of transport (eg, a wheelchair) may be desirable for traversing long distances.

Energy expenditure is influenced by the level of amputation, walking surface, etiology of the amputation, patient's age and overall health, and components of the prosthesis. Although published investigations report on small samples, the conclusions confirm clinical experience.

TRANSTIBIAL AMPUTATION

Comparison of able-bodied men and those with transtibial amputation not caused by vascular disease indicates that the latter had a 16% greater oxygen consumption and a freely chosen ambulation pace 11% slower. Those with longer amputation limbs used less oxygen.[1] A higher cost may be attributed to the increased mechanical work performed when the walker transfers weight from the prosthesis to the sound limb.[2] The surface also influences energy usage. On asphalt and mown lawn, the wearers used more oxygen than the control subjects; walking on high grass was the most arduous, as demonstrated by a greater energy cost and a slower speed.[3]

Prosthetic components may influence the energy cost of walking. One comparison of subjects walking with energy-storing feet and with solid ankle, cushion heel (SACH; Otto Bock, Minneapolis, Minnesota) feet revealed slightly lower oxygen usage with the dynamic C-Walk (Otto Bock) and Flex-Foot (Ossur, Aliso Viejo, California), and a lower percentage of age-predicted maximum heart rate.[4] An earlier comparison did not show an appreciable difference.[5] Other investigators measured the performance of subjects who had traumatic amputations and those with vascular disease. People who had vascular amputation did not walk faster or more efficiently with energy-storing feet.[6] Although manufacturers seek lighter weight components, weight difference of as much as 908 g (2 pounds) did not have an appreciable effect on energy consumption.[7-10] Contradicting these results is a study in which the mass of the prosthesis was matched to the sound limb; the energy cost was significantly greater, and step length, swing time, and stance time were more asymmetrical.[11]

TRANSFEMORAL AMPUTATION

In contrast with able-bodied adults whose comfortable walking speed is the same as the most efficient walking speed, those with transfemoral amputation selected a slower, more comfortable walking speed than the most efficient walking speed. Energy expenditure per second did not differ between the 2 groups; however, expenditure per distance was greater among those wearing prostheses.[12,13]

Prosthetic components may also influence the energy cost of walking. People walking with energy-storing

Edelstein JE, Muroz A.
Lower-Limb Prosthetics and Orthotics: Clinical Concepts (pp 113-118).
© 2011 Taylor & Francis Group.

feet used less energy than when wearing the SACH foot.[14] As research with adults with transtibial amputation shows, those wearing transfemoral prostheses also had approximately the same energy cost regardless of the weight of the prosthesis.[15] Although no appreciable difference exists between walking with a locked and an unlocked knee unit, when subjects walked with the knee they customarily used, they were more efficient.[16] Young patients given a choice between prostheses having sliding friction or pneumatic knee units generally preferred the pneumatic swing phase control, even though the energy cost was actually higher than with the mechanical knee unit.[17] Comparison of performance with the CaTech hydraulic knee unit and the Adaptive (both units are from Endolite, Miamisburg, Ohio) microprocessor-controlled pneumatic and hydraulic unit demonstrated no significant difference in metabolic cost.[18] Several investigations of the Intelligent (Endolite) microprocessor-controlled knee unit concur that these components are associated with slightly less oxygen consumption than when subjects walked with nonmicroprocessor units.[19-22] Similar results have been obtained when adults used the C-Leg (Otto Bock).[23-25] Though differences in oxygen usage were small, subjects did increase their physical activity with the newer components.[23,25]

Socket design may also affect the metabolic cost of walking. Compared with the quadrilateral socket, subjects who walked with prostheses that had an ischial containment socket used less oxygen and walked faster; differences were more pronounced when they walked faster.[26]

COMPARISONS OF SUBJECTS WITH TRANSTIBIAL AND TRANSFEMORAL AMPUTATION

Several investigators reported on studies comparing adults with transtibial amputation with those wearing transfemoral prostheses. The energy expenditure rate was 0% to 15% greater in the transtibial group than in able-bodied adults. Those with transfemoral amputation needed 30% to 60% more oxygen than the able-bodied subjects.[27] Adults with dysvascular transtibial amputation used about the same energy as those with traumatic transfemoral amputation when walking at a self-selected speed.[28] Compared with control subjects, others demonstrated that walking with a transtibial prosthesis increases oxygen consumption by about 25%, and with a transfemoral prosthesis the increase is 55% to 65%. Vascular etiology of amputation increases energy consumption on the order of at least 20%. Prosthetic alignment, particularly changing ankle angle, also changes oxygen use. With transfemoral prostheses, shifting the knee axis forward increased the energy requirement.[29]

HIP DISARTICULATION AND TRANSPELVIC AMPUTATION

Small sample studies of adults who wore hip disarticulation (HD) and transpelvic (TP) prostheses walked at approximately half the velocity of able-bodied adults. The energy cost per distance was 80% to 125% greater than normal for HD and TP, respectively.[30] Adults with HD prostheses equipped with microprocessor-controlled pneumatic swing-phase controlled knee units consumed less oxygen than when they used prostheses having a friction brake.[31]

BILATERAL AMPUTATIONS

Young adults with bilateral transfemoral amputation walked 21% slower and had 49% higher energy cost compared with able-bodied adults, possibly because balance and maneuvering with prostheses is more arduous.[32] One patient wearing C-Legs walked farther and faster with less oxygen consumption than with other knee units.[33] Another person was tested while walking with regular length prostheses and with stubbies (ie, short, nonarticulated prostheses). With stubbies, the individual used 24% less oxygen than with long prostheses; control subjects, however, were 47% and 79% more efficient.[34] Both people with bilateral transfemoral and those with bilateral transtibial amputation consumed much less oxygen when propelling a wheelchair compared to walking.[35,36] The difference is particularly striking at the higher amputation levels, where oxygen cost ranges from 466% to 707% of wheeling, with velocity ranging from one-quarter to one-third of wheelchair travel.[36] A recent study of people with various combinations of bilateral amputations demonstrated the complexity of comparing individuals having one level of amputation with others having different levels. Energy consumption did not necessarily follow the expectation that those with bilateral transtibial amputation would use the least oxygen and walk the fastest. Obesity was a major determinant of walking economy.[37]

OTHER OBJECTIVE FUNCTIONAL MEASURES

Gait analysis in a small sample of people with transfemoral amputation indicated that if the femur is at least 57% of the length of the contralateral femur, length does not dramatically alter gait.[38]

Walking velocity reflects the individual's duration of static weight bearing on the prosthesis. On average, those with transtibial amputation walked at the rate of 1.70 m/s, whereas subjects wearing transfemoral prostheses averaged 0.78 m/s.[39] Others reported similar velocity results comparing people walking with transtibial and transfemoral prostheses.[40] Heart rate among men with traumatic transtibial amputation is similar to that of able-bodied men.[41]

Physical examination is an essential element in predicting functional outcome. Amputation creates skeletal, articular, and muscular imbalance which may lead to osteoarthritis,[42] osteoporosis, and other disorders.[43] In addition to those with vascular disease, patients who sustained traumatic amputation are vulnerable to cardiovascular disease, possibly because of insulin resistance, smoking, excessive alcohol consumption, and fatty diet.[44] Predictors of poor functional outcome among adults with unilateral dysvascular amputation include advanced age at amputation, limited balance on the sound leg, and cognitive impairment.[45,46]

A review of 31 adults with dysvascular transfemoral/transtibial bilateral amputation revealed generally poor outcome; patients whose initial amputation was transtibial were unlikely to be fitted with a transfemoral prosthesis after the contralateral amputation. Those who were able to walk with 2 prostheses were so slow that they could not cross a street in time with the traffic light.[47] In contrast, three-quarters of patients with bilateral amputation, primarily those wearing bilateral transtibial prostheses, walked. Half were community ambulators.[48]

The ability of the patient to balance on the prosthesis has a major bearing on the individual's likelihood of walking with a prosthesis. Those with poorer balance are older; more apt to be female; and more likely to use an assistive device, have poor perceived health, be depressed, and fear falling.[49-52]

The ultimate determinant of outcome is survival. A retrospective longitudinal cohort study of 2616 veterans revealed that the 6-month survival rate depended on the function of the individual. For those who required total assistance, 73% were alive at 6 months; 91% of the maximal assistance group survived. Amputation level was not a significant factor in survival.[53] Another study of a large number of patients demonstrated that survival was influenced by amputation level, with people who sustained transfemoral amputation at greater jeopardy; diabetes and renal disease are other negative factors.[54] Diabetes was also implicated in diminishing survival among a cohort of 734 people with amputations performed over a decade. Men had a high incidence of amputation but did not exceed women with regard to survival.[55] Other investigators reported a median survival of 4 years, with diabetes conferring a poorer prognosis.[56] Similar results have also been reported elsewhere.[57] Adults with diabetes died at significantly younger ages than people who did not have diabetes and were more likely to sustain revision of the amputation limb.[58] Of patients who underwent amputation after failed revascularization, 59% were alive at 5 years. Approximately half of the survivors wore prostheses.[59]

Two recent reviews describe patients who sustained bilateral amputation. In the first, survival was about 4 years, with 85% walking.[60] The other study determined mortality after 5 years as 69%, and only 38% of patients walked.[61]

Prosthetic use is another objective indicator of outcome. Younger age, employment, marriage, distal amputation, traumatic etiology, and the absence of phantom limb pain all distinguish people who continue to wear their prostheses.[62] Those with transtibial amputation were more apt to use their prostheses if the amputation limb was at least 4.75 inches (12 cm) long.[63] Other studies confirm that patients younger than 50 are likely to achieve community mobility, regardless of amputation level.[64-66] Individuals with amputation and hemiparesis were more apt to walk with a prosthesis if both affected the same side and if the paresis was relatively mild.[67]

The antithesis of independence is institutionalization. Adults who are relatively old, live alone, and have unilateral transfemoral amputation or bilateral amputation are least able to live at home.[68]

Returning to work is a most favorable outcome. One research team reported that two-thirds of patients returned to work, although many changed jobs.[69] Another positive outcome is resumption of automobile driving, achieved by more than 80% of subjects in one study.[70]

SUBJECTIVE RESPONSES

Many questionnaires are designed to enable recording the subjective responses of patients and clinicians' appraisals,[71-74] including L Test of Functional Mobility,[75] Amputee Mobility Predictor,[76] Craig Hospital Inventory of Environmental Factors,[77] Lower Limb Amputee Measurement Scale,[78] and Frenchay Activities Index.[79] They attempt to define quality of life, perhaps the ultimate expression of rehabilitation outcome.

Middle-aged men reported high quality of life.[80] Another sample expressed a wide range of opinions regarding their life satisfaction; depression and participation in daily living are key elements influencing their responses.[81] Several studies of men who sustained amputation while in military service confirmed relatively high quality of life.[82-86]

Neuropsychological factors play a role in the functional outcome of people with amputations. Visual memory, verbal fluency, age, amputation level, and pain predict functional outcome.[87] Fostering the patient's self-management skills has a major positive effect on the quality of life of people with amputations, particularly younger adults and those with recent amputation.[88] Patients who believe in the efficacy of rehabilitation have more positive outcomes.[89]

REFERENCES

1. Gailey RS, Wenger MA, Raya M, Kirk N. Energy expenditure of transtibial amputees during ambulation at self-selected pace. *Prosthet Orthot Int.* 1994;18:84-91.

2. Houdijk H, Pollmann E, Groenewold M, et al. The energy cost for the step-to-step transition in amputee walking. *Gait Posture.* 2009;30:35-40.

3. Paysant J, Brevaert C, Datie AM, et al. Influence of terrain on metabolic and temporal gait characteristics of unilateral transtibial amputees. *J Rehabil Res Dev.* 2006;43:153-160.

4. Hsu MJ, Nielsen DH, Lin-Chan SJ, Shurr D. The effects of prosthetic foot design on physiologic measurements, self-selected walking velocity, and physical activity in people with transtibial amputation. *Arch Phys Med Rehabil.* 2006;87:123-129.

5. Torburn L, Powers CM, Guitierrez R, et al. Energy expenditure during ambulation in dysvascular and traumatic below-knee amputees: a comparison of five prosthetic feet. *J Rehabil Res Dev.* 1995;32:111-119.

6. Casillas JM, Dulieu V, Cohen M, Marcer I. Bioenergetic comparison of a new energy-storing foot and SACH foot in traumatic below-knee vascular amputations. *Arch Phys Med Rehabil.* 1995;76:39-44.

7. Lin-Chan SJ, Nielsen DH, Yack HJ, et al. The effects of added prosthetic mass on physiologic responses and stride frequency during multiple speeds of walking in persons with transtibial amputation. *Arch Phys Med Rehabil.* 2003;84:1865-1871.

8. Gailey RS, Nash MS, Atchley TA, et al. The effects of prosthesis mass on metabolic cost of ambulation in non-vascular transtibial amputees. *Prosthet Orthot Int.* 1997;21:9-16.

9. Lehmann JF, Price R, Okumura R, et al. Mass and mass distribution of below-knee prostheses: effects on gait efficiency and self-selected walking speed. *Arch Phys Med Rehabil.* 1998;79:162-168.

10. Lin S-J, Bose N. Six-minute walk test in persons with transtibial amputation. *Arch Phys Med Rehabil.* 2008;89:2354-2359.

11. Mattes SJ, Martin PE, Royer TD. Walking symmetry and energy cost in persons with unilateral transtibial amputations: matching prosthetic and normal limb inertial properties. *Arch Phys Med Rehabil.* 2000;81:561-856.

12. Jaegers SM, Vos LD, Rispens P, et al. The relationship between comfortable and most metabolically efficient walking speed in persons with unilateral above knee amputation. *Arch Phys Med Rehabil.* 1993;74:521-525.

13. Hagberg K, Häggström E, Brånemark R. Physiological cost index (PCI) and walking performance in individuals with transfemoral prostheses compared to healthy controls. *Disabil Rehabil.* 2007;29:643-649.

14. Graham LE, Datta D, Heller B, Howitt J. A comparative study of oxygen consumption for conventional and energy-storing prosthetic feet in transfemoral amputees. *Clin Rehabil.* 2008;22:896-901.

15. Czerniecki JM, Gitter A, Weaver K. Effects of alterations in prosthetic shank mass on the metabolic cost of ambulation in above-knee amputees. *Arch Phys Med Rehabil.* 1994;73:348-352.

16. Isakov E, Susak Z, Becker E. Energy expenditure and cardiac response in above-knee amputee while using prosthesis with open and locked knee mechanisms. *Scand J Rehabil Med.* 1985;12(suppl):108-111.

17. Boonstra AM, Schrama J, Fidler V, Eisma WH. Energy cost during ambulation in transfemoral amputees: a knee joint with a mechanical swing phase control vs a knee joint with pneumatic swing phase control. *Scand J Rehabil Med.* 1995;27:77-81.

18. Jepson F, Datta D, Harris I, et al. A comparative evaluation of the Adaptive knee and CaTech knee joints: a preliminary study. *Prosthet Orthot Int.* 2008;32:84-92.

19. Chin T, Machida K, Sawamura S, et al. Comparison of different microprocessor controlled knee joints on the energy consumption during walking in transfemoral amputees: Intelligent knee prosthesis (IP) versus C-Leg. *Prosthet Orthot Int.* 2006;30:73-80.

20. Taylor MB, Clark E, Offord EA, Baxter C. A comparison of energy expenditure by a high level transfemoral amputee using the Intelligent prosthesis and conventionally damped prosthetic limbs. *Prosthet Orthot Int.* 1996;20:116-121.

21. Buckley JG, Spence WD, Solomonidis SE. Energy cost of walking: comparison of Intelligent prosthesis with conventional mechanism. *Arch Phys Med Rehabil.* 1997;78:330-333.

22. Datta D, Heller B, Howitt J. A comparative evaluation of oxygen consumption and gait pattern in amputees using Intelligent prostheses and conventionally damped knee swing-phase control. *Clin Rehabil.* 2005;19:398-403.

23. Seymour R, Engbretson B, Kott K, et al. Comparison between the C-Leg microprocessor-controlled prosthetic knee and non-microprocessor control prosthetic knees: a preliminary study of energy expenditure, obstacle course performance, and quality of life survey. *Prosthet Orthot Int.* 2007;31:51-61.

24. Orendurff MS, Segal AD, Klute GK, et al. Gait efficiency using the C-Leg. *J Rehabil Res Dev.* 2006;43:239-246.

25. Kaufman KR, Levine JA, Brey RH, et al. Energy expenditure and activity of transfemoral amputees using mechanical and microprocessor-controlled prosthetic knees. *Arch Phys Med Rehabil.* 2008;89:1380-1385.

26. Gailey RS, Lawrence D, Barditt C. The CAT-CAM socket and quadrilateral socket: a comparison of energy cost during ambulation. *Prosthet Orthot Int.* 1993;17:95-100.

27. Genin JJ, Bastien GJ, Franck B, et al. Effect of speed on the energy cost of walking in unilateral traumatic lower limb amputees. *Eur J Appl Physiol.* 2008;103:655-663.

28. Detrembleur C, Vanmarsenille JM, De Cuyper F, Dierick F. Relationship between energy cost, gait speed, vertical displacement of centre of body mass and efficiency of pendulum-like mechanism in unilateral amputee gait. *Gait Posture.* 2005;21:333-340.

29. Schmalz T, Blumentritt S, Jarasch R. Energy expenditure and biomechanical characteristics of lower limb amputee gait: the influence of prosthetic alignment and different prosthetic components. *Gait Posture.* 2002;16:255-263.

30. Nowroozi F, Salvanelli ML, Gerber LH. Energy expenditure in hip disarticulation and hemipelvectomy. *Arch Phys Med Rehabil.* 1983;64:300-303.

31. Chin T, Sawamura S, Shiba R, et al. Energy expenditure during walking in amputees after disarticulation of the hip: a microprocessor-controlled swing-phase control knee versus a mechanical-controlled stance-phase control knee. *J Bone Joint Surg.* 2005;87B:117-119.

32. Hoffman MD, Sheldahl LM, Buley KJ, Sandford PR. Physiological comparison of walking among bilateral above-knee amputee and able-bodied subjects, and a model to account for the differences in metabolic cost. *Arch Phys Med Rehabil.* 1997;78:385-392.

33. Perry J, Burnfield JM, Newsam CJ, Conley P. Energy expenditure and gait characteristics of a bilateral amputee walking with C-Leg prostheses compared with stubby and conventional articulating prostheses. *Arch Phys Med Rehabil.* 2004;85:1711-1717.

34. Crouse SF, Lessard CS, Rhodes J, et al. Oxygen consumption and cardiac response of short-leg and long-leg prosthetic ambulation in a patient with bilateral above-knee amputation: comparisons with able-bodied men. *Arch Phys Med Rehabil.* 1990;71:313-317.

35. DuBow LL, Witt PL, Kadaba MP, et al. Oxygen consumption of elderly persons with bilateral below-knee amputations: amputation vs wheelchair propulsion. *Arch Phys Med Rehabil.* 1983;64:255-259.

36. Wu YJ, Chen SY, Lin MC, et al. Energy expenditure of wheeling and walking during prosthetic rehabilitation in a woman with bilateral transfemoral amputations. *Arch Phys Med Rehabil.* 2001;82:265-269.

37. Wright DA, Marks L, Payne RC. A comparative study of the physiological costs of walking in ten bilateral amputees. *Prosthet Orthot Int.* 2008;32:57-67.

38. Baum BS, Schnall BL, Tis JE, Lipton JS. Correlation of residual limb length and gait parameters in amputees. *Injury.* 2008;39:728-733.

39. Jones ME, Bashford GM, Mann JM. Weight bearing and velocity in transtibial and transfemoral amputees. *Prosthet Orthot Int.* 1997;21:183-186.

40. MacKenzie EJ, Bosse MJ, Castillo RC, et al. Functional outcomes following trauma-related lower-extremity amputation. *J Bone Joint Surg Am.* 2004;86A:1636-1645.

41. Bussmann JB, Schrauwen HJ, Stam HJ. Daily physical activity and heart rate response in people with a unilateral traumatic transtibial amputation. *Arch Phys Med Rehabil.* 2008;89:430-434.

42. Struyf PA, van Heugten CM, Hitters MW, Smeets RJ. The prevalence of osteoarthritis of the intact hip and knee among traumatic leg amputees. *Arch Phys Med Rehabil.* 2009;90:440-446.

43. Gailey R, Allen K, Castles J, et al. Review of secondary physical conditions associated with lower-limb amputation and long-term prosthesis use. *J Rehabil Res Dev.* 2008;45:15-29.

44. Naschitz JE, Lenger R. Why traumatic leg amputees are at increased risk for cardiovascular diseases. *QJM.* 2008;101:251-259.

45. Schoppen T, Boonstra A, Groothoff JW, et al. Physical, mental, and social predictors of functional outcome in unilateral lower-limb amputees. *Arch Phys Med Rehabil.* 2003;84:803-811.

46. Sansam K, Neumann V, O'Connor R, Bhakta B. Predicting walking ability following lower limb amputation: a systematic review of the literature. *J Rehabil Med.* 2009;41:593-603.

47. Bhangu S, Devlin M, Pauley T. Outcomes of individuals with transfemoral and contralateral transtibial amputation due to dysvascular etiologies. *Prosthet Orthot Int.* 2009;33:33-40.

48. Shin JC, Kim EJ, Park CI, Park ES, Shin KH. Clinical features and outcomes following bilateral lower limb amputation in Korea. *Prosthet Orthot Int.* 2006;30:155-164.

49. Miller WC, Deathe AB. A prospective study examining balance confidence among individuals with lower limb amputation. *Disabil Rehabil.* 2004;26:875-881.

50. Miller WC, Speechley M, Deathe AB. Balance confidence among people with lower-limb amputations. *Phys Ther.* 2002;82:856-865.

51. Miller WC, Speechley M, Deathe B. The prevalence and risk factors of falling and fear of falling among lower extremity amputees. *Arch Phys Med Rehabil.* 2001;82:1031-1037.

52. Miller WC, Deathe AB, Speechley M, Koval J. The influence of falling, fear of falling, and balance confidence on prosthetic mobility and social activity among individuals with a lower extremity amputation. *Arch Phys Med Rehabil.* 2001;82:1238-1244.

53. Stineman MG, Kurichi JE, Kwong PL, et al. Survival analysis in amputees based on physical independence grade achievement. *Arch Surg.* 2009;144:543-551.

54. Aulivola B, Hile CN, Hamdan AD, et al. Major lower extremity amputation: outcome of a modern series. *Arch Surg.* 2004;139:395-399.

55. Heikkinen M, Saarinen J, Suominen VP, et al. Lower limb amputations: differences between the genders and long-term survival. *Prosthet Orthot Int.* 2007;31:277-286.

56. Kulkarni J, Pande S, Morris J. Survival rates in dysvascular lower limb amputees. *Int J Surg.* 2006;4:217-221.

57. Dillingham TR, Pezzin LE, MacKenzie EJ, Burgess AR. Use and satisfaction with prosthetic devices among persons with trauma-related amputations: a long-term outcome study. *Am J Phys Med Rehabil.* 2001;80:563-571.

58. Nehler MR, Coll JR, Hiatt WR, et al. Functional outcome in a contemporary series of major lower extremity amputations. *J Vasc Surg.* 2003;38:7-14.

59. Reed AB, Delvecchio C, Giglia JS. Major lower extremity amputation after multiple revascularizations: was it worth it? *Ann Vasc Surg.* 2008;22:335-340.

60. MacNeill B, Devlin M, Pauley T, Yudin A. Long-term outcomes and survival of patients with bilateral transtibial amputations after rehabilitation. *Am J Phys Med Rehabil.* 2008;87:189-196.

61. Inderbitzi R, Buettiker M, Enzler M. The long-term mobility and mortality of patients with peripheral arterial disease following bilateral amputation. *Eur J Vasc Endovasc Surg.* 2003;26:59-64.

62. Raichle KA, Hanley MA, Molton I, et al. Prosthesis use in persons with lower- and upper-limb amputation. *J Rehabil Res Dev.* 2008;45:961-972.

63. Arwert HJ. Residual-limb quality and functional mobility 1 year after transtibial amputation caused by vascular insufficiency. *J Rehabil Res Dev.* 2007;44:717-722.

64. Davies B, Datta D. Mobility outcome following unilateral lower limb amputation. *Prosthet Orthot Int.* 2003;27: 186-190.

65. Munin MC, Espejo-De Guzman MC, Boninger ML, et al. Predictive factors for successful early prosthetic ambulation among lower-limb amputees. *J Rehabil Res Dev.* 2001;38:379-384.

66. Fletcher DD, Andrews KL, Butters MA, et al. Rehabilitation of the geriatric vascular amputee patient: a population-based study. *Arch Phys Med Rehabil.* 2001;82:776-779.

67. Brunelli S, Averna T, Porcacchia P, et al. Functional status and factors influencing the rehabilitation outcome of people affected by above-knee amputation and hemiparesis. *Arch Phys Med Rehabil.* 2006;87:995-1000.

68. Remes L, Isoaho R, Vahlberg T, et al. Predictors for institutionalization and prosthetic ambulation after major lower extremity amputation during an eight-year follow-up. *Aging Clin Exp Res.* 2009;21:129-135.

69. Burger H, Marincek C. Return to work after lower limb amputation. *Disabil Rehabil.* 2007;29:1323-1329.

70. Boulias C, Meikle B, Pauley T, Devlin M. Return to driving after lower-extremity amputation. *Arch Phys Med Rehabil.* 2006;87:1183-1188.

71. Rommers GM, Vos LD, Groothoff JW, Eisma WH. Mobility of people with lower limb amputations: scales and questionnaires: a review. *Clin Rehabil.* 2001;15:92-102.

72. Deathe AB, Wolfe DL, Devlin M, et al Selection of outcome measures in lower extremity amputation rehabilitation: ICF activities. *Disabil Rehabil.* 2009;31:1455-1473.

73. Hebert JS, Wolfe DL, Miller WC, et al. Outcome measures in amputation rehabilitation: ICF body functions. *Disabil Rehabil.* 2009;19:1-14.

74. Kohler F, Cieza A, Stucki G, et al. Developing core sets for persons following amputation based on the International Classification of Functioning, Disability, and Health as a way to specify functioning. *Prosthet Orthot Int.* 2009;33: 117-129.

75. Deathe AB, Miller WC. The L test of functional mobility: measurement properties of a modified version of the timed "up & go" test designed for people with lower-limb amputations. *Phys Ther.* 2005;85:626-635.

76. Gailey RS, Roach KE, Applegate EB, et al. The Amputee Mobility Predictor: an instrument to assess determinants of the lower-limb amputee's ability to ambulate. *Arch Phys Med Rehabil.* 2002;83:613-627.

77. Ephraim PL, MacKenzie EJ, Wegener ST, et al. Environmental barriers experienced by amputees: the Craig Hospital Inventory of Environmental Factors—Short Form. *Arch Phys Med Rehabil.* 2006;87:328-333.

78. Cheifetz O, Bayley M, Grad S, et al. The Lower Limb Amputee Measurement Scale: reliability and predictive validity. *Prosthet Orthot Int.* 2007;31:300-312.

79. Miller WC, Deathe AB, Harris J. Measurement properties of the Frenchay Activities Index among individuals with a lower limb amputation. *Clin Rehabil.* 2004;18: 414-422.

80. Zidarov D, Swaine B, Gauthier-Gagnon C. Quality of life of persons with lower-limb amputation during rehabilitation and at 3-month follow-up. *Arch Phys Med Rehabil.* 2009;90:634-645.

81. Asano M, Rushton P, Miller WC, Deathe BA. Predictors of quality of life among individuals who have a lower limb amputation. *Prosthet Orthot Int.* 2008;32:231-243.

82. Tekin L, Safaz Ý, Göktepe AS, Yazýcýodlu K. Comparison of quality of life and functionality in patients with traumatic unilateral below knee amputation and salvage surgery. *Prosthet Orthot Int.* 2009;33:17-24.

83. Dougherty PJ. Transtibial amputees from the Vietnam War. Twenty-eight-year follow-up. *J Bone Joint Surg Am.* 2001;83:383-389.

84. Dougherty PJ. Long-term follow-up of unilateral transfemoral amputees from the Vietnam war. *J Trauma.* 2003;54:718-723.

85. Dougherty PJ. Long-term follow-up study of bilateral above-the-knee amputees from the Vietnam War. *J Bone Joint Surg Am.* 1999;81:1384-1390.

86. Sherman RA. Utilization of prostheses among US veterans with traumatic amputation: a pilot survey. *J Rehabil Res Dev.* 1999;36:100-108.

87. O'Neill BF, Evans JJ. Memory and executive function predict mobility rehabilitation outcome after lower-limb amputation. *Disabil Rehabil.* 2009;11:1-9.

88. Wegener ST, Mackenzie EJ, Ephraim P, et al. Self-management improves outcomes in persons with limb loss. *Arch Phys Med Rehabil.* 2009;90:373-378.

89. Callaghan B, Condie E, Johnston M. Using the common sense self-regulation model to determine psychological predictors of prosthetic use and activity limitations in lower limb amputees. *Prosthet Orthot Int.* 2008;32: 324-336.

Chapter 17

Orthotic Principles

Orthoses are appliances worn on the body for therapeutic reasons. Those devices that encompass one or more parts of the lower limb are known as lower-limb orthoses. Foot orthoses (FOs) may be an insert worn inside the shoe, an internal modification glued inside the shoe, or an external modification secured to the shoe sole or heel. An ankle-foot orthosis (AFO) includes a FO and a proximal portion that extends over the lower leg. The knee-ankle-foot orthosis (KAFO) encompasses the thigh, leg, and foot. A hip-knee-ankle-foot orthosis (HKAFO) extends from the pelvis to the foot, and a trunk-hip-knee-ankle-foot orthosis (THKAFO) starts at the upper trunk and covers the thighs, legs, and feet. These orthoses are described in subsequent chapters.

Knee orthoses (KOs), which cover the knee, and hip orthoses (HOs), which surround one or both hips, are variations of KAFOs and HKAFOs.

PURPOSES OF ORTHOSES

The basic purpose of all orthoses is to apply force to the body. The therapeutic benefit of force application may be to accomplish the following:

> *Resist motion:* Rigid components prevent motion at the joint that is covered by the orthosis and, in some designs, affect an adjacent joint. For example, an individual with quadriceps paralysis who wears a KAFO with a mechanical lock engaged will avoid the risk of knee collapse when the person stands and walks. Someone else with knee paralysis may be fitted with an AFO that applies posteriorly directed force near the knee to resist knee flexion. Support is sometimes used to describe motion resistance. Resisting motion may be intended to maintain more normal joint alignment, as in the case of a person with genu recurvatum who wears a KAFO that resists the abnormal position.

> *Assist motion:* The most common example of orthotic motion assistance is an AFO that has a plastic or metal spring at the ankle to compensate for dorsiflexor weakness by assisting ankle dorsiflexion during swing phase. Such an orthosis prevents foot drop in swing phase, which may otherwise lead to tripping.

> *Transfer force:* A FO with a metatarsal bar that shifts load from painful metatarsophalangeal joints to the midfoot exemplifies an orthosis that transfers force.

COMFORT

Comfort is the primary requirement of any orthosis, regardless of its purpose. An uncomfortable orthosis will result either in the patient not wearing it, thus wasting money and professional time, or skin irritation. The key to comfort is pressure minimization and distribution. Pressure is reduced by increasing the contact area, reducing the force, or a combination of both strategies. Force is reduced by an orthosis that has relatively great leverage through which the longitudinal segments of the orthosis apply force. Too long an orthosis, however, may impinge on adjacent joints. The area of the body comfortably covered by the orthosis depends, in part, on the amount of subcutaneous fat and muscle tissue in the braced body part. A patient with atrophy requires greater skin coverage to ensure comfort. The drawback of covering a large area of the skin is that the underlying skin cannot dissipate heat or perspiration readily.

Some portion of an orthosis always touches the body. Snug contact without constriction is essential. Tight bands compress superficial blood vessels, causing pain and potentially tissue breakdown. Nevertheless, contact should not be excessively loose; too loose an orthosis tends to rub the skin as the patient moves.

Edelstein JE, Muroz A.
Lower-Limb Prosthetics and Orthotics: Clinical Concepts (pp 119-122).
© 2011 Taylor & Francis Group.

THREE-POINT FORCE APPLICATION

Orthoses apply pressure systems (ie, a series of forces and counterforces to implement the purposes described previously). The 3-point force system is basic. A principal force acts in 1 direction and 2 counterforces located proximal and distal to the principal force act in the opposite direction. For example, a patient with genu varum will have the deformity controlled by wearing an orthosis that exerts medially directed force on the lateral aspect of the knee and laterally directed counterforces on the lateral aspect of the thigh and leg.

The floor (ground) reaction (ie, the force applied by the floor to the patient in response to the force the person exerts on the floor) is another force that aids an orthosis to perform its function. When the wearer stands or walks, all lower-limb orthoses interact with the floor reaction.

MATERIALS

Contemporary orthoses are made of many materials, which differ in strength, flexibility, ease of forming, weight, appearance, durability, and cost. The type of material influences the effectiveness of the orthosis for a given patient.

Strength is the ability of a material to resist forces. An obese person exerts more force on an orthosis than does a frail patient. *Stress* refers to the effect of force on or within a material. *Pressure* refers to the amount of force applied per unit surface area. A narrow calf band on an AFO, for example, applies high local pressure to the wearer's leg and high stress within the band. To alleviate this situation, either the contact area must be increased or the orthosis must be made of very strong material to resist high force.

Materials can be strengthened by increasing the thickness; corrugating the midsection or rolling the edges; or reinforcing the material with a stronger material, such as carbon fiber. A given material curved with an acute angle will bend more readily than will the same material with a wider curve. Breakage is more apt to occur at the site of a nick or hammer mark than in a smooth, uncurved portion.

Compressive stress exists when force squeezes the material; the walker compresses the shoe heel during the early stance phase of gait. *Tensile stress* refers to pulling the material; a coil spring in an AFO pulls the shoe upward during swing phase of gait. *Shear* is the third primary type of stress; planes of the material slide over each other; the components of an overlapping knee joint in a KAFO exert shear stress on one another.

Strain is the change in shape of a material as a result of stress. *Stiffness* is the amount of stress that must be applied to a material to cause strain, whether for intentionally shaping or unintentionally deforming or breaking the material. *Brittleness* refers to breakage when relatively low force is applied. Cold metal becomes more brittle; thus, the patient is more likely to damage a brace in the winter. *Fatigue resistance* is the ability of the material to withstand repetitive loading. An active child, for example, subjects his orthoses to frequent repetitive loading, which may cause the joints to fail due to material fatigue.

Elasticity is the ratio of stress to strain, the ability of a material to recover its original dimensions. *Plasticity* describes a material that changes shape without cracking; a malleable material reshapes under compression, whereas a ductile material alters shape under tension. *Corrosion resistance* refers to chemical deterioration; some materials, such as leather, are vulnerable to corrosion by urine and perspiration.

Plastics and metals predominate in contemporary orthoses,[1] although some orthoses have leather, rubber, wood, or cloth elements. The physical and aesthetic properties of each material influence design, durability, and cost, as well as the patient's acceptance of the orthosis.

Plastics are synthetic organic (carbon-containing) materials. The huge variety of plastics results from the near infinite ways in which molecules can be combined. The properties of a given plastic depend on its molecular arrangement. As a group, plastics are relatively lightweight, easily shaped, strong, easily cleaned, corrosion resistant, and available in many colors.

Thermoplastics, such as polyethylene[2] and polypropylene,[3] are popular materials for orthoses. When heated, thermoplastic becomes malleable; it can be reshaped and it then retains the new shape upon cooling. Usually, thermoplastics can be reheated and reshaped indefinitely, allowing the orthotist to alter the fit of the appliance by heating the plastic, as well as by removing or adding material. The temperature at which thermoplastics become malleable varies. Most lower-limb orthoses are made of thermoplastics that require a high temperature to become malleable. The material is usually formed over a plaster model of the body part. The model may be obtained by wrapping the limb with a wet plaster bandage; then, when the plaster dries, removing it, filling the hollow replica of the limb with liquid plaster to create a model of the body part, and molding the plastic over the model. Alternatively, plastic may be molded over a model obtained by using computer-aided design and computer-aided manufacture (CAD-CAM). Many thermoplastics are relatively weak, easily stained, and flammable.

Alternate molecular arrangements produce thermosetting plastics, such as polyester and epoxy. Thermosetting plastics cannot be reshaped, under most circumstances, after they are molded and the chemical reaction is complete. An orthosis made of thermosetting plastic can be altered by removing plastic or by adding pads or other material. In general, thermosetting plastics are strong, impervious to heat, and readily colored.

Hydrogen, nitrogen, and other gases can be forced into plastics to create resilient material, useful as padding.[2] Closed-cell foam material is relatively firm and heavy, whereas open-cell foam is soft, porous, and tends to compress permanently, losing its resilience. Some viscoelastic plastics are used to absorb shock, as in shoe soles.[4-7]

A chemical element that is lustrous, opaque, and ductile is termed a *metal*. Most metals are strong, stiff, fatigue resistant, and impervious to the effects of environmental heat. For orthotic purposes, metals are generally in the form of alloys, a combination of elements, at least 1 of which is a metal. Combining a metal with other elements usually improves strength, wear resistance, and corrosion resistance. Fundamentally, the mechanical properties of metals depend on their chemical structure.

Aluminum alloys with the addition of copper, manganese, or other elements are often used in orthoses. Aluminum is radiolucent, more malleable, and much lighter than steel. To achieve equivalent rigidity, the aluminum components of an orthosis need to be thicker but are still lighter than comparable steel parts. Aluminum is unsuitable for hinges in orthoses because it is subject to fatigue failure.

Stainless steel, an alloy of iron, nickel, and chromium, is the most common form of steel in orthoses. Nickel increases corrosion resistance, and chromium improves ductility. Stainless steel is heavier, stiffer, and stronger than most other materials and is radiopaque.

Titanium is much lighter than steel, is corrosion resistant, and has high strength-to-weight ratio; however, it is more expensive than steel or aluminum. Magnesium is another lightweight, strong material sometimes used in the uprights of lower-limb orthoses.

Some elements, such as carbon and silicone, have properties that are similar to both metals and nonmetals, and are known as *metalloids*. Silicone offers little friction resistance but is not malleable or ductile and is a poor conductor of heat. It is an excellent interface between the orthosis and tender portions of skin. Carbon,[8-11] considered both a metal and a metalloid, is often used to reinforce an orthosis; the material is stiff, light, and strong but not very malleable. Carbon ribbons, however, enable carbon fiber to be used to reinforce weaker material.

Leather is animal skin that has been tanned, a chemical process that toughens the skin and makes it more flexible, stronger, and more porous. The specific skin and the type of tanning determine the physical properties of a given leather. Leather is porous and incompressible and can be molded over a model of a body part. Someone who is allergic to a particular leather may tolerate another leather or the same leather that has been tanned with different chemicals. Alternatively, a fabric or plastic interface may be placed between the patient's skin and the leather.

Cowhide is very strong and is therefore frequently used for straps and the upper portion of shoes. Kidskin and deerskin are very soft and suitable for shoe uppers for patients who have hammer toes and other tender areas on the dorsum of the foot. The texture of horsehide is particularly comfortable next to the skin, making it a popular lining for bands, such as a calf band.

Among various woods, cork is the most common wood used in orthoses. The bark of the cork oak tree is exceptionally lightweight and resilient, making it appropriate for shoe lifts and arch supports. Sometimes, cork is ground and mixed with rubber or other materials to achieve greater flexibility or economy. *Cushion cork* is a combination of cork and rubber or cork and ethyl vinyl acetate. *Thermomold cork* includes polyolefin to create a material that is easy to mold. Other woods are occasionally used in shoe construction. For example, balsa wood is sometimes used for shoe elevations because it is even lighter than cork yet has comparable strength and resilience.

Rubber is the sap of rubber trees that has been cured, usually by heating, to remove sulfur. Rubber has considerable elasticity, shock absorbency, and toughness. Less expensive and more resistant to corrosion than natural rubber, synthetic rubber, such as *neoprene*, may be less elastic than natural rubber. Whether natural or synthetic, rubber provides excellent traction on shoe soles and is a good padding material. Rubber strands may be woven with cotton or other fabric to create elastic straps and inserts. Open-cell (sponge) rubber is made with sodium bicarbonate, which creates carbon dioxide bubbles that create the tiny bubble-like cells in sponge rubber. This type of rubber recovers quickly when compressive stress is removed and is washable, soft, and very resilient. Cells, however, compress permanently after a relatively brief period of use. Closed-cell (expanded) rubber is manufactured by forcing nitrogen into rubber. It resists shear force and moisture and responds more slowly than open cell rubber to compressive stress.

Fabric, whether cotton, wool, or synthetic materials, is commonly used in orthoses. The properties of the fabric depend on the material itself and the way it is formed.[12] Cotton is strong, absorbs perspiration readily, and is hypoallergenic; thus, it is very suitable for socks. Knitted cotton conforms readily to the body and is often used as a liner worn under an orthosis. Wool has excellent resilience. Some foot orthoses are made of felt, wool, and other fibers matted together by steam and pressure. The higher the wool content, the more durable the felt. Felt is lightweight and porous but compresses readily.

Polyester and nylon are synthetic fabrics that can be used in orthoses. Polyester fibers may be combined with cotton to create a relatively inexpensive material that is strong and dries easily. A very popular application of nylon is hook and pile fasteners, which are easier to engage than buckles, snaps, buttons, or laces.

Most orthoses contain several materials. The materials may be sewn, riveted, or glued to one another. Riveting involves joining material by a rigid fastener. Gluing depends on the chemical characteristics of the surfaces to be joined, inasmuch as no universal adhesive exists. Synthetic resin glues, whether thermoplastic or thermosetting, are widely used because they bond many surfaces, such as joining a strap to the shell of an AFO. Rubber-based adhesives resist impact loads, making them suitable for many FOs.

DESIGN

In addition to the properties of the materials in the orthosis, its design has a marked effect on the performance of the patient who wears it. For each person, the orthosis must provide a unique combination of rigidity and flexibility to suit the therapeutic purpose. Trim lines[13] that cover more of the limb provide greater rigidity. Patients who are very concerned about the appearance of the orthosis may insist on particular colors, as well as streamlined contour. Others may value ease of donning or maintenance, both of which can be addressed in the design. Often, a given clinical condition can be managed with alternate designs and materials.

REFERENCES

1. Trower TA. Changes in lower extremity prosthetic practice. *Phys Med Rehabil Clin N Am*. 2006;17:23-30.
2. Kuncir EJ, Wirta RW, Golbranson FL. Load-bearing characteristics of polyethylene foam: an examination of structural and compression properties. *J Rehabil Res Dev*. 1990;27:229-238.
3. Convery P, Greig RJ, Ross RS, Sockalingam S. A three centre study of the variability of ankle foot orthoses due to fabrication and grade of polypropylene. *Prosthet Orthot Int*. 2004;28:175-182.
4. Withnall R, Eastaugh J, Freemantle N. Do shock absorbing insoles in recruits undertaking high levels of physical activity reduce lower limb injury? A randomized controlled trial. *J R Soc Med*. 2006;99:32-37.
5. Gillespie KA, Dickey JP. Determination of the effectiveness of materials in attenuating high frequency shock during gait using filterbank analysis. *Clin Biomech (Bristol, Avon)*. 2003;18:50-59.
6. Windle CM, Gregory SM, Dixon SJ. The shock attenuation characteristics of four different insoles when worn in a military boot during running and marching. *Gait Posture*. 1999;9:31-37.
7. Cinats J, Reid DC, Haddow JB. A biomechanical evaluation of sorbothane. *Clin Orthop Relat Res*. 1987;222:281-288.
8. Hachisuka K, Arai K, Arai M. Carbon fibre reinforced plastic knee-ankle-foot orthosis with a partially flexible thigh cuff: a modification for comfort while sitting on a toilet seat. *Prosthet Orthot Int*. 2007;31:133-137.
9. Hachisuka K, Makino K, Wada F, et al. Clinical application of carbon fibre reinforced plastic leg orthosis for polio survivors and its advantages and disadvantages. *Prosthet Orthot Int*. 2006;30:129-135.
10. Steinfeldt F, Seifert W, Günther KP. Modern carbon fibre orthoses in the management of polio patients—a critical evaluation of the functional aspects. *Z Orthop Ihre Grenzgeb*. 2003;141:357-361.
11. Heim M, Yaacobi E, Azaria M. A pilot study to determine the efficiency of lightweight carbon fibre orthoses in the management of patients suffering from post-poliomyelitis syndrome. *Clin Rehabil*. 1997;11:302-305.
12. Sanders JE, Greve JM, Mitchell SB, Zachariah SG. Material properties of commonly-used interface materials and their static coefficients of friction with skin and socks. *J Rehabil Res Dev*. 1998;35:161-176.
13. Sumiya T, Suzuki Y, Kasahara T. Stiffness control in posterior-type plastic ankle-foot orthoses: effect of ankle trimline. Part 2: orthosis characteristics and orthosis/patient matching. *Prosthet Orthot Int*. 1996;20:132-137.

Chapter 18

Shoes and Foot Orthoses

Patients with foot disorders require suitably designed, well-fitting shoes. Depending on the clinical problem, the individual may also benefit from shoe modifications, foot orthoses, or a combination of both.

SHOE DESIGNS

Although shoe designs are myriad, they can virtually all be analyzed in terms of 4 basic components, each of which has clinical relevance (Figure 18-1).

Upper

The portion of the shoe that covers the dorsum of the foot is designated as the *upper*. Two critical features of the upper are its height and the style of closure. Most patients are well served by a pair of shoes having a low upper (one that terminates below the malleoli). Shoes with a low upper are usually less expensive, faster to don, and provide sufficient foot support; they may also be augmented with a foot or an ankle-foot orthosis. A high upper covers the malleoli (Figure 18-2).

Many people with foot deformities or weakness require a shoe with an adjustable closure. The conventional closure is lacing through 5 or more pairs of eyelets. *Lace stays* are flaps on the upper that contain the eyelets. This facilitates adjusting the fit of the shoe. The Blucher closure features lace stays with the distal margins separate from each other (Figure 18-3). This style is attributed to Gebhard von Blucher (1742-1819), Field Marshal of Prussia, who sought a readily adjustable shoe style for his troops. The Blucher closure permits the greatest adjustability to accommodate foot deformities and changes in foot volume; it also allows one to open the shoe to the maximum extent. An alternative to the Blucher closure is the Bal, or Balmoral upper, named after the shoe introduced in Balmoral Castle, Scotland, in the 1850s (Figure 18-4). This upper style has the distal margins sewn together or is made of a single piece of leather or other material. The Bal upper is suitable for patients who do not need much adjustability in shoe snugness and who have no difficulty donning the shoe. Versions of both the Blucher and Bal upper are available with straps that permit opening the shoe and changing its fit.

Sole

The portion of the shoe under the foot is the *sole*. The *outsole* contacts the walking surface, and above the outsole is the *insole*, which contacts the plantar surface of the foot. For patients with balance impairment, the outsole should offer sufficient traction so the wearer can avoid slipping on the walking surface. The insole should also be resilient enough to absorb the shock generated as the individual walks.[1] If maximum shock absorption is required, both the insole and the outsole should be resilient.

Heel

The shoe *heel* is located under the anatomic heel and aids weight transfer through the stance phase of gait. A resilient base provides the shoe heel with enough traction to prevent the shoe from sliding on the floor. A higher heel transfers more weight to the forefoot, as compared with a low heel, and is associated with uncomfortable weight shift to the forefoot[2] as well as greater impact force.[3,4] Older women wearing high-heeled shoes climbed stairs more slowly with more trunk lateral bending, hip internal rotation, and hip abduction.[5] A broad heel reduces pressure on the anatomic heel by increasing the bearing area.

Reinforcements

Shoe reinforcements protect the foot and can make the shoe suitable for particular orthotic designs (Figure 18-5). The *counter* reinforces the posterior portion of the upper and should lie snugly against the anatomic heel. A loose counter can permit the shoe to slide on the foot and may cause heel blisters. The *toe box*, or *boxing*,

Edelstein JE, Muroz A.
Lower-Limb Prosthetics and Orthotics: Clinical Concepts (pp 123-128).

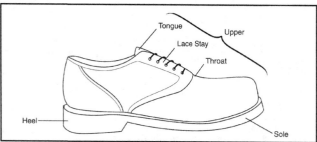

Figure 18-1. Parts of a shoe. (Reprinted with permission from Edelstein JE, Bruckner J. *Orthotics: A Comprehensive Clinical Approach.* Thorofare, NJ: SLACK Incorporated; 2002.)

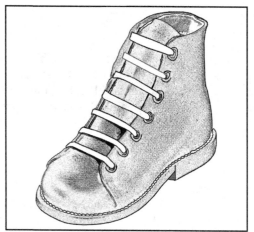

Figure 18-2. High upper. (Reprinted with permission from Edelstein JE, Bruckner J. *Orthotics: A Comprehensive Clinical Approach.* Thorofare, NJ: SLACK Incorporated; 2002.)

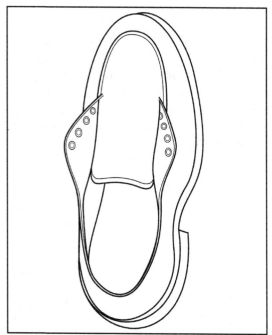

Figure 18-3. Blucher closure. (Reprinted with permission from Edelstein JE, Bruckner J. *Orthotics: A Comprehensive Clinical Approach.* Thorofare, NJ: SLACK Incorporated; 2002.)

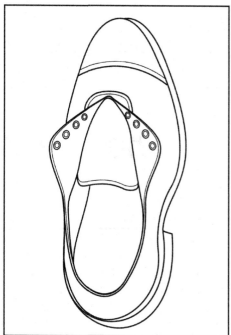

Figure 18-4. Bal closure. (Reprinted with permission from Edelstein JE, Bruckner J. *Orthotics: A Comprehensive Clinical Approach.* Thorofare, NJ: SLACK Incorporated; 2002.)

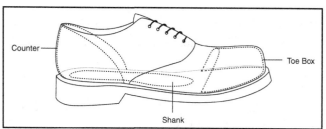

Figure 18-5. Reinforcements. (Reprinted with permission from Edelstein JE, Bruckner J. *Orthotics: A Comprehensive Clinical Approach.* Thorofare, NJ: SLACK Incorporated; 2002.)

protects the patient's toes. The toe box should be spacious enough to accommodate any toe deformities that may be present. If the shoe is to be riveted to a stirrup, as part of an ankle-foot orthosis, the shoe requires a steel shank piece located in the midportion of the shoe.

SHOE FIT

The shoe should be as wide as the widest part of the foot, usually at the metatarsophalangeal joints. A shoe that is too wide may allow the foot to slide, diminishing the patient's control of the shoe. A shoe that is too narrow will squeeze the foot and confine sole erosion to the longitudinal midline; sometimes, the narrow shoe will show abrasion of the medial and lateral portions of the upper.

Adequate length is also important for optimal foot function. The shoe should be approximately 0.5-inch

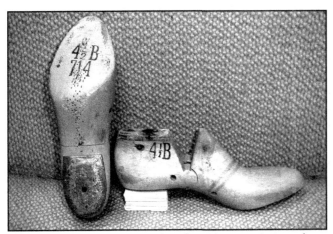

Figure 18-6. Lasts. (Reprinted with permission from Edelstein JE, Bruckner J. *Orthotics: A Comprehensive Clinical Approach*. Thorofare, NJ: SLACK Incorporated; 2002.)

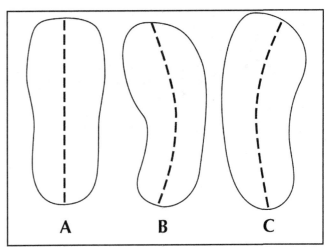

Figure 18-7. Flared lasts. (A) Straight last. (B) Inflared right last. (C) Outflared right last. (Reprinted with permission from Edelstein JE, Bruckner J. *Orthotics: A Comprehensive Clinical Approach*. Thorofare, NJ: SLACK Incorporated; 2002.)

(1 cm) longer than the longest toe. A shoe that is too long interferes with the propulsive phase of gait, whereas a shoe that is too short can bruise the toes. Wearing shoes that are too short is common among women in nursing homes and is associated with ulceration and foot pain.[6] The *last* determines the length, width, and volume within the shoe (Figure 18-6). Flared lasts are occasionally needed, particularly for children with congenital foot deformities (Figure 18-7).

SHOES FOR OLDER ADULTS

In addition to proper size, other considerations contribute to lessening the risk of falls among older people, particularly women. Balance and gait are best when subjects wear shoes with low heels, resilient soles, and secure fastening on the dorsum; and poorest when they wear firm-soled, slip-on shoes, slippers, or were barefoot.[7-14] High-heeled shoes also were associated with greater muscular activity when subjects walked.[15]

FOOT ORTHOSES

Conservative management of the foot and ankle, whether by inserts or shoe modifications, is used to improve gait in the treatment of patients with arthritis, diabetes, other neuropathies, trauma, and congenital deformities. Orthoses may be classified as accommodative (shock absorbing), semi-rigid (redistributes weight), or rigid (supportive).[16] They may be inside the shoe or on the outsole or heel. Evidence for the effectiveness of specific orthoses is based largely on subjective reports with little objective reliability or validity.[17]

Inserts and Internal Modifications

Presumably, the most popular foot orthoses are inserts worn inside the shoe. They are readily available at a modest price in drug stores and similar establishments. Modifications are orthoses, often custom made, that are attached to the shoe. Both internal modifications and inserts apply force close to the foot and are inconspicuous. Modifications ensure that if the patient wears the modified shoe, the intended shoe design and fit, as well as the modification, will be used. Because these orthoses occupy space within the shoe, they may convert a well-fitting shoe into one that is uncomfortable, especially distally. Inserts usually can be worn with several shoes made over the same last.

A *heel insert* or internal modification lies under the anatomic heel. Made of resilient material, such as neoprene, polyurethane, or silicone, the heel insert absorbs shock at the time of heel contact and may prevent the anatomic heel from sliding inside the shoe. Limited evidence suggests that prefabricated heel inserts are more effective in relieving heel pain than custom-made ones.[18]

The most common insert or internal modification is the three-quarter insert (Figure 18-8A) or modification, extending from the posterior margin of the shoe to the area beneath the proximal border of the metatarsal heads. If made of resilient material, it absorbs shock during midstance. If, however, the insert is made of firm material, such as polypropylene, nylon acrylic, or metal, it can be shaped to support the longitudinal arch, the transverse metatarsal arch, or both arches. The three-quarter insert is usually less expensive than other inserts and does not crowd the toes within the shoe.

A full-length insert or modification (Figure 18-8B) extends from the posterior margin of the shoe to the distal margin. It is unlikely to slide within the shoe, unlike the three-quarter insert. Total contact-resilient insoles reduce high heel and metatarsal head pressures, redistributing the pressure to the midfoot.[19] Effectiveness

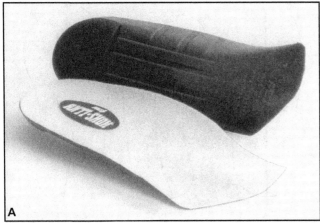
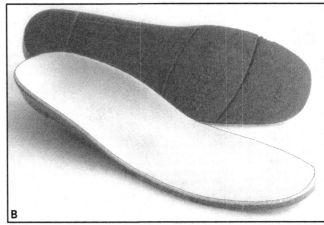

Figure 18-8. Inserts. (A) Three-quarter inserts. (B) Full-length inserts. (Reprinted with permission from Edelstein JE, Bruckner J. *Orthotics: A Comprehensive Clinical Approach.* Thorofare, NJ: SLACK Incorporated; 2002.)

of and compliance with custom-made inserts may be greater with mass-produced ones.[20-22] Others found that prefabricated orthoses were equally effective in the short term,[23] whereas long-term benefits were controversial.[22,24]

Longitudinal arch supports are a common example of a shoe insert. The University of California Biomechanics Laboratory insert is custom made to correct flexible pes valgoplanus (Figure 18-9).

A *metatarsal pad* is a convexity located under the fore-foot, between the first and fifth metatarsals, posterior to the metatarsal heads (Figure 18-10).[25] The pad transfers pressure from the sensitive metatarsophalangeal joints to the relatively insensitive metatarsal shafts.[26]

External Modifications

The orthotist or pedorthist may secure material to the plantar surface of the outsole or between the insole and the outsole, creating an external modification.

A *heel wedge*, also called a *post*, applies oblique force to the rear foot. A lateral heel wedge, usually 6 degrees,[27] shifts weight bearing medially and increases rear foot pronation. A medial wedge has the opposite effect. Objective evidence of their effects on proximal joints appears to be minimal,[28] although electromyographic studies of subjects wearing medial wedges demonstrated both increased tibialis anterior and peroneus longus activity, regardless of the height of the wedge.[29] Results of wearing heel wedges may relate more to their proprioceptive influence than to biomechanical effects.[30]

Other heel modifications include the beveled heel, the resilient heel, and the heel lift. The *beveled heel* has material removed from the posterior portion of the heel, whereas the *resilient heel* retains the posterior portion. Both heel designs facilitate the transition from heel contact to foot flat in the early part of stance phase, thereby reducing or eliminating the flexion floor reaction affecting the knee. A *heel lift* is a flat piece of material added to the heel.

Figure 18-9. University of California Biomechanics Laboratory insert.

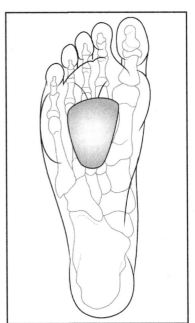

Figure 18-10. Metatarsal pad. (Reprinted with permission from Edelstein JE, Bruckner J. *Orthotics: A Comprehensive Clinical Approach.* Thorofare, NJ: SLACK Incorporated; 2002.)

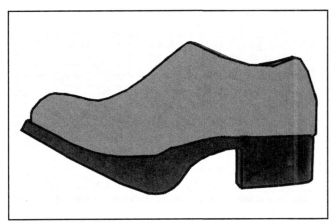

Figure 18-11. Rocker bar. (Reprinted with permission from Edelstein JE, Bruckner J. *Orthotics: A Comprehensive Clinical Approach*. Thorofare, NJ: SLACK Incorporated; 2002.)

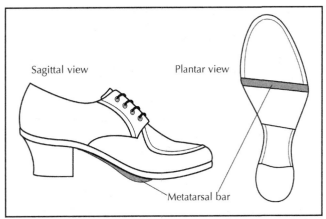

Figure 18-12. Metatarsal bar. (Reprinted with permission from Edelstein JE, Bruckner J. *Orthotics: A Comprehensive Clinical Approach*. Thorofare, NJ: SLACK Incorporated; 2002.)

The most common sole modifications are the rocker bar (Figure 18-11) and the metatarsal bar (Figure 18-12). The *rocker bar* is a convexity with the apex located posterior to the metatarsal heads. It reduces the distance on the sole that the patient must traverse during stance phase. Various designs of rocker bar are used, and all reduce forefoot pressure by shifting pressure posteriorly[31,32] and simulate forefoot hyperextension.[33]

The *metatarsal bar* is a flat piece of material secured on the sole in the area beneath the proximal borders of the metatarsal heads. It transfers stress from the metatarsophalangeal joints to the metatarsal shafts and reduces mediolateral forefoot motion. Both bars facilitate the wearer's transition through the late stance phase of gait.

The *sole lift* is flat material added to the sole and is usually used in combination with a heel lift.

REFERENCES

1. Perry SD, Radtke A, Goodwin CR. Influence of footwear midsole material hardness on dynamic balance control during unexpected gait termination. *Gait Posture.* 2007;25:94-98.

2. Hong WH, Lee YH, Chen HC, et al. Influence of heel height and shoe insert on comfort perception and biomechanical performance of young female adults during walking. *Foot Ankle Int.* 2005;26:1042-1048.

3. Yung-Hui L, Wei-Hsien H. Effects of shoe inserts and heel height on foot pressure, impact force, and perceived comfort during walking. *Appl Ergon.* 2005;36:355-362.

4. Wang YT, Pascoe DD, Kim CK, Xu D. Force patterns of heel strike and toe off on different heel heights in normal walking. *Foot Ankle Int.* 2001;22:486-492.

5. Hsue BJ, Su FC. Kinematics and kinetics of the lower extremities of young and older women during stair ascent while wearing low and high-heeled shoes. *J Electromyogr Kinesiol.* 2009;19:1071-1078.

6. Burns SL, Leese GP, McMurdo ME. Older people and ill fitting shoes. *Postgrad Med J.* 2002;78:344-346.

7. Menant JC, Steele JR, Menz HB, et al. Optimizing footwear for older people at risk of falls. *J Rehabil Res Dev.* 2008;45:1167-1181.

8. Menz HB, Morris ME, Lord SB. Footwear characteristics and risk of indoor and outdoor falls in older people. *Gerontology.* 2006;52:174-180.

9. Tencer AF, Koepsell TD, Wolf ME, et al. Biomechanical properties of shoes and risk of falls in older adults. *J Am Geriatr Soc.* 2004;52:1840-1846.

10. Sherrington C, Menz HB. An evaluation of footwear worn at the time of fall-related hip fracture. *Age Ageing.* 2003;32:192-203.

11. Arnadottir SA, Mercer VS. Effects of footwear on measurements of balance and gait in women between the ages of 65 and 93 years. *Phys Ther.* 2000;80:17-27.

12. Koepsell TD, Wolf ME, Buchner DM, et al. Footwear style and risk of falls in older adults. *J Am Geriatr Soc.* 2004;52:1495-1501.

13. Horgan NF, Crehan F, Bartlett E, et al. The effects of usual footwear on balance amongst elderly women attending a day hospital. *Age Ageing.* 2009;38:62-67.

14. Menant JC, Steele JR, Menz HB, et al. Effects of walking surfaces and footwear on temporo-spatial gait parameters in young and older people. *Gait Posture.* 2009;29:392-397.

15. Murley GS, Landorf KB, Menz HB, Bird AR. Effect of foot posture, foot orthoses, and footwear on lower limb muscle activity during walking and running: a systematic review. *Gait Posture.* 2009;29:172-187.

16. Janisse DJ, Janisse E. Shoe modification and the use of orthoses in the treatment of foot and ankle pathology. *J Am Acad Orthop Surg.* 2008;16:152-158.

17. Ball KA, Afheldt MJ. Evolution of foot orthotics—part 1: coherent theory or coherent practice? *J Manipulative Physiol Ther.* 2002;25:116-124.

18. Crawford F, Thomson C. Interventions for treatment plantar heel pain [serial on CD-ROM]. *Cochrane Database Syst Rev.* 2003;3:CD000416.

19. Chen WP, Ju CW, Tang FT. Effects of the total contact insoles on the plantar stress redistribution: a finite element analysis. *Clin Biomech.* 2003;18:17-24.

20. Trotter LC, Pierrynowski MR. Changes in gait economy between full-contact custom-made foot orthoses and prefabricated inserts in patients with musculoskeletal pain: a randomized clinical trial. *J Am Podiatr Med Assoc.* 2008;98:429-435.

21. Martin JE, Hosch JC, Goforth WP, et al. Mechanical treatment of plantar fasciitis: a prospective study. *J Am Podiatr Med Assoc.* 2001;91:55-62.

22. Landorf KB, Keenan AM, Herbert RD. Effectiveness of foot orthoses to treat plantar fasciitis: a randomized trial. *Arch Intern Med.* 2006;166:1305-1310.

23. Baldassin V, Gomes CR, Beraldo PS. Effectiveness of prefabricated and customized foot orthoses made from low-cost foam for noncomplicated plantar fasciitis: a randomized controlled trial. *Arch Phys Med Rehabil.* 2009;90: 701-706.

24. Roos E, Engström M, Söderberg B. Foot orthoses for the treatment of plantar fasciitis. *Foot Ankle Int.* 2006; 27:606-611.

25. Hsi WL, Kang JH, Lee XX. Optimum position of metatarsal pad in metatarsalgia for pressure relief. *Am J Phys Med Rehabil.* 2005;84:514-520.

26. Brodtkorb TH, Kogler GWE, Arndt A. The influence of metatarsal support height and longitudinal axis position on plantar foot load. *Clin Biomech (Bristol, Avon).* 2008;23:640-647.

27. Kakihana W, Torii S, Akai M, et al. Effect of a lateral wedge on joint moments during gait in subjects with recurrent ankle sprain. *Am J Phys Med Rehabil.* 2005;84:858-864.

28. Nester CJ, van der Linden ML, Bowker P. Effect of foot orthoses on the kinematics and kinetics of normal walking gait. *Gait Posture.* 2003;17:180-187.

29. Murley GS, Bird AR. The effect of three levels of foot orthotic wedging on the surface electromyographic activity of selected lower limb muscles during gait. *Clin Biomech (Bristol, Avon).* 2006;21:1074-1080.

30. Ball KA, Afheldt MJ. Evolution of foot orthotics—part 2: research reshapes long-standing theory. *J Manipulative Physiol Ther.* 2002;25:125-134.

31. Brown D, Wertsch JJ, Harris GF, et al. Effect of rocker soles on plantar pressures. *Arch Phys Med Rehabil.* 2004;85: 81-86.

32. van Schie C, Ulbrecht JS, Becker MB, Cavanagh PR. Design criteria for rigid rocker shoes. *Foot Ankle Int.* 2000;21:833-844.

33. Wu WL, Rosenbaum D, Su FC. The effects of rocker sole and SACH heel on kinematics in gait. *Med Eng Phys.* 2004;26:639-646.

Chapter 19

Ankle-Foot Orthoses

Ankle-foot orthoses (AFOs) are often prescribed for patients who require assistance to prevent toe drag during swing phase, with or without foot and ankle stabilization during stance phase. Most people who wear these orthoses are able to walk without them; however, gait may be clumsy and fatiguing. The basic components of AFOs are a foundation, ankle control, foot control, and superstructure. The shoe is always part of the lower-limb orthotic prescription.

FOUNDATION

The distal portion of the AFO is either a shoe *insert* or a steel component secured to the shoe. Contemporary AFOs usually have an insert (Figure 19-1) that fits inside the wearer's shoe. The insert is frequently made of plastic or carbon fiber, molded to a cast of the patient's foot. The shoe must fasten high on the dorsum of the foot, either with laces or straps, to secure the orthosis to the leg. Advantages of an insert foundation include an ease in donning because the shoe is not attached to the AFO; the possibility of incorporating a longitudinal arch support, metatarsal pad, and similar orthoses in the insert; a lighter weight; the opportunity to wear various shoes of the same heel height; and reduced conspicuousness of the orthosis. The few patients who are not candidates for an insert foundation are generally those who have used a steel attachment for many years or those who are not expected to wear appropriate shoes.

A *stirrup* is an alternate foundation (Figure 19-2). It is a steel "U"-shaped fixture with a central portion riveted to the midportion of the shoe through the shank piece; a steel shank is required. Stirrups ensure that if the orthosis is worn, it will be used with an appropriate shoe. Because the stirrup and the shank are steel, this foundation adds more weight to the orthosis than an insert foundation. The orthotic ankle joint must be aligned precisely with the anatomic ankle to avoid unwanted shifting of the proximal portion of the orthosis.

The solid stirrup is one piece (Figure 19-3). It provides maximum stability to the orthosis; however, donning takes more time and the patient is limited to wearing only the shoe having the stirrup.

A split stirrup consists of 3 pieces (Figure 19-4); namely, a central portion riveted to the shoe through the shank and 2 side pieces that fit into a channel in the central portion. The split stirrup facilitates donning because the uprights of the orthosis can be detached from the shoe. The patient may have several shoes fitted with the central portion to enable interchanging shoes for aesthetic and hygienic reasons. Disadvantages include greater weight and bulk than the solid stirrup and the risk that one or both side pieces may inadvertently dislodge, particularly if the wearer walks with marked torsional movements.

A few AFOs have a *caliper foundation*. It requires that the shoe heel have a transverse channel drilled into it, into which a steel cylindrical tube is fitted. Unilateral or bilateral side bars fit into the tube. The major advantage of the caliper is the ease of fitting the round side bar into the tube. A serious shortcoming is the distal displacement of the axis of ankle movement, which may cause the proximal portion of the AFO to slide on the leg and cause abrasion. As with the split stirrup, the caliper may subject the wearer to the possibility of having the side bar unintentionally slip out of the shoe attachment.

ANKLE (SAGITTAL PLANE) CONTROL

Most AFOs are prescribed for patients who have insufficient dorsiflexion control during swing phase. The resulting toe drag may cause the patient to trip. The simplest intervention is a pick-up strap from the anterior portion of the shoe to a cuff around the ankle. The strap prevents the foot from plantar flexing. It is conspicuous, and the cuff may chafe the posterior aspect of the leg.

Edelstein JE, Muroz A.
Lower-Limb Prosthetics and Orthotics: Clinical Concepts (pp 129-140).
© 2011 Taylor & Francis Group.

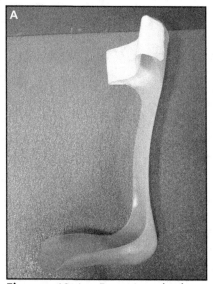
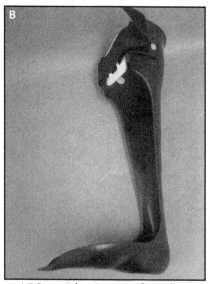
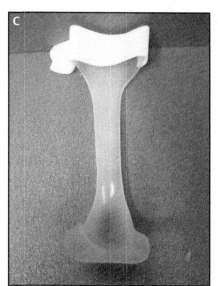

Figure 19-1. Posterior leaf spring AFO with insert foundation. (A) Lateral view, polypropylene. (B) Lateral view, carbon fiber. (C) Anterior view, polypropylene.

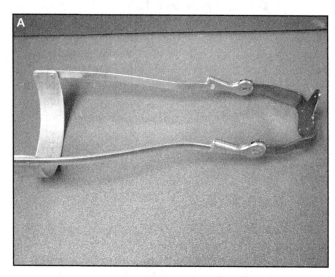

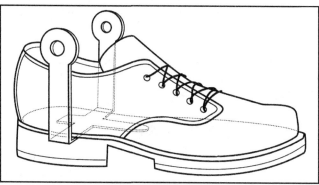

Figure 19-3. Solid stirrup. (Reprinted with permission from Edelstein JE, Bruckner J. *Orthotics: A Comprehensive Clinical Approach*. Thorofare, NJ: SLACK Incorporated; 2002.)

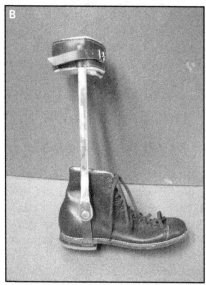

Figure 19-2. Stirrup. (A) Component. (B) Stirrup in AFO.

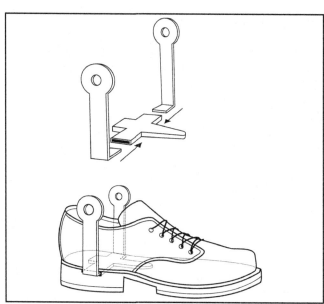

Figure 19-4. Split stirrup. (Reprinted with permission from Edelstein JE, Bruckner J. *Orthotics: A Comprehensive Clinical Approach*. Thorofare, NJ: SLACK Incorporated; 2002.)

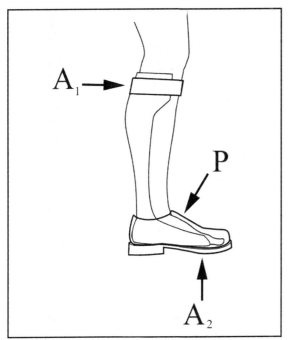

Figure 19-5. Three-point force system. A_1 and A_2: Anteriorly-directed force. P: Posteriorly directed force. (Reprinted with permission from Edelstein JE, Bruckner J. *Orthotics: A Comprehensive Clinical Approach*. Thorofare, NJ: SLACK Incorporated; 2002.)

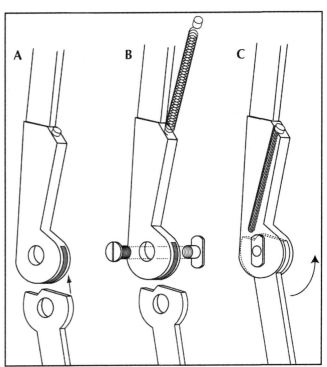

Figure 19-6. Dorsiflexion spring assist. (A) Stirrup fits into joint. (B) Screw secures stirrup to joint; spring over channel. (C) Spring within channel. (Reprinted with permission from Edelstein JE, Bruckner J. *Orthotics: A Comprehensive Clinical Approach*. Thorofare, NJ: SLACK Incorporated; 2002.)

The posterior leaf spring AFO is an insert orthosis made of semiflexible plastic, typically polypropylene, or carbon fiber (see Figure 19-1). The orthosis has a posterior upright that plantar flexes slightly during early stance and recoils during swing phase, keeping the foot in a neutral position. The upright may be a thin vertical strip or an "X"-shaped extension of the shoe insert. Flexibility of the orthosis can be increased by removing some material from the upright. The 3-point force system in this orthosis maintains ankle position (Figure 19-5). A disadvantage of this design is that once removed, material cannot be restored.

A dorsiflexion spring assist also prevents toe drag (Figure 19-6). This component is the proximal termination of a solid or split stirrup. It consists of a chamber that contains a coil spring. The chamber is the distal portion of an upright. The spring compresses during late stance as the wearer transfers weight forward and recoils during swing phase, thereby lifting the foot and shoe. The degree of spring compression can be adjusted by tightening or loosening a screw at the top of the chamber. Consequently, the amount of assistance can be modified repeatedly. The disadvantages of the dorsiflexion spring assist are that it is part of a stirrup and is rather bulky.

An alternative for patients who require swing phase control is a posterior stop (Figure 19-7). A posterior stop is a simple component that is usually a part of a stirrup or caliper foundation. It restricts plantar flexion in both

swing phase and stance phase. Consequently, the full length of the sole cannot contact the floor after heel contact unless the patient flexes the knee. The person also is unable to plantar flex during late stance to provide maximum propulsive force. The posterior stop joint does not restrict dorsiflexion.

A solid ankle (Figure 19-8) in a plastic AFO and a limited motion ankle (Figure 19-9) in an orthosis with a stirrup foundation restrict all foot and ankle motions. The bichannel adjustable ankle lock (BiCAAL; Kingsley, Costa Mesa, California; Becker Orthopedic, Troy, Michigan; Fillauer, Chattanooga, Tennessee) joint is a variation of the limited motion ankle (Figure 19-10). It consists of anterior and posterior spring-filled chambers, permitting adjustment of the ankle angle of the orthotic upright. These joints restrict motion at the foot and ankle in all planes. During early stance, the knee is normally subjected to a marked flexion moment of force; if the individual's knee extensor strength is adequate, then the knee will not collapse. In the presence of extensor paralysis, however, orthotic restraint of ankle dorsiflexion reduces the tendency of the knee to flex. Ankle control imposes difficulties when the wearer encounters stairs. The person should place the entire foot on the step rather than tip-toeing up and down. Similarly, squatting and other activities normally performed with marked dorsiflexion are compromised. Loosening the strap on the shell reduces the difficulty.

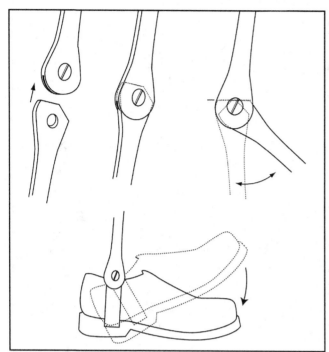

Figure 19-7. Plantar flexion stop. (Reprinted with permission from Edelstein JE, Bruckner J. *Orthotics: A Comprehensive Clinical Approach*. Thorofare, NJ: SLACK Incorporated; 2002.)

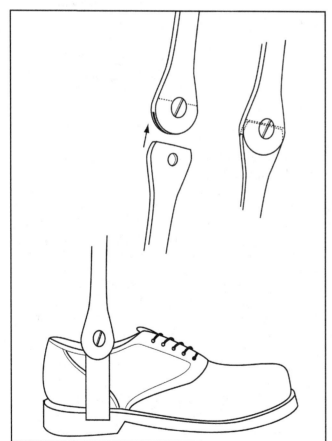

Figure 19-9. Limited motion stop. (Reprinted with permission from Edelstein JE, Bruckner J. *Orthotics: A Comprehensive Clinical Approach*. Thorofare, NJ: SLACK Incorporated; 2002.)

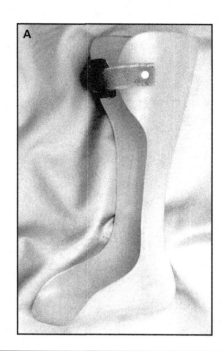

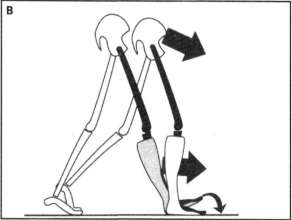

Figure 19-8. Solid ankle. (A) Orthosis. (B) Restricting plantar flexion, the orthosis transfers flexion force to the knee and hip. (Reprinted with permission from Perry J, Burnfield JM. *Gait Analysis: Normal and Pathological Function*. 2nd ed. Thorofare, NJ: SLACK Incorporated; 2010; Edelstein JE, Bruckner J. *Orthotics: A Comprehensive Clinical Approach*. Thorofare, NJ: SLACK Incorporated; 2002.)

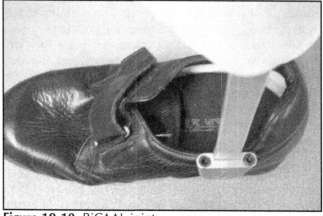

Figure 19-10. BiCAAL joint.

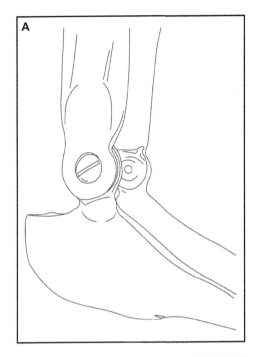

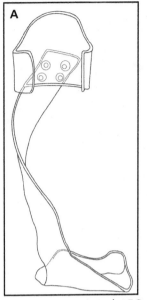

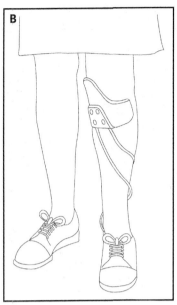

Figure 19-12. Spiral AFO.

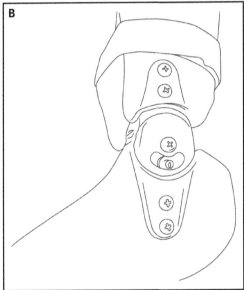

Figure 19-11. Hinged AFOs. (A) Basic hinge. (B) Adjustable excursion hinge.

The hinged ankle in a plastic AFO permits ankle motion (Figure 19-11). Many hinge designs are manufactured, some of which permit adjustment of ankle excursion. Hinged ankles which permit plantar flexion reduce the flexion stress on the knee and facilitate stair climbing and squatting. The drawback of a hinged ankle is evident in patients who need maximum motion control in the presence of pain or marked ankle instability.

FOOT (FRONTAL AND TRANSVERSE PLANE) CONTROL

Restricting all foot and ankle motions is most feasible with a plastic solid ankle AFO (Figure 19-8A). To assist the patient during early stance, the shoe worn with a solid ankle AFO should have a resilient heel; a rocker bar will assist late stance. A steel alternative is a limited motion ankle joint that blocks sagittal motion and tends to reduce frontal and transverse plane movement. A spiral AFO is a plastic or carbon fiber orthosis that includes a curved upright (Figure 19-12). The distal termination is at the medial side of the foot plate. The upright curves around the leg, ending at the proximomedial aspect of the leg. The springy upright reduces pes varus, assists propulsion in late stance, and resists plantar flexion in swing phase. A hemispiral AFO is similar; its distal termination is on the lateral side of the foot plate, and the orthosis is more rigid (Figure 19-13). A valgus correction strap can be added to the limited motion ankle joint; the strap is attached to the medial portion of the shoe upper near the sole and is buckled around the lateral upright (Figure 19-14). The strap applies a laterally directed force to the foot. Conversely, a varus correction strap attached to the lateral portion of the shoe and buckled around the medial upright applies a medially directed force to the shoe. Drawbacks of the straps include reliance on the wearer to select the appropriate snugness. A loose strap fails to apply the desired force and an overly tight strap is uncomfortable and may irritate the skin.

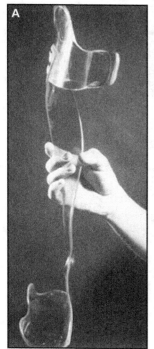
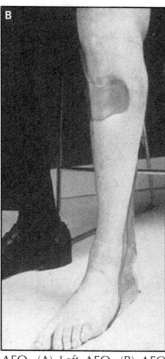

Figure 19-13. Hemispiral AFO. (A) Left AFO. (B) AFO on left leg. (Reprinted with permission from Edelstein JE, Bruckner J. *Orthotics: A Comprehensive Clinical Approach*. Thorofare, NJ: SLACK Incorporated; 2002.)

SUPERSTRUCTURE

The proximal portion of an AFO is the superstructure, consisting of a vertical and a horizontal component. The vertical portion of an AFO may be a plastic or carbon fiber single posterior upright; anterior shell (Figure 19-15); spiral upright; hemispiral or diagonal upright; or aluminum or steel bilateral uprights (Figure 19-16), lateral upright, or medial upright.

The posterior upright is relatively flexible, providing dorsiflexion assist during swing phase. An anterior upright or shell restricts dorsiflexion. A posterior shell encompasses the posterior half of the leg, providing a wide area on which to distribute force (Figure 19-17). Because the trim lines of the shell of the solid AFO extend slightly anterior to the malleoli, the shell limits all rearfoot, midfoot, and ankle motion. A flange may be added to the medial edge of the shell to exert a laterally directed force, thereby limiting pes valgus. A hinged shell is joined to the footplate by a pair of hinges. Many hinge designs are available, some of which permit adjusting the range of motion (see Figure 19-11B). The spiral and hemispiral also provide slight flexibility to the orthosis, particularly the spiral. Metal uprights, whether unilateral or bilateral, contribute to stability of the AFO.

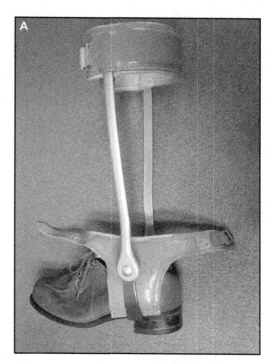

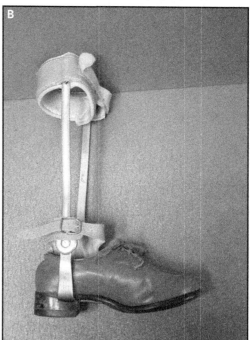

Figure 19-14. Valgus control strap on right AFO. (A) Medial view. (B) Lateral view.

Although a single upright is less conspicuous, weight reduction, compared with bilateral uprights, is negligible because the steel shoe attachment must be reinforced to avoid breakage.

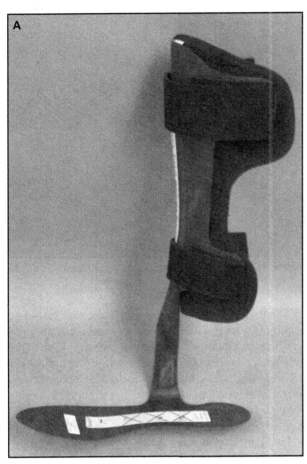
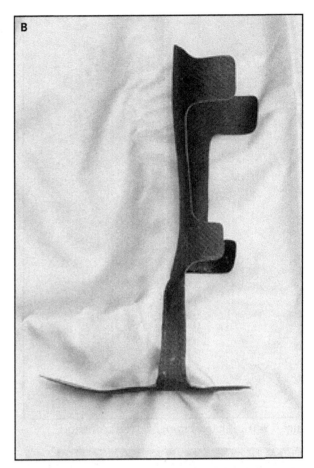
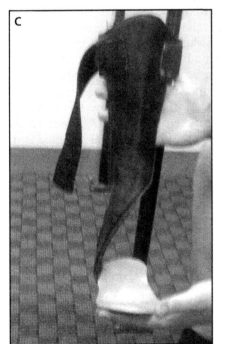
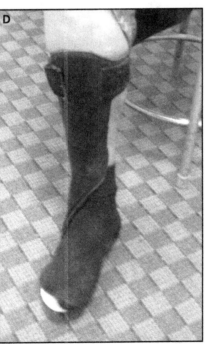
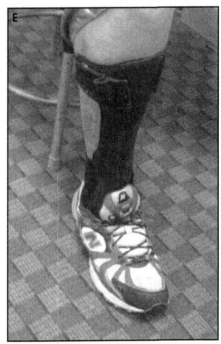

Figure 19-15. AFO with anterior upright. (A) Left AFO, medial view. (B) Left AFO, lateral view. (C) Right AFO, anterior view. (D) AFO on right leg. (E) AFO in shoe on right leg. (A and B Reprinted with permission from Edelstein JE, Bruckner J. *Orthotics: A Comprehensive Clinical Approach*. Thorofare, NJ: SLACK Incorporated; 2002.)

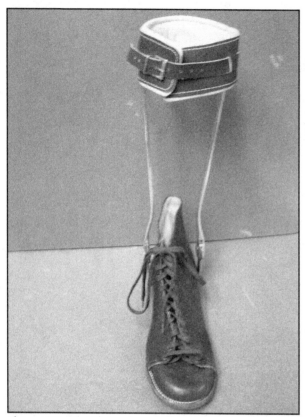

Figure 19-16. Bilateral uprights with calf band.

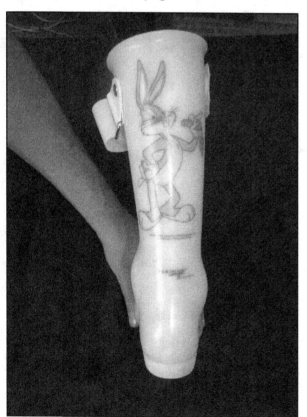

Figure 19-17. Solid ankle with cartoon.

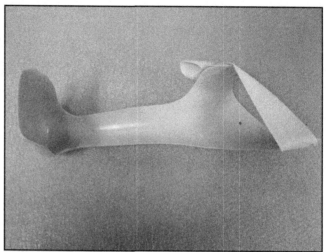

Figure 19-18. Posterior upright with proximal extension.

The trim line of the shell or upright may be extended proximally on the medial side to exert a laterally directed force at the knee to control genu valgum (Figure 19-18). In a similar fashion, extending the lateral side of the trim line will control genu varum. An orthosis that terminates immediately above the malleoli is known as a *supramalleolar orthosis* (Figure 19-19), ordinarily prescribed only for young children with foot instability.

Horizontal options for the AFO are a posterior calf band, anterior band (Figure 19-20), or weight-reducing brim (Figure 19-21). All options stabilize the upright(s). Most AFOs have a calf band, either rigid plastic or leather and felt-upholstered aluminum. The calf band applies an anteriorly directed force near the knee. An anterior band applies a posteriorly directed force, stabilizing the knee particularly in the presence of quadriceps weakness. A weight-reducing brim resembles the proximal portion of a transtibial prosthesis. Ordinarily, the brim is used with bilateral uprights and solid ankle, limited motion, or BiCAAL ankle to support some weight, reducing the weight-bearing load on the distal leg and foot. Because the patient's foot is on the floor, the brim does not eliminate distal weight bearing. A patten bottom prevents the foot from touching the floor, and thus the orthosis supports all weight proximally (Figure 19-22).

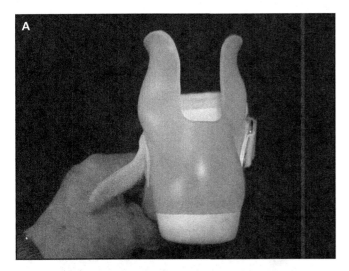

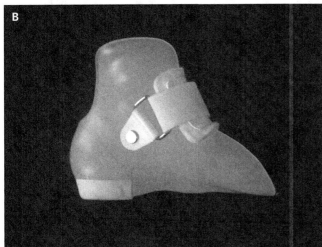

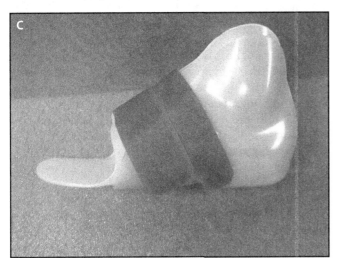

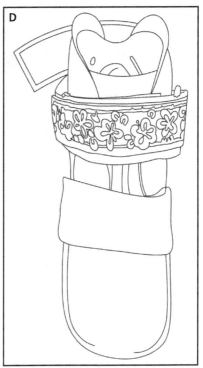

Figure 19-19. Supramalleolar AFO. (A) Posterior view. (B) Medial view. (C) Lateral view. (D) Anterior view.

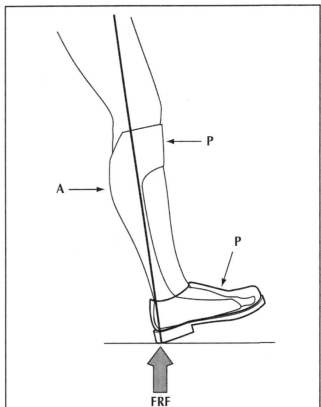

Figure 19-20. AFO with anterior band. A: Anteriorly directed force. P: Posteriorly directed force. FRF: Floor reaction force. (Reprinted with permission from Edelstein JE, Bruckner J. *Orthotics: A Comprehensive Clinical Approach.* Thorofare, NJ: SLACK Incorporated; 2002.)

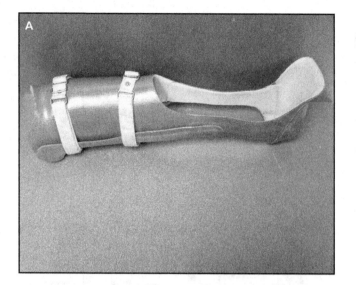

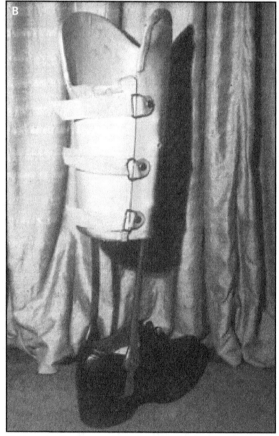

Figure 19-21. Weight-relieving brim. (A) Uprights covered with laminate. (B) Posterolateral view.

BIOMECHANICAL ANALYSES OF ANKLE-FOOT ORTHOSES

Objective evaluations of the forces generated by AFOs are relatively few. Force transducers can be installed in orthoses to determine the amount of load applied by the wearer. Optoelectronic gait analysis can be used to

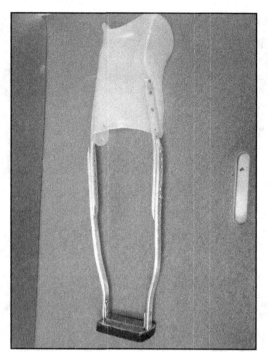

Figure 19-22. Weight-reducing AFO with patten bottom.

calculate the joint loading when subjects wore various brace designs.[1] Another approach involves a replicated human leg that continuously registers joint configuration and force exerted by the orthosis.[2] Mathematical analysis of forces between the AFO and the leg suggests that forces in the orthosis are greatest when the AFO compensates for plantar flexor insufficiency in late stance phase, and least when the orthosis supports the foot, in the absence of dorsiflexion power in swing phase.[3] Consequently, a lighter weight AFO will suffice to prevent foot drag. Several research teams have investigated the effect of various types of plastic, particularly polypropylene.[4,5] Material testing reveals that carbon fiber springs significantly increase energy return in late stance, compared with joints made from other materials.[6] Footwear also influences gait kinematics.[7]

Many AFOs are prescribed to control untoward motion or assist motion of the ankle and foot. Posterior leaf spring AFOs are popular for dorsiflexion assistance. The amount of assistance increases with greater height of the walls of the orthosis, more narrow width of the ankle joint area, and thinner plastic.[8] Although a narrow ankle width increases the flexibility of the orthosis, it also increases the risk of breakage in this area.[9]

The instantaneous center of rotation of these orthoses converges at the junction between the posterior upright and the shoe insert. The axis shifts posteriorly from the anatomical ankle axis, causing the proximal portion of the orthosis to shift up and down when the wearer walks.[10] AFOs with mechanical ankle joints also exhibit shifting, particularly if the axis of the orthotic joint is misaligned.[11] The movement of the AFO emphasizes the need for the patient to wear hose between the skin and the orthosis to avoid chafing.

Solid ankle AFOs are worn to stabilize the ankle and foot, particularly in the presence of global paralysis, instability, or pain. Several biomechanical studies of orthotic restraint confirm that resistance depends on how well the AFO conforms to the contour of the leg and foot and the properties of the material from which the orthosis is made.[12,13] Trimming the AFO around the malleoli to improve comfort may eventually cause failure of the orthosis.[14,15] Alternatively, removing material from the proximal portion of the shell may be indicated to reduce the weight of the orthosis and expose more of the skin for purposes of ventilation.[16]

Virtually all people who wear AFOs do so in order to walk more easily. A solid ankle AFO increases force in the Achilles tendon while reducing triceps surae activity[17] and reducing the ground reaction force.[18] Comparison of a solid ankle AFO and a posterior leaf spring AFO demonstrated that the rigid AFO disturbed velocity, step length, and step time, whereas the flexible AFO only affected stance phase, regardless of its stiffness.[19] A lateral sole wedge added to a solid ankle AFO reduced the frontal plane moment of force at the knee, whereas a medial wedge had the opposite effect.[20] Because walking involves more than traversing level surfaces, investigations of the effect of orthoses as subjects rise from chairs is relevant. Solid ankle AFOs restrain ankle dorsiflexion, thus compelling greater hip and trunk motion.[21] Stair ascent and descent are most disturbed by solid ankle AFOs, compared with orthoses with ankle hinges.[22]

SUMMARY

Although orthotic prescription should be influenced by the interaction of the biomechanical attributes of a given orthosis and the patient's clinical status, other considerations should be recognized to maximize the possibility that the patient will actually wear the orthosis. If the deficit is severe, a conspicuous orthosis is usually well accepted. Alternatively, if the orthosis is uncomfortable, interferes excessively with the patient's daily function, or is unattractive, the individual is more likely to reject it.[23]

REFERENCES

1. Johnson GR, Ferrarin M, Harrington M, et al. Performance specification for lower limb orthotic devices. *Clin Biomech (Bristol, Avon).* 2004;19:711-718.

2. Bregman DJ, Rozumalski A, Koops D, et al. A new method for evaluating ankle foot orthosis characteristics: BRUCE. *Gait Posture.* 2009;30:144-149.

3. McHugh B. Analysis of body-device interface forces in the sagittal plane for patients wearing ankle-foot orthoses. *Prosthet Orthot Int.* 1999;23:75-81.

4. Convery P, Greig RJ, Ross RS, Sockalingam S. A three centre study of the variability of ankle foot orthoses due to fabrication and grade of polypropylene. *Prosthet Orthot Int.* 2004;28:175-182.

5. Ross RS, Greig RJ, Convery P. Comparison of bending stiffness of six different colours of copolymer polypropylene. *Prosthet Orthot Int.* 1999;23:63-71.

6. Alimusaj M, Knie I, Wolf S, et al. Functional impact of carbon fiber springs in ankle-foot orthoses. *Orthopade.* 2007;36:752-756.

7. Churchill AJ, Halligan PW, Wade DT. Relative contribution of footwear to the efficacy of ankle-foot orthoses. *Clin Rehabil.* 2003;17:553-557.

8. Nagaya M. Shoehorn-type ankle-foot orthoses: prediction of flexibility. *Arch Phys Med Rehabil.* 1997;78:82-84.

9. Chu TM, Reddy NP. Stress distribution in the ankle-foot orthosis used to correct pathological gait. *J Rehabil Res Dev.* 1995;32:349-360.

10. Sumiya T, Suzuki Y, Kasahara T, Ogata H. Instantaneous centers of rotation in dorsi/plantar flexion movements of posterior-type plastic ankle-foot orthoses. *J Rehabil Res Dev.* 1997;34:279-285.

11. Fatone S, Hansen AH. A model to predict the effect of ankle joint misalignment on calf band movement in ankle-foot orthoses. *Prosthet Orthot Int.* 2007;31:76-87.

12. Raikin SM, Parks BG, Noll KH, Schon LC. Biomechanical evaluation of the ability of casts and braces to immobilize the ankle and hindfoot. *Foot Ankle Int.* 2001;22:214-219.

13. Kadakia AR, Espinosa N, Smerek J, et al. Radiographic comparison of sagittal plane stability between cast and boots. *Foot Ankle Int.* 2008;29:421-426.

14. Braund M, Kroontje D, Brooks J, et al. Analysis of stiffness reduction in varying curvature ankle foot orthoses. *Biomed Sci Instrum.* 2005;41:19-24.

15. Sumiya T, Suzuki Y, Kasahara T. Stiffness control in posterior-type plastic ankle-foot orthoses: effect of ankle trimline. Part 2: orthosis characteristics and orthosis/patient matching. *Prosthet Orthot Int.* 1996;20:132-137.

16. Nowak MD, Abu-Hasaballah KS, Cooper PS. Design enhancement of a solid ankle-foot orthosis: real-time contact pressures evaluation. *J Rehabil Res Dev.* 2000;37:273-281.

17. Fröberg A, Komi P, Ishikawa M, et al. Force in the Achilles tendon during walking with ankle foot orthosis. *Am J Sports Med.* 2009;37:1200-1207.

18. Kitaoka HB, Crevoisier XM, Harbst K, et al. The effect of custom-made braces for the ankle and hindfoot on ankle and foot kinematics and ground reaction forces. *Arch Phys Med Rehabil.* 2006;87:130-135.

19. Guillebastre B, Calmels P, Rougier P. Effects of rigid and dynamic ankle-foot orthoses on normal gait. *Foot Ankle Int.* 2009;30:51-56.

20. Schmalz T, Blumentritt S, Drewitz H, Fresilier M. The influence of sole wedges on frontal plane knee kinetics, in isolation and in combination with representative rigid and semi-rigid ankle-foot-orthoses. *Clin Biomech (Bristol, Avon).* 2006;21:631-639.

21. King LA, Van Sant AF. The effect of solid ankle-foot orthoses on movement patterns used in a supine-to-stand rising task. *Phys Ther.* 1995;75:952-964.

22. Radtka SA, Oliveira GB, Lindstrom KE, Borders MD. The kinematic and kinetic effects of solid, hinged, and no ankle-foot orthoses on stair locomotion in healthy adults. *Gait Posture.* 2006;24:211-218.

23. Basford JR, Johnson SJ. Form may be as important as function in orthotic acceptance: a case report. *Arch Phys Med Rehabil.* 2002;83:433-435.

Chapter 20

Knee-Ankle-Foot Orthoses

Knee-ankle-foot orthoses (KAFOs) are usually intended for people who have knee instability, particularly when the quadriceps muscle group is paralyzed. The patient risks knee collapse during early stance phase.

Compliance with wearing a KAFO is poorer than with an ankle-foot orthosis (AFO). KAFOs contact more of the skin, exposing the wearer to discomfort from heat retention and potential chafing. Compared with travel in a wheelchair, gait with KAFOs tends to be slower and more awkward. Cosmetic issues confound the likelihood of the patient's accepting the orthosis. Besides adding bulk to the limb, the knee hinges alter the drape of trousers or a skirt when the wearer sits and may fray the overlying fabric. Noise when the knee lock engages may be disconcerting. Donning a larger orthosis is more time consuming. Consequently, every effort should be made to achieve functional goals with an AFO or other means, if at all possible.

The basic components of a KAFO are a shoe, foundation, ankle and foot control, knee control, and superstructure.[1-3]

FOUNDATION

The KAFO has the same choice of foundations as the AFO; namely, an insert (Figure 20-1) or a riveted attachment, such as a stirrup (Figure 20-2).

ANKLE AND FOOT CONTROL

Many contemporary KAFOs include a solid ankle, which restricts all ankle, rearfoot and midfoot motion. If the orthosis has metal uprights, a bichannel adjustable ankle lock (BiCAAL; Kingsley, Costa Mesa, California; Becker Orthopedic, Troy, Michigan; Fillauer, Chattanooga, Tennessee), limited motion ankle joint, or a posterior stop may be included and a valgus or varus correction strap added. Most KAFOs have bilateral leg and thigh uprights for maximum orthotic stability.

KNEE SAGITTAL CONTROL

Basic knee control is provided by a pair of single-axis knee joints attached to bilateral leg uprights distally and bilateral thigh uprights proximally. Single-axis joints that are offset with the pivot posterior to the anatomic knee axis resist knee flexion when the wearer stands. Such offset joints do not restrict knee flexion during swing phase and when the individual sits. If the wearer ascends a ramp steep enough to displace the weightline posterior to the orthotic joint axis, then the knee will no longer be stable.

Knee stability is usually provided by some type of lock. The simplest is the *drop ring lock*. When the leg and thigh uprights are in straight alignment, a metal rectangular ring encircles portions of the uprights, preventing orthotic motion; the ring drops into the locked position. A spring-loaded retention button in the lock (Figure 20-3) prevents inadvertent knee flexion; the user must force the ring over the button in order to engage the lock. The retention button prevents inadvertent locking, which might otherwise occur when the patient prepares to sit. Both medial and lateral uprights should have locks for maximum orthotic stability. For the individual who has poor balance, a thigh-level release (Figure 20-4) may be added to the lock so that the person can operate the locks by pulling a lever at the upper thigh. The drop ring lock is contraindicated in the presence of knee flexion contracture.

An alternate knee lock is the *pawl lock*, which usually has a bail release (Figure 20-5). The pawl has a projecting tooth that lodges in a receptacle to lock the joint. A *bail* is a semicircular metal bar attached posteriorly to the medial and lateral pawl locks. The lock engages automatically, either by a coil spring within the locking mechanism or by an elastic webbing strap attached proximally to the bail and distally to the calf band. The wearer unlocks the pawl lock by either compressing the coil spring by means of a short lever or pulling

Edelstein JE, Muroz A.
Lower-Limb Prosthetics and Orthotics: Clinical Concepts (pp 141-148).
© 2011 Taylor & Francis Group.

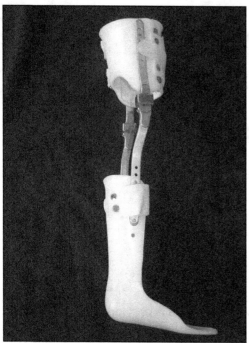

Figure 20-1. KAFO: solid ankle, bilateral drop ring locks.

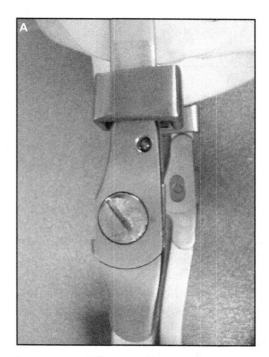

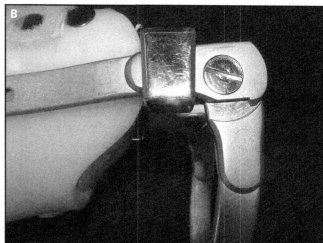

Figure 20-3. Drop ring lock with retention spring. (A) Extension. Note the spring-loaded button. (B) Flexion.

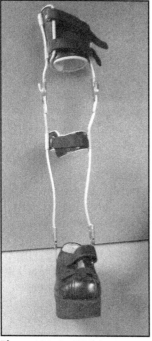

Figure 20-2. KAFO: Stirrup and bilateral drop ring locks.

upward on the bail. The bail is easier to manage, although it adds to the bulk of the braced leg. As with the drop ring lock, the pawl lock can only be worn by an individual who has full passive range of knee motion.

In the presence of knee flexion contracture, the KAFO must include a knee joint that accommodates the deformity. The *fan lock* has a hinge with several holes into which a screw is fitted; the hinge is adjusted to match the angle of the anatomic knee. A drop ring lock completes the assembly. A *serrated lock* is similar (Figure 20-6). Its hinge has a saw-toothed plate that can be placed in a mating ring to suit the angle of the patient's knee. As with the fan lock, a drop ring ensures knee stability. A ratchet lock is another option (Figure 20-7). The mechanism has a series of notches into which a pin can lodge, depending on the angle of the knee. When the pin is in place, the lock is secure, without the need for a drop ring. The ratchet lock also provides stability as the wearer moves from the seated to the standing position.

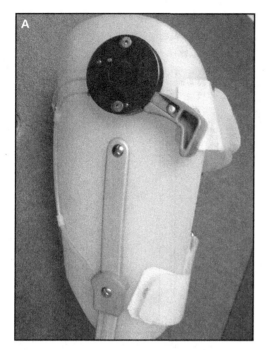

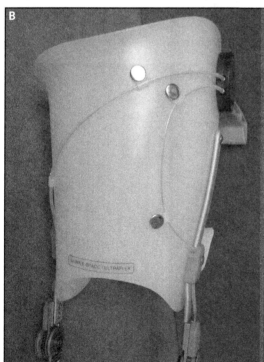

Figure 20-4. Thigh-level release. (A) Lateral view. (B) Posterior view.

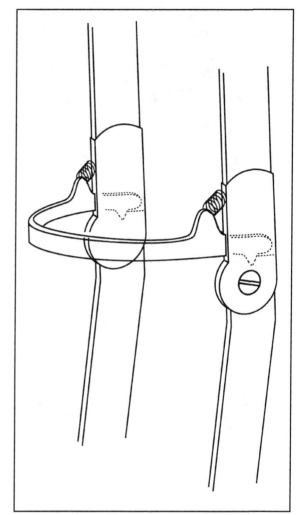

Figure 20-5. Pawl lock with bail release.

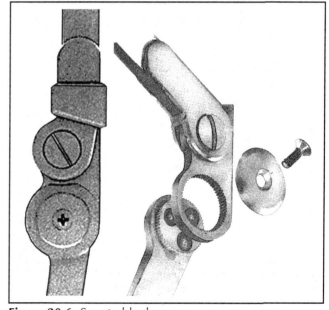

Figure 20-6. Serrated lock.

The KAFO for the patient with knee weakness usually requires a plastic suprapatellar (Figure 20-8) or pretibial band (Figure 20-9), or a leather patellar pad (Figure 20-10). The bands apply a posteriorly directed force above or below the anatomic knee, resisting any tendency toward knee flexion when the knee lock is engaged. The pad provides a posteriorly directed force on the patella. Although adjustable, the pad is much less

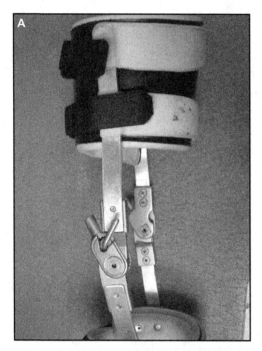

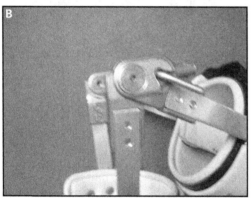

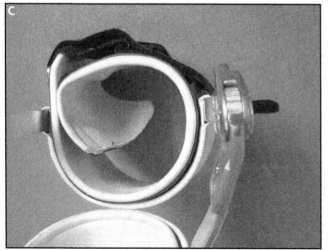

Figure 20-7. Ratchet lock. (A) Lateral view, lock engaged. (B) Lateral view, lock disengaged. (C) Superior view.

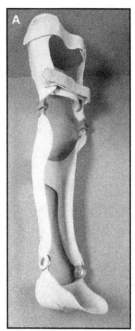
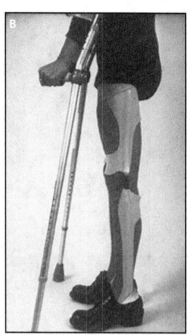

Figure 20-8. Suprapatellar band. (A) KAFO. (B) KAFO on a patient. (Reprinted with permission from Edelstein JE, Bruckner J. *Orthotics: A Comprehensive Clinical Approach*. Thorofare, NJ: SLACK Incorporated; 2002.)

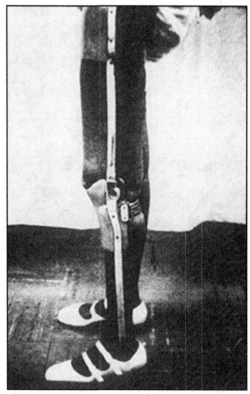

Figure 20-9. Pretibial band. (Reprinted with permission from Edelstein JE, Bruckner J. *Orthotics: A Comprehensive Clinical Approach*. Thorofare, NJ: SLACK Incorporated; 2002.)

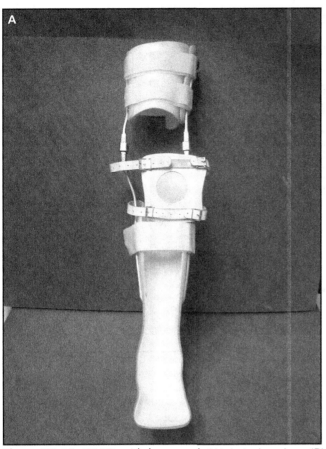
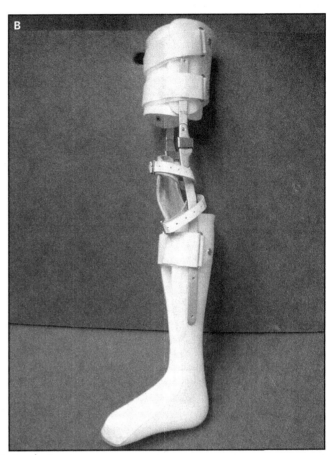

Figure 20-10. KAFO with knee pad. (A) Anterior view. (B) Lateral view.

convenient. It is secured to the orthosis with 4 straps: above and below the orthotic knee joint on the medial side and above and below the joint on the lateral side. Consequently, donning the orthosis takes additional time to buckle the straps. If the straps are snug enough to prevent knee flexion, then when the wearer wishes to sit, the medial (or lateral) straps must be loosened. They need to be tightened again when the patient stands.

The stance control KAFO provides knee stability during early stance yet allows the orthotic knee joint to flex during swing phase when the wearer is not bearing weight on the braced limb.[4-8] Most units are contraindicated in the presence of hip or knee flexion contracture or marked obesity. Stance control is achieved in several ways. The Free Walk (Otto Bock, Minneapolis, Minnesota; HealthCare, Plymouth, Minnesota) and the UTX (Becker Orthopedic, Troy, Michigan) have a single lateral tubular upright from the foot plate to the proximal thigh cuff. A control cable inside the upright connects the foot plate to the knee lock. The unit is unlocked by 10 degrees of dorsiflexion. In addition to the general contraindications, these mechanisms are contraindicated in the presence of ankle fusion. On the lateral upright, the Swing Phase Lock (Figure 20-11; Fillauer, Chattanooga, Tennessee) incorporates a pendulum-operated lock stabilizing the knee joint at heel contact; during late stance, the

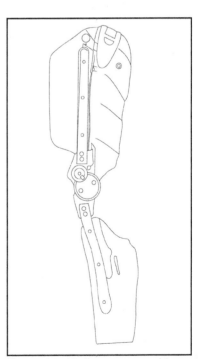

Figure 20-11. Stance control knee joint.

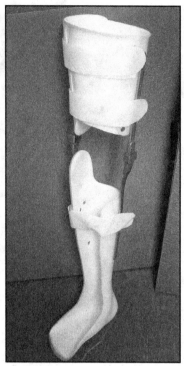

Figure 20-12. Calf shell lateral extension.

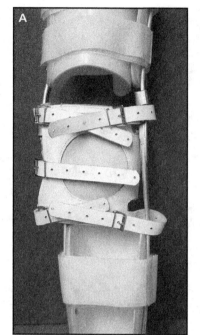

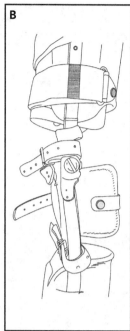

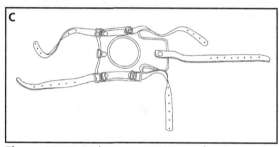

Figure 20-13. Valgus correction pad. (A) Anterior view. (B) Lateral view. (C) Valgus correction pad with medial extension.

pendulum swings forward, unlocking the unit. The medial upright has a friction-controlled unit regulating knee flexion during swing phase. The wearer can select manual lock, manual unlock, or automatic locking mode. Besides those noted above, the unit is also contraindicated if the patient has hip flexor paralysis or knee deformity. The Load Response Knee Joint (Becker) has a spiral spring in the knee joint; the unit allows slight knee flexion during early stance, providing shock absorption. FullStride (Becker) automatically unlocks during swing phase and can be worn by the patient who has genu varum or valgum; the individual must have slight passive ankle dorsiflexion. SafetyStride (Becker) provides mechanical locking, regardless of knee angle, and is designed for the patient who does not have full passive knee extension. As with FullStride, ankle dorsiflexion excursion is needed. A pneumatic spring unit can be added to aid knee extension. UltraSafeStep (Ultraflex Systems, Downingtown, Pennsylvania) provides stance control through 30 degrees of knee flexion for stability and shock absorption, swing phase assist, and a cam lock for positive stabilization. It also has a ratchet to stabilize the knee as the wearer rises from a chair.

Electronic control involving a sensor that detects the position of the leg during the gait cycle is a more sophisticated option. E-MAG Active (Otto Bock) operates independently of the ankle. In contrast, the E-Knee KAFO (Becker) has a foot sensor in the foot plate that determines whether the wearer is bearing weight; if so, the knee joint locks in any degree of flexion. The patient does not need active muscle contraction at the hip, knee, or ankle, although marked genu valgum and varum are contraindications. The Rehab E-Knee (Becker) is an adjustable KAFO intended to enable the clinician to assess the patient's suitability for a stance control joint.

A survey of wearers of stance control knee orthoses resulted in positive responses, although weight, appearance, and ease of donning and doffing were complaints.[7]

KNEE FRONTAL CONTROL

All orthotic knee joints restrict mediolateral motion of the anatomic knee to some extent. The patient with genu valgum may benefit from a KAFO with a plastic calf band extending proximally on the medial side (Figure 20-12). Genu varum is addressed with a laterally extended calf band. The plastic extensions are not adjustable by the patient.

Several alternatives in contemporary practice present difficulties. A patellar pad with 5 straps has the fifth strap attached to an extension of the pad (Figure 20-13).

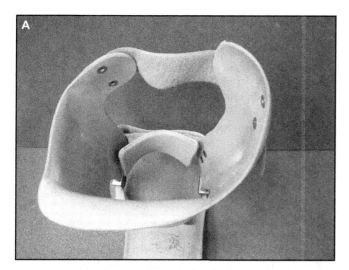

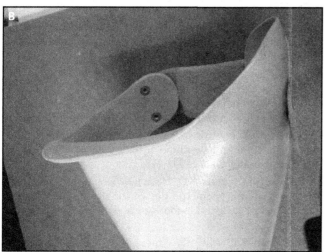

Figure 20-14. Ischial bearing brim. (A) Superior view. (B) Posterolateral view.

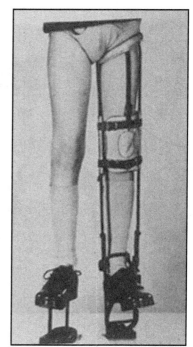

Figure 20-15. Weight-relieving knee-ankle-foot orthosis (KAFO), ischial ring, knee locks, patten bottom, contralateral lift. (Reprinted with permission from Edelstein JE, Bruckner J. *Orthotics: A Comprehensive Clinical Approach.* Thorofare, NJ: SLACK Incorporated; 2002.)

For genu valgum, the pad extension is medial, with the fifth strap buckled around the lateral upright. The strap tends to impinge uncomfortably in the popliteal fossa. In place of the 5-strap knee pad, the KAFO may have a circular padded disc; for genu valgum, the pad is located on the medial upright in the vicinity of the orthotic knee joint. The disc avoids popliteal impingement but offers relatively little area for force distribution. A spreader bar is a metal bar between medial uprights of bilateral KAFOs. It prevents frontal movement.

SUPERSTRUCTURE

The KAFO is completed with bilateral or unilateral thigh uprights and 1 or 2 thigh bands. The proximal thigh band may provide an ischial-bearing brim (Figure 20-14) if the orthosis is intended to reduce or eliminate weight from the braced limb. The brim has a horizontal shelf under the ischial tuberosity.

Full weight relief is achieved with a KAFO that has, in addition to a weight-bearing brim or ischial ring, a locked knee joint and a patten bottom (Figure 20-15), which ensures that the foot on the braced side cannot touch the floor. Bilateral uprights terminate distally in the patten bottom. The uprights have a ring on each side to which the shoe is attached, so that the shod foot dangles beneath the orthosis. The contralateral shoe requires a lift to maintain a level pelvis.

Linking the proximal ends of the medial uprights of a pair of KAFOs (Figure 20-16) may enable some patients with low thoracic or lumbar paraplegia to ambulate more easily than they might with more cumbersome orthoses.[9,10] A recent alternative involves linking both ankle joints and hinging the proximomedial uprights. The orthosis allows users to keep both feet always parallel to the floor while walking and assists leg swinging.[11]

BIOMECHANICAL ANALYSES OF KNEE-ANKLE-FOOT ORTHOSES

As with all orthoses, few objective investigations have been published. Installing force transducers in the orthosis is more costly than utilizing kinematic and kinetic data obtained in a gait laboratory.[12,13] One

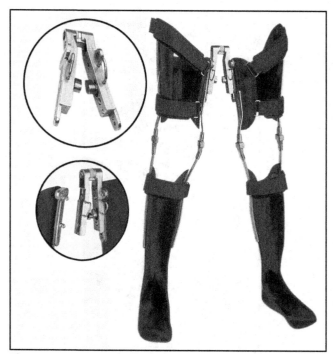

Figure 20-16. Medially linked KAFOs. (Reprinted with permission from Cascade Prosthetics & Orthotics.)

avenue of analysis that may yield immediate benefit is a technique for standardizing the sizes of orthoses to facilitate mass production of the plastic portions of the orthosis.[14] Forces applied by KAFOs to the wearer and forces within the orthosis are influenced by the materials used in orthotic fabrication and the designs of the devices.[15,16]

Studies of subjects walking with KAFOs focus on stance control knee orthoses.[17-20] Limited samples demonstrated improved gait kinematics. Gait analysis of medially linked KAFOs demonstrated their efficacy with a small group of research subjects.[21]

REFERENCES

1. American Academy of Orthotists and Prosthetists. Findings of a state of the science conference on knee-ankle-foot orthoses for ambulation. *J Prosthet Orthot.* 2006;18:137-208.

2. Fatone S. A review of the literature pertaining to KAFOs and HKAFOs for ambulation. *Proc Amer Acad Orthot Prosthet.* 2006;7:P137-P168.

3. Merritt JL, Yoshida K. Knee-ankle-foot orthoses: indications and practical applications of long leg braces. *Phys Med Rehabil.* 2000;14:395-420.

4. Yakimovich T, Lemaire ED, Kofman J. Engineering design review of stance-control knee-ankle-foot orthoses. *J Rehabil Res Dev.* 2009;46:257-267.

5. Zissimopoulos A, Fatone S, Gard SA. Biomechanical and energetic effects of a stance-control orthotic knee joint. *J Rehabil Res Dev.* 2007;44:503-513.

6. McMillan AG, Kendrick K, Michael JW, et al. Preliminary evidence for effectiveness of a stance control orthosis. *J Prosthet Orthot.* 2004;16:6-13.

7. Suga T, Kameyama O, Ogawa R, et al. Newly designed computer controlled knee-ankle-foot orthosis (Intelligent Orthosis). *Prosthet Orthot Int.* 1998;22:230-239.

8. Bernhardt KA, Irby SE, Kaufman KR. Consumer opinions of a stance control knee orthosis. *Prosthet Orthot Int.* 2006;30:246-256.

9. Middleton JW, Sinclair PJ, Smith RM, Davis GM. Postural control during stance in paraplegia: effects of medially linked versus unlinked knee-ankle-foot orthoses. *Arch Phys Med Rehabil.* 1999;80:1558-1565.

10. Abe K. Comparison of static balance, walking velocity, and energy consumption with knee-ankle-foot orthosis, Walkabout orthosis, and reciprocating gait orthosis in thoracic-level paraplegic patients. *J Prosthet Orthot.* 2006;18:87-91.

11. Genda E, Oota K, Suzuki Y, et al. A new walking orthosis for paraplegics: hip and ankle linkage system. *Prosthet Orthot Int.* 2004;28:69-74.

12. Andrysek J, Redekop S, Matsui MC, et al. A method to measure the accuracy of loads in knee-ankle-foot orthoses using conventional gait analysis, applied to persons with poliomyelitis. *Arch Phys Med Rehabil.* 2008;89:1372-1379.

13. Johnson GR, Ferrarin M, Harrington M, et al. Performance specification for lower limb orthotic devices. *Clin Biomech (Bristol, Avon).* 2004;19:711-718.

14. Dwivedi M, Shetty KD, Nath LN. Design and development of anthropometric device for the standardization of sizes of knee-ankle-foot orthoses. *J Med Eng Technol.* 2009;33:87-94.

15. Kaufman KR, Irby SE. Ambulatory KAFOs: a biomechanical engineering perspective. *Proc Amer Acad Orthot Prosthet.* 2006;7:P175-P182.

16. Michael JW. KAFOs for ambulation: an orthotist's perspective. *Proc Amer Acad Orthot Prosthet.* 2006;7:P187-P191.

17. Hwang S, Kang S, Cho K, Kim Y. Biomechanical effect of electromechanical knee-ankle-foot-orthosis on knee joint control in patients with poliomyelitis. *Med Biol Eng Comput.* 2008;46:541-549.

18. Moreno JC, Brunetti F, Rocon E, Pons JL. Immediate effects of a controllable knee ankle foot orthosis for functional compensation of gait in patients with proximal leg weakness. *Med Biol Eng Comput.* 2008;46:43-53.

19. Yakimovich T, Lemaire ED, Kofman J. Preliminary kinematic evaluation of a new stance-control knee-ankle foot orthosis. *Clin Biomech (Bristol, Avon).* 2006;21:1081-1089.

20. Hebert JS, Liggins AB. Gait evaluation of an automatic stance-control knee orthosis in a patient with postpoliomyelitis. *Arch Phys Med Rehabil.* 2005;86:1676-1680.

21. Suzuki T, Sonoda S, Saitoh E, et al. Prediction of gait outcome with the knee-ankle-foot orthosis with medial hip joint in patients with spinal cord injuries: a study using recursive partitioning analysis. *Spinal Cord.* 2007;45:57-63.

Chapter 21

Hip-Knee-Ankle-Foot and Higher Orthoses

The knee-ankle-foot orthosis (KAFO) can be augmented to increase control of the hips and trunk.

HIP CONTROL

The addition of a pelvic band with unilateral or bilateral hip joints converts the KAFO to a hip-knee-ankle-foot orthosis (HKAFO; Figures 21-1 and 21-2). The usual band is a bilateral pelvic band that covers the posterior half of the lower torso and is attached to each lateral upright of the KAFO by means of a hip joint. Rarely is a unilateral pelvic band appropriate because the single orthosis tends to rotate on the lower limb. If the patient requires a single orthosis, a more stable alternative is a double pelvic band, also known as a *Hessing band,* which is anchored on the pelvis by 2 horizontal bands.

The single-axis hip joint, in combination with the pelvic band, restricts frontal and transverse hip motion. The hip joint may include a drop ring lock to restrict motion in all directions (Figure 21-3). The 2-position hip joint permits locking the hips in flexion to aid in sitting, or neutral position for standing stability. Usually, the orthotic knee joints are locked. Less commonly prescribed is an abduction hip joint, which allows abduction but restricts adduction. A steel abduction bar attaches to the medial uprights of an HKAFO to prevent the orthoses from adducting.

Alternatives to a rigid pelvic band and hip joints are rotation control straps attached to a pair of KAFOs. To control internal rotation, a pair of straps is used (Figure 21-4). The patient wears a webbing waist belt. In the back of the belt, the straps are riveted. Each strap extends from the midposterior belt to the lateral upright of the KAFO. To control external rotation, a single strap suffices (Figure 21-5). The strap is attached to 1 lateral upright, passes anterior at the level of the groin, and is secured to the other lateral upright. Unlike a rigid band

and hip joints, the webbing strap(s) can be removed for laundering and offer much less interference during toileting.

HIP AND TRUNK CONTROL

The individual who requires more orthotic control may be fitted with a trunk-hip-knee-ankle-foot orthosis (THKAFO), which consists of an HKAFO surmounted by a lumbosacral orthosis (Figure 21-6). The trunk orthosis may include a pair of lateral uprights, a pair of posterior uprights, a thoracic band in the back, and a fabric abdominal front. The pelvic band of the THKAFO serves as the inferior termination of the trunk orthosis. Alternatively, the trunk orthosis may be a semirigid plastic jacket to which lateral upright(s) are attached. The orthosis enables the patient with trunk and leg paralysis to stand. Nevertheless, THKAFOs are very restrictive, particularly if the orthotic hip joints are locked. The orthosis is heavy, bulky, and difficult to don.

Alternative orthoses include various standing frames (Figure 21-7), the parapodium, and several designs of reciprocating gait orthoses[1-4] (Figure 21-8). *Standing frames* and *parapodia* are mass produced for children. They incorporate a base, a means of attaching to the wearer's shoes, bilateral uprights to which chest and knee pads are attached in the front, and a posterior dorsolumbar pad. The standing frame has no orthotic joints; consequently, as the child grows, the same frame will fit for several years. The swivel walker has foot plates which swivel a few degrees as the wearer shifts weight. The parapodium is a more complex version of the standing frame. It has hip and knee joints that the child can cause to flex or extend by rotating each lateral upright. Both the standing frame and the parapodium must be worn over trousers.

Edelstein JE, Muroz A.
Lower-Limb Prosthetics and Orthotics: Clinical Concepts (pp 149-154).
© 2011 Taylor & Francis Group.

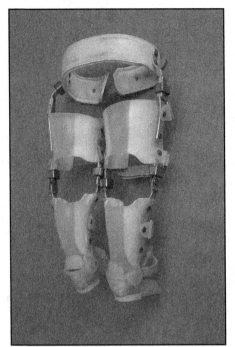

Figure 21-1. Plastic-metal HKAFOs.

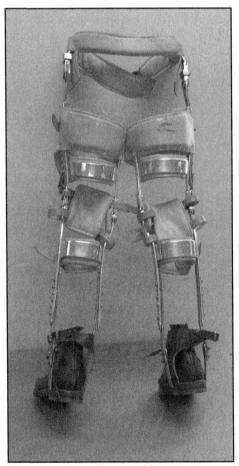

Figure 21-2. Leather-metal HKAFOs.

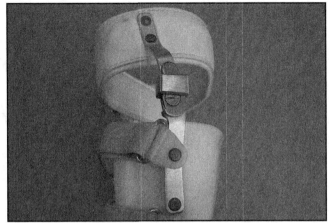

Figure 21-3. Hip drop ring lock.

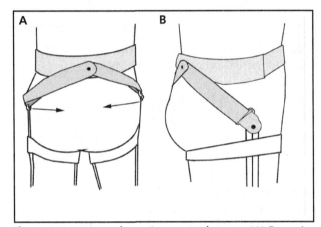

Figure 21-4. Internal rotation control straps. (A) Posterior view. (B) Lateral view. (Reprinted with permission from Edelstein JE, Bruckner J. *Orthotics: A Comprehensive Clinical Approach.* Thorofare, NJ: SLACK Incorporated; 2002.)

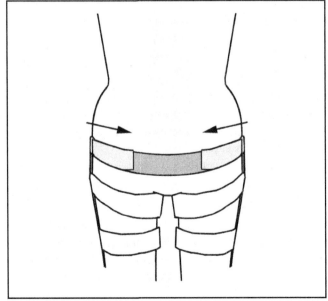

Figure 21-5. External rotation control strap, anterior view. (Reprinted with permission from Edelstein JE, Bruckner J. *Orthotics: A Comprehensive Clinical Approach.* Thorofare, NJ: SLACK Incorporated; 2002.)

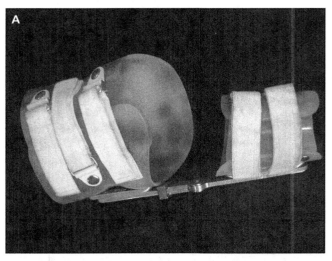

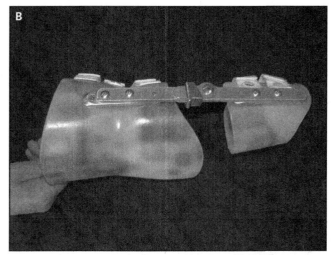

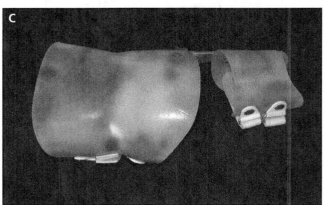

Figure 21-6. THKAFO with drop ring lock. (A) Anterior view. (B) Posterior view. (C) Lateral view.

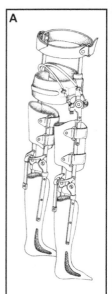

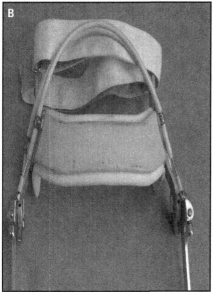

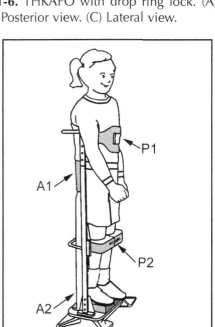

Figure 21-7. Swivel walker. A1 and A2: Anteriorly directed forces. P1 and P2: Posteriorly directed forces. (Reprinted with permission from Edelstein JE, Bruckner J. *Orthotics: A Comprehensive Clinical Approach*. Thorofare, NJ: SLACK Incorporated; 2002.)

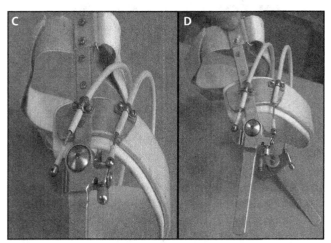

Figure 21-8. Reciprocating gait orthosis. (A) Posterolateral view. (Reprinted with permission from Fillauer, Inc.) (B) Posterior view. (C) Lateral view, hip extended. (D) Lateral view, left hip flexed, right hip extended.

Reciprocating gait orthoses are composed of a pair of KAFOs with solid ankles and locked knees. The KAFOs are surmounted by a reciprocating gait mechanism that links the lateral uprights of the 2 orthoses. The original version of the mechanism has 2 steel cables. Newer versions feature a single cable or a linkage system. When the wearer advances the right leg, the left leg is stabilized by tension in the cable or the link. Because the hips are not locked, the individual can perform a 2- or 4-point reciprocal gait with the aid of crutches or a walker. The gait sequence is as follows:

1. *Shift*: Shift weight onto the stance leg by upper trunk lateral motion.
2. *Tuck*: Extend the neck and upper trunk to stabilize the hips.
3. *Push*: Exert downward force through the hands on the crutches or walker to raise the body off the floor.
4. *Kick*: Leaning posteriorly causes the braced leg to swing forward.
5. *Repeat*: Repeat using the opposite leg.

Slow, laborious gait with heavy loading of the upper limbs[5] accounts for the high level of rejection of the reciprocating gait orthosis.[6]

The ParaWalker, also known as the Hip Guidance Orthosis (Orthotic Reseach and Locomotor Assessment Unit, The Robert Jones and Agnes Hunt Orthopaedic Hospital, Oswestry, England; Figure 21-9), is a similar device. Rather than linking the 2 KAFOs, the ParaWalker is an HKAFO with a rigid pelvic band. The orthotic hip joints provide limited flexion and extension. The gait sequence is similar to that described for the reciprocating gait orthosis.

BIOMECHANICAL ANALYSES OF HIP-KNEE-ANKLE-FOOT ORTHOSES AND TRUNK-HIP-KNEE-ANKLE-FOOT ORTHOSES

Gait analyses of patients wearing reciprocating gait orthoses confirm their slow, awkward performance.[7,8] Design modification may improve the wearer's function. Among the suggested improvements are changing the hip joints from single axis to multiple axis to allow rotational movement. Allowing internal and external rotation should increase stride length and improve the durability of the orthosis.[9] Reducing the stiffness of the hip joints may reduce the patient's dependence on compensatory rotation of the upper trunk and shoulder girdle.[10]

Comparing the reciprocating gait orthoses with medially linked KAFOs indicates that adults with low thoracic paraplegia wearing the latter were able to rise and sit faster, whereas the reciprocating gait orthoses facilitated faster gait on level and sloped surfaces.[11]

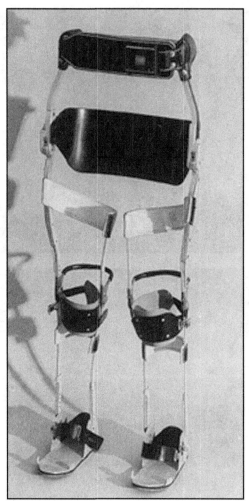

Figure 21-9. ParaWalker. (Reproduced from Jefferson RJ, Whittle MW. Performance of three walking orthoses: a case study using gait analysis. *Prosthet Orthot Int.* 1990;14:104 with permission from Informa Medical and Pharmaceutical Science–Journals.)

REFERENCES

1. Campbell JH. Linked hip-knee-ankle-foot orthoses designed for reciprocal gait. *Proc Amer Acad Orthot Prosthet.* 2006;7:P204-P208.
2. Baardman G, IJzerman MJ, Hermens HJ, et al. The influence of the reciprocal hip joint link in the Advanced Reciprocating Gait Orthosis on standing performance in paraplegia. *Prosthet Orthot Int.* 1997;21:210-221.
3. IJzerman MJ, Baardman G, Hermens HJ, et al. The influence of the reciprocal cable linkage in the advanced reciprocating gait orthosis on paraplegic gait performance. *Prosthet Orthot Int.* 1997;21:52-61.
4. Phillips DL, Field RE, Broughton NS, Menelaus MB. Reciprocating orthoses for children with myelomeningocele: a comparison of two types. *J Bone Joint Surg Br.* 1995;77:110-113.

5. Johnson WB, Fatone S, Gard SA. Walking mechanics of persons who use reciprocating gait orthoses. *J Rehabil Res Dev.* 2009;46:435-446.

6. Sykes L, Edwards J, Powell ES, Ross ER. The reciprocating gait orthosis: long-term usage patterns. *Arch Phys Med Rehabil.* 1995;76:779-783.

7. Dall PM, Muller B, Stallard I, et al. The functional use of the reciprocal hip mechanism during gait for paraplegic patients walking in the Louisiana State University reciprocating gait orthosis. *Prosthet Orthot Int.* 1999;23: 152-162.

8. Tashman S, Zajac FE, Perkash I. Modeling and simulation of paraplegic ambulation in a reciprocating gait orthosis. *J Biomech Eng.* 1995;117:300-308.

9. Mazur JM, Sienko-Thomas S, Wright N, Cummings RJ. Swing-through vs. reciprocating gait patterns in patients with thoracic-level spina bifida. *Z Kinderchir.* 1990;45(suppl 1):23-25.

10. van der Spek JH, Veltink PH, Hermens HJ, et al. Static and dynamic evaluation of the influence of supplementary hip-joint stiffness on crutch-supported paraplegic stance. *IEEE Trans Neural Syst Rehabil Eng.* 2003;11: 452-462.

11. Harvey LA, Smith MB, Davis GM, Engel S. Functional outcomes attained by T9-12 paraplegic patients with the Walkabout and the isocentric reciprocal gait orthoses. *Arch Phys Med Rehabil.* 1997;78:706-711.

Chapter 22

Orthotic Static Evaluation

The orthotic evaluation procedure is similar to that described for transtibial and transfemoral prosthetic evaluation. Prior to gait training, the patient and the orthosis should be assessed at the initial evaluation. The clinical team will determine whether the orthosis should be granted a *pass, provisional pass* (indicating minor problems), or *fail* (indicating major problems that would interfere with training). At the time of discharge, the clinical team should repeat the evaluation. The outcome of the final evaluation is either pass or fail.

To expedite the evaluation, the clinician should have a checklist listing the following questions, as well as an unupholstered chair and secure environment (eg, parallel bars) for the patient. A ribbon is needed if the orthosis has a weight-relieving component.

ORTHOSIS OFF OF THE PATIENT

Check the patient's skin, noting any blemishes and other abnormalities. If possible, ask the patient to wear shoes and walk without the orthosis. Observe any gait abnormalities.

1. Is the orthosis as prescribed? Verify that the shoe, foundation, ankle control, foot control, and superstructure of the ankle-foot orthosis (AFO), the knee unit, and superstructure of the knee-ankle-foot orthosis (KAFO) are the same as in the prescription. Very occasionally, the clinical team determines that the patient would benefit from different component(s); if the change(s) are reflected in an amended prescription, then the orthosis is satisfactory. If not, the orthosis must include the prescribed components. In a child's orthosis, is there adequate provision for lengthening the orthosis?

➤ Observe the patient walking without the orthosis. Note any abnormalities and any complaints of pain or instability.

2. Can the patient don the orthosis easily with little or no assistance? Although the patient has not been trained to don the orthosis, the individual should be able to insert the foot and leg into the shoe and orthosis with minimal difficulty. At the time of the final evaluation, the person should be able to don the orthosis accurately, independently, and rapidly. If not, the orthosis may need an adjustment or further training as indicated.

STANDING

The patient should stand within parallel bars or another secure environment.

3. Is the patient comfortable when standing with the heel midlines 6 inches (15 cm) apart? Question the patient regarding comfort and observe any movement or facial expression indicative of discomfort. Note the sites of any complaints of discomfort.

4. Are the shoe construction and design satisfactory and does the shoe fit properly with the appropriate length, width, and snugness at the heel? Examine the upper, including the shoe closure, the sole, the heel, and the snugness of the counter. The shoe should be longer than the longest toe and as wide as the metatarsophalangeal width of the foot. The sole and heel of the shoe should be flat on the floor except for the distal portion, which should curve upward slightly. The sole (except for the distal portion) and heel should be flat whether or not wedges or lifts have been added.

5. If the orthosis has an insert foundation, is there minimal rocking between the insert and the shoe? Ask the patient to shift weight mediolaterally and anteroposteriorly and note whether the insert remains stationary. A loose insert may irritate the skin or interfere with optimal gait.

Edelstein JE, Muroz A.
Lower-Limb Prosthetics and Orthotics: Clinical Concepts (pp 155-158).
© 2011 Taylor & Francis Group.

6. Do mechanical joints lie over the corresponding anatomical joints? The orthotic ankle joint should lie at the distal tip of the medial malleolus to avoid vertical motion of the orthosis on the leg when the patient walks. The mechanical knee joints should be approximately 0.75-inch (2 cm) above the medial tibial plateau. The orthotic hip joint should be slightly higher and anterior to the greater trochanter, to compensate for the lower and posterior position of the greater trochanter relative to the acetabulum. Misplaced mechanical joints can restrict the patient's motion.

7. Is there adequate clearance between mechanical and anatomic joints? Insufficient clearance risks skin breakdown, whereas excessive clearance makes the orthosis unduly bulky.

8. With a valgus or varus correction strap, is the foot position adequately controlled? Check the snugness of the valgus correction strap that buckles around the lateral upright or the varus correction strap that is fastened around the medial upright.

9. Do the shells, bands, and uprights conform to the contours of the leg, thigh, and trunk? Confirm that the rigid portions of the orthosis do not pinch the skin or gap.

10. Is there adequate clearance between the calf shell or band and the head of the fibula? The calf band should terminate below the fibular head to avoid impingement on the peroneal nerve.

11. With a weight-relieving brim, is there adequate reduction in weight bearing through the orthosis? Place a ribbon in the shoe prior to having the patient don the shoe. One end of the ribbon should be at the midpoint of the shoe interior and the other end should protrude from the back of the shoe. The patient then dons the orthosis and stands facing forward with body weight equally distributed between the two legs. The evaluator pulls the ribbon from the shoe, confirming that the patient is not bearing full weight through the lower limb.

➤ If full weight relief is sought, the required orthosis is a KAFO with an ischial bearing brim and a patten bottom. The shoe on the braced side should not touch the floor. An AFO with a weight-bearing brim suffices for partial unweighting of the braced limb.

12. Are locks secure and easy to operate? If the orthosis has a knee lock, with or without a hip lock, these should engage easily and securely. Otherwise, the patient risks inadvertent collapse.

13. Is there adequate clearance (usually 2 inches [5 cm]) between the proximal margin of the thigh shell or band and the perineum? Verify that the orthosis is not excessively high. Too high a margin will be painful and will compel an abducted gait.

14. Is any flesh roll above the thigh shell or band minimal? Check the circumference of the thigh shell or band to make certain that soft tissue does not overhang the band. A flesh roll is uncomfortable, can irritate the underlying skin, and will cause the patient to walk with an abducted gait.

15. Is the proximolateral aspect of the thigh shell or thigh band below the greater trochanter but at least 1 inch (2.5 cm) higher than the medial aspect of the thigh shell or medial upright? Optimum orthotic control can be achieved by a sufficiently high proximal band without irritating the skin over the greater trochanter.

16. Are the uprights at the midline of the leg and thigh? View the patient from the side to determine whether the band(s) or shell is contoured so that the uprights are at the midline. Relatively flat bands shift the uprights anteriorly; overly concave bands displace the uprights posteriorly. If the patient has genu recurvatum, an orthosis with concave bands will fail to control the knee position.

17. Does the quadrilateral brim have adequate relief for the adductor longus tendon? The anteromedial aspect of the brim should have a relief to avoid undue compression of the adductor longus tendon, which is a sensitive structure.

18. Does the quadrilateral brim have a sufficient seat for the ischial tuberosity? The posterior brim should have an adequately horizontal shelf for the ischial tuberosity so that the patient can be comfortable when bearing weight on the orthosis.

19. With a quadrilateral brim, does the ischial tuberosity rest on the ischial seat? Ask the patient to lean forward slightly while the examiner slides the index finger between the ischial tuberosity and the ischial seat. One should be able to palpate the tuberosity and the ischial seat with the finger. The tuberosity should lie on the seat for maximum comfort.

20. Does the pelvic band lie flat on the trunk, between the trochanters and the iliac crests? Check the upper and lower margins of the band to confirm that it is not pressing into the wearer's soft tissue.

SITTING

21. Can the patient sit comfortably with hips and knees flexed 90 degrees? The patient should sit on an unupholstered chair with feet flat on the floor. Note any complaints of discomfort. The bottom of the thigh shell or distal thigh band and the top of the calf shell or band should be equidistant from the knee, to avoid impingement in the popliteal fossa.

WALKING

22. Does the patient walk on a level surface with less abnormal movement with the orthosis than without it? Compare the observation of the patient's gait with the orthosis with the previous observation of walking without the orthosis. Note any complaints voiced by the patient regarding discomfort and instability. Support and motion control are achieved primarily by the rigidity of the orthosis. Although the individual who receives his or her first orthosis will not have had much gait training, the orthotist will have guided the person through a few steps in order to complete the alignment procedure. Judgments made at the initial evaluation are tentative; however, any gross gait abnormalities should be recorded.

23. Is the patient's performance on stairs and ramps satisfactory? This item can be omitted at the initial evaluation. If the patient has marginal functional prognosis, the item is irrelevant. Otherwise, the patient should demonstrate confidence on stairs and ramps. The individual who is unable to traverse stairs and ramps safely may require additional training.

24. Does the orthosis operate quietly? Listen for metallic noises or other indications that the orthosis is unstable.

ORTHOSIS OFF OF THE PATIENT

25. Is the skin free of abrasions or other discolorations attributable to the orthosis? Inspect the skin to detect any irritations attributable to the orthosis. Compare the skin after orthotic wear with the examination conducted prior to donning the orthosis, looking for any new color changes. Redness persisting for more than 10 minutes necessitates a possible adjustment of the orthosis.

26. Is the construction neat without faulty plastic molding, hammer marks, unfinished stitching, or other imperfections? Check for uniformity of the stitching. Determine whether the plastic portions are uniform and all rivets and other fasteners are secured smoothly. Move the joints slowly to check range of motion. *Binding* refers to tilting of the distal portion of the joint in relation to the proximal member so as to interfere with movement. If the medial and lateral stops do not contact their respective stops at the same time, the stop that contacts first will erode more rapidly and may contribute to twisting of the orthosis.

27. Do all components function satisfactorily? Check all locks, fasteners and other hardware on the orthosis. Malfunction of any part of the orthosis may prevent the patient from wearing it.

28. Does the patient consider the orthosis satisfactory as to comfort, function, and appearance? Solicit the patient's opinion, noting any favorable and unfavorable comments. If the patient is dissatisfied, referral to the multidisciplinary clinic team for reevaluation is indicated. Problems that are identified should be resolved.

Chapter 23

Pathological Gait Analysis

A principal purpose of lower-limb orthoses is to improve the individual's gait. Abnormal gait may be characterized by slower velocity, fatigue, and pain in joints that are overly stressed.[1-5] If the individual wears an orthosis, walking reflects both the underlying pathology and the modifications imposed by the orthosis. The gait pattern may reflect a compromise between anatomic deficiency addressed by the orthosis and the device itself, which may introduce negative changes. For example, the patient with paralyzed knee extensors may benefit from a knee-ankle-foot orthosis (KAFO) with a knee lock that prevents knee collapse; however, the locked knee prevents the usual knee flexion during swing phase. Orthoses that do not fit properly or malfunction will also change the way the wearer walks.

The following discussion identifies the most common gait problems, the ways they disturb gait, and the physiologic causes, as well as the positive and negative effects of orthoses on each abnormality. In addition, typical gait patterns associated with various pathologies are described.

EARLY STANCE

1. *Foot slap*: Flail foot. Forefoot slaps the ground quickly and noisily (Figure 23-1).
   - Decreases tibial advancement
   - Decreases shock absorption by limiting knee flexion
   - Physiologic causes:
     - Weak dorsiflexors, sometimes associated with toe drag during swing phase; foot slap is most likely to occur when the patient is fatigued
   - Orthotic causes:
     - Inadequate dorsiflexion spring assist
     - Inadequate plantar stop

2. *Toe contact*: Forefoot makes initial contact; tip-toe posture may or may not be maintained throughout stance phase (Figure 23-2).
   - Loses heel rocker; dorsiflexors normally pull tibia forward
   - Decreases tibial advancement
   - Decreases shock absorption by limiting knee flexion
   - Physiologic causes:
     - Weak dorsiflexors, associated with toe drag during swing phase
     - Pes equinus
     - Knee flexion contracture greater than 30 degrees
     - Extensor synergy
     - Heel pain
     - Short ipsilateral leg
   - Patient requires:
     - Dorsiflexion spring assist or plantar stop if dorsiflexors are weak
     - Contralateral heel lift with or without sole lift to compensate for knee flexion contracture or extensor synergy
     - Heel lift to compensate for pes equinus or leg shortening
     - Resilient heel insert in the shoe to reduce impact on the painful heel

3. *Flat foot contact*: Entire foot contacts the floor at initial contact.
   - Decreases tibial advancement
   - Decreases shock absorption
   - Decreases contralateral step length
   - Physiologic causes:
     - Weak quadriceps; keep weight line anterior to knee

Edelstein JE, Muroz A.
Lower-Limb Prosthetics and Orthotics: Clinical Concepts (pp 159-168).
© 2011 Taylor & Francis Group.

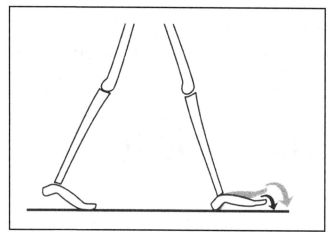

Figure 23-1. Foot slap. (Reprinted with permission from Perry J, Burnfield JM. *Gait Analysis: Normal and Pathological Function*. 2nd ed. Thorofare, NJ: SLACK Incorporated; 2010.)

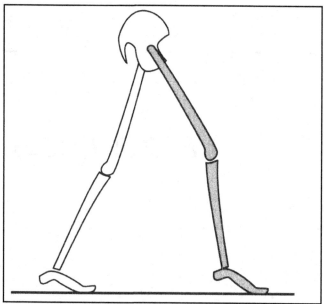

Figure 23-2. Toe contact. (Reprinted with permission from Perry J, Burnfield JM. *Gait Analysis: Normal and Pathological Function*. 2nd ed. Thorofare, NJ: SLACK Incorporated; 2010.)

- ¤ Pain anywhere in limb
- ¤ Impaired proprioception and/or balance
- ➤ Orthotic cause:
  - ¤ Inadequate traction from shoe sole
- ➤ Patient requires:
  - ¤ Ankle-foot orthosis (AFO) with anterior band to stabilize knee
  - ¤ KAFO with stance control
  - ¤ KAFO with knee lock
  - ¤ Assistive device to reduce load on lower limb and augment proprioception
4. *Medial border contact*: Medial border of the foot contacts the floor at initial contact.
   - ➤ Reduces support surface
   - ➤ Decreases shock absorption
   - ➤ Physiologic causes:
     - ¤ Pes planovalgus (hyperpronation)
     - ¤ Achilles tendon contracture
   - ➤ Orthotic cause:
     - ¤ Malalignment of uprights or stirrup in leather-metal orthosis
   - ➤ Patient requires:
     - ¤ Medial heel wedge with or without medial sole wedge
     - ¤ Longitudinal arch support
     - ¤ Solid ankle AFO to control valgus
     - ¤ Valgus correction strap
5. *Lateral border contact*: Lateral border of the foot contacts the floor at initial contact.
   - ➤ Reduces support surface
   - ➤ Decreases shock absorption
   - ➤ Physiologic causes:
     - ¤ Pes varus
     - ¤ Pes equinovarus
     - ¤ Extensor synergy
   - ➤ Orthotic cause:
     - ¤ Malalignment of uprights or stirrup in leather-metal orthosis
   - ➤ Patient requires:
     - ¤ Lateral heel wedge with or without lateral sole wedge
     - ¤ Solid ankle AFO to control varus
     - ¤ Varus correction strap
6. *Toe-in*: Forefoot points inward.
   - ➤ Undue stress on lateral ankle and knee ligaments
   - ➤ Physiologic causes:
     - ¤ Internal tibial torsion
     - ¤ Hip anteversion
   - ➤ Orthotic cause:
     - ¤ Malalignment of uprights or stirrup in leather-metal orthosis
7. *Toe-out*: Forefoot points outward.
   - ➤ Undue stress on medial ankle and knee ligaments
   - ➤ Physiologic causes:
     - ¤ External tibial torsion
     - ¤ Hip retroversion
     - ¤ Overcorrected anteversion
     - ¤ Weak knee extensors; knee axis not in line of progression

➢ Orthotic causes:
  ¤ Malalignment of uprights or stirrup in leather-metal orthosis
  ¤ Requires AFO with anterior band or KAFO with stance control in the presence of weak knee extensors

8. *Wide walking base*: Heel centers are more than 4 inches (10 cm) apart.
  ➢ Fatigue as distance the center of gravity shifts increases
  ➢ Physiologic causes:
    ¤ Poor balance
    ¤ Hip abduction contracture
    ¤ Long leg (short contralateral leg)
  ➢ Orthotic causes:
    ¤ Insufficient heel lift
    ¤ KAFO; High medial upright
    ¤ Hip-knee-ankle-foot orthosis (HKAFO); abducted hip joint
    ¤ Patient requires walking aid

9. *Narrow walking base*: Base is less than 5 cm; if one foot crosses in front of the other, the gait is known as *scissoring*.
  ➢ Unstable walking base
  ➢ Physiologic causes:
    ¤ Adductor spasticity
  ➢ Orthotic cause:
    ¤ KAFO; may benefit from a spreader bar; however, the bar limits gait options to drag-to, swing-to, and swing-through gait patterns

10. *Excessive knee flexion*: Knee flexes excessively when the foot contacts the floor (Figure 23-3).
  ➢ Risks falling
  ➢ Increases demand on knee and hip extensors
  ➢ Physiologic causes:
    ¤ Weak knee extensors
    ¤ Knee flexion contracture
    ¤ Hip flexion contracture
    ¤ Short contralateral leg
    ¤ Flexor spasticity
    ¤ Knee pain[6-10]
  ➢ Orthotic causes:
    ¤ Solid ankle or limited motion stop prevents plantar flexion
    ¤ KAFO; inadequate knee lock
  ➢ Patient requires:
    ¤ A walking aid
    ¤ AFO with anterior band or KAFO with stance control in the presence of weak knee extensors
    ¤ Contralateral shoe lift in the presence of short leg

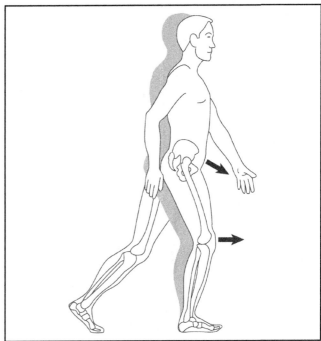

Figure 23-3. Excessive knee flexion.

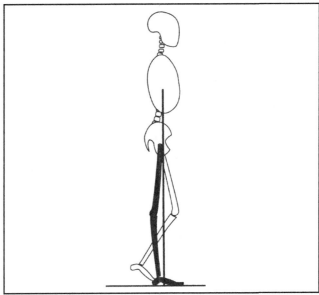

Figure 23-4. Hyperextended knee. (Reprinted with permission from Perry J, Burnfield JM. *Gait Analysis: Normal and Pathological Function.* 2nd ed. Thorofare, NJ: SLACK Incorporated; 2010.)

11. *Hyperextended knee*: Knee hyperextends as weight is transferred to leg (Figure 23-4).
  ➢ Painful knee
  ➢ Physiologic causes:
    ¤ Genu recurvatum
    ¤ Weak knee extensors
    ¤ Lax knee ligaments
    ¤ Extensor synergy
    ¤ Pes equinus

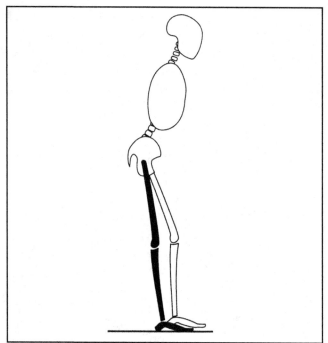

Figure 23-5. Anterior trunk bending. (Reprinted with permission from Perry J, Burnfield JM. *Gait Analysis: Normal and Pathological Function*. 2nd ed. Thorofare, NJ: SLACK Incorporated; 2010.)

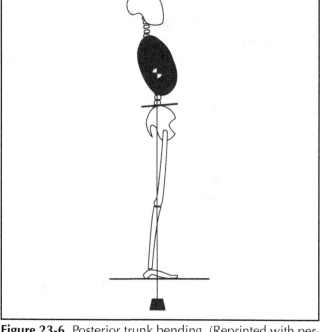

Figure 23-6. Posterior trunk bending. (Reprinted with permission from Perry J, Burnfield JM. *Gait Analysis: Normal and Pathological Function*. 2nd ed. Thorofare, NJ: SLACK Incorporated; 2010.)

> - Orthotic causes:
>   - ¤ Excessively concave calf band
>   - ¤ Pes equinus uncompensated by contralateral shoe lift
>   - ¤ Inadequate knee lock

12. *Anterior trunk bending*: Patient leans forward as weight is transferred to the stance leg, thereby shifting line of gravity in front of the knee (Figure 23-5).
    - ➤ Undue stress on low back
    - ➤ Physiologic causes:
      - ¤ Hip flexion contracture
      - ¤ Knee flexion contracture
      - ¤ Flexor spasticity
      - ¤ Knee extensor weakness or paralysis
    - ➤ Orthotic cause:
      - ¤ Inadequate knee lock
    - ➤ Patient requires:
      - ¤ Resilient or beveled heel to reduce knee flexion moment of force
      - ¤ AFO with anterior band or KAFO with stance control or knee lock

13. *Posterior trunk bending*: Patient leans backward as weight is transferred to the stance leg to avoid uncontrolled hip flexion (Figure 23-6).
    - ➤ Undue stress on low back
    - ➤ Physiologic causes:
      - ¤ Limited hip mobility

- ¤ Weak hip extensors
- ¤ Extensor synergy
- ➤ Orthotic causes:
  - ¤ Patient requires assistive device
  - ¤ Inadequate hip lock
  - ¤ Knee lock

14. *Lateral trunk bending*: Patient leans to the side at initial contact (Figure 23-7).
    - ➤ Unilateral; lean toward affected side
    - ➤ Bilateral; waddle
      - ¤ Fatigue as lateral shift of center of gravity increases
      - ¤ Undue stress on low back
    - ➤ Physiologic causes:
      - ¤ Weak hip abductors (Trendelenburg gait)
      - ¤ Hip abductor contracture
      - ¤ Hip pain; antalgic gait
      - ¤ Dislocated hip
      - ¤ Long leg; abduct and lean
      - ¤ Short leg
    - ➤ Orthotic causes:
      - ¤ KAFO; high medial upright
      - ¤ HKAFO; abducted hip joint
      - ¤ Insufficient heel lift
      - ¤ Patient requires walking aid

15. *Internal rotation*: Entire lower limb is rotated internally.
    - ➤ Decreases forward progression

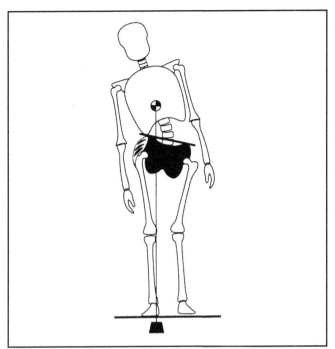

Figure 23-7. Lateral trunk bending. (Reprinted with permission from Perry J, Burnfield JM. *Gait Analysis: Normal and Pathological Function*. 2nd ed. Thorofare, NJ: SLACK Incorporated; 2010.)

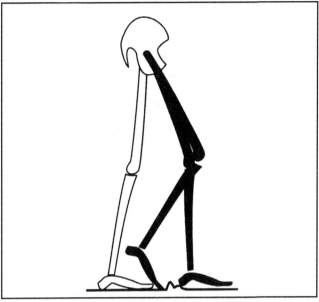

Figure 23-8. Toe drag. (Reprinted with permission from Perry J, Burnfield JM. *Gait Analysis: Normal and Pathological Function*. 2nd ed. Thorofare, NJ: SLACK Incorporated; 2010.)

- ➤ Physiologic causes:
  - ¤ Weak external rotators
  - ¤ Spastic internal rotators; scissors gait
  - ¤ Anteversion
- ➤ Patient requires:
  - ¤ Rotation control straps
  - ¤ HKAFO
16. *External rotation*: Entire lower limb is rotated externally.
- ➤ Increases limb stability
- ➤ Reduces length of forefoot lever
- ➤ Physiologic causes:
  - ¤ Weak knee extensors
  - ¤ Hip retroversion
  - ¤ Weak internal rotators
- ➤ Patient requires:
  - ¤ Rotation control straps
  - ¤ HKAFO

LATE STANCE

1. *Insufficient propulsion*: Calcaneal gait, Syme's gait; delayed or weak transfer of weight over the forefoot.
- ➤ Decreases forefoot rocker
- ➤ Decreases contralateral step length
- ➤ Decreases propulsion

- ➤ Physiologic causes:
  - ¤ Weak plantar flexors
  - ¤ Metatarsalgia
  - ¤ Ankle fusion
- ➤ Orthotic causes:
  - ¤ Solid ankle or limited motion ankle joint prevents plantar flexion
  - ¤ Patient requires a rocker bar on shoe sole

SWING

1. *Toe drag/drop foot*: Toes maintain contact with the floor (Figure 23-8).
- ➤ Inadequate clearance, risks tripping
- ➤ Decreases step length
- ➤ Physiologic causes:
  - ¤ Paralyzed dorsiflexors
  - ¤ Extensor synergy
  - ¤ Weak hip flexors
  - ¤ Pes equinus
  - ¤ Contralateral short leg
- ➤ Orthotic causes:
  - ¤ Inadequate dorsiflexion assist
  - ¤ Inadequate plantar flexion stop
  - ¤ Patient requires contralateral shoe lift in the presence of short leg
2. *Steppage*: Exaggerated hip and knee flexion to clear the foot (Figure 23-9).
- ➤ Fatigue
- ➤ Risk of tripping

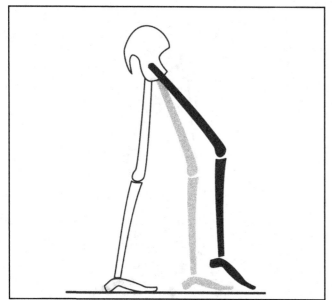

Figure 23-9. Steppage. (Reprinted with permission from Perry J, Burnfield JM. *Gait Analysis: Normal and Pathological Function*. 2nd ed. Thorofare, NJ: SLACK Incorporated; 2010.)

> Physiologic causes:
>> ¤ Weak, rather than completely paralyzed, dorsiflexors
> Orthotic causes:
>> ¤ Inadequate dorsiflexion assist
>> ¤ Inadequate plantar flexion stop

3. *Hip hiking*: Pelvic elevation to enable the limb to swing forward (Figure 23-10).
> Low back stress
> Risk of tripping
> Physiologic causes:
>> ¤ Extensor synergy
>> ¤ Weak dorsiflexors
>> ¤ Weak hip flexors
>> ¤ Pes equinus
> Orthotic causes:
>> ¤ Knee lock
>> ¤ Inadequate dorsiflexion assist
>> ¤ Inadequate plantar flexion stop

4. *Circumduction*: Limb moves outward in a semicircular arc.
> Asymmetrical rhythm
> Slow velocity
> Risks tripping
> Physiologic causes:
>> ¤ Extensor synergy
>> ¤ Weak dorsiflexors
>> ¤ Weak hip flexors
>> ¤ Pes equinus

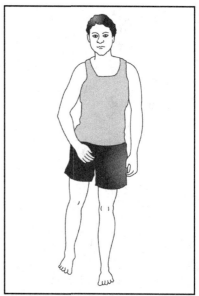

Figure 23-10. Hip hiking.

> Orthotic causes:
>> ¤ Knee lock
>> ¤ Inadequate dorsiflexion assist
>> ¤ Inadequate plantar flexion stop

5. *Vaulting*: Exaggerated plantar flexion of contralateral leg to enable the ipsilateral limb to swing forward.
> Fatigue in contralateral leg
> Asymmetrical rhythm
> Risks tripping
> Physiologic causes:
>> ¤ Extensor synergy
>> ¤ Weak dorsiflexors
>> ¤ Weak hip flexors
>> ¤ Pes equinus
> Orthotic causes:
>> ¤ Knee lock
>> ¤ Inadequate dorsiflexion assist
>> ¤ Inadequate plantar flexion stop

EFFECTS OF ANATOMIC AND PHYSIOLOGICAL ABNORMALITIES

> Weak dorsiflexors
>> ¤ Foot slap
>> ¤ Toe contact
>> ¤ Toe drag/drop foot
>> ¤ Steppage
>> ¤ Hip hiking
>> ¤ Circumduction
>> ¤ Vaulting

- ➤ Weak plantar flexors
  - ¤ Insufficient propulsion
- ➤ Pes equinus
  - ¤ Toe contact
  - ¤ Hyperextended knee
  - ¤ Toe drag/drop foot
  - ¤ Steppage
  - ¤ Hip hiking
  - ¤ Circumduction
  - ¤ Vaulting
- ➤ Pes planovalgus (hyperpronation)
  - ¤ Medial border contact
- ➤ Pes varus, equinovarus
  - ¤ Lateral border contact
- ➤ Achilles tendon contracture
  - ¤ Medial border contact
  - ¤ Hyperextended knee
- ➤ Metatarsalgia
  - ¤ Insufficient propulsion
- ➤ Heel pain
  - ¤ Toe contact
- ➤ Ankle fusion
  - ¤ Insufficient propulsion
- ➤ Knee extensor weakness
  - ¤ Flat foot contact
  - ¤ Toe-out
  - ¤ Excessive knee flexion
  - ¤ Anterior trunk bending
  - ¤ External rotation
- ➤ Knee flexion contracture
  - ¤ Toe contact
  - ¤ Excessive knee flexion
  - ¤ Anterior trunk bending
- ➤ Genu recurvatum
  - ¤ Hyperextended knee
- ➤ Knee ligamentous laxity
  - ¤ Hyperextended knee
- ➤ Internal tibial torsion
  - ¤ Toe-in
- ➤ External tibial torsion
  - ¤ Toe-out
- ➤ Hip extensor weakness
  - ¤ Posterior trunk bending
- ➤ Hip flexor weakness
  - ¤ Toe drag/drop foot
  - ¤ Hip hiking
  - ¤ Circumduction
- ➤ Hip abductor weakness (Trendelenburg gait)[3]
  - ¤ Lateral trunk bending/waddling

- ➤ Hip external rotator weakness
  - ¤ Internal rotation
- ➤ Hip internal rotator weakness
  - ¤ External rotation
- ➤ Hip flexion contracture
  - ¤ Excessive knee flexion
  - ¤ Anterior trunk bending
- ➤ Hip abduction contracture
  - ¤ Wide walking base
  - ¤ Lateral trunk bending/waddling
- ➤ Hip anteversion
  - ¤ Toe-in
  - ¤ Internal rotation
- ➤ Hip retroversion
  - ¤ External rotation
- ➤ Limited hip mobility
  - ¤ Posterior trunk bending
- ➤ Dislocated hip
  - ¤ Lateral trunk bending/waddling
- ➤ Extensor synergy
  - ¤ Toe contact
  - ¤ Lateral border contact
  - ¤ Hyperextended knee
  - ¤ Posterior trunk bending
  - ¤ Toe drag/foot drop
  - ¤ Hip hiking
  - ¤ Circumduction
  - ¤ Vaulting
- ➤ Flexor spasticity
  - ¤ Excessive knee flexion
  - ¤ Anterior trunk bending
- ➤ Adductor spasticity
  - ¤ Narrow walking base
- ➤ Internal rotator spasticity
  - ¤ Internal rotation: scissors gait
- ➤ Short ipsilateral leg
  - ¤ Toe contact
  - ¤ Lateral trunk bending
- ➤ Short contralateral leg
  - ¤ Wide walking base
  - ¤ Excessive ipsilateral knee flexion
  - ¤ Lateral trunk bending
  - ¤ Toe drag/drop foot
  - ¤ Hip hiking
  - ¤ Steppage
  - ¤ Ipsilateral circumduction
  - ¤ Vaulting

> Impaired proprioception and/or balance
  ¤ Flat foot contact
  ¤ Wide walking base
> Hip pain
  ¤ Lateral trunk bending/waddling
> Pain anywhere in limb[6-10]
  ¤ Flat foot contact

EFFECTS OF OPTIMAL AND INADEQUATE ORTHOSES

> Solid ankle AFO
  ¤ Excessive knee flexion
  ¤ Insufficient propulsion
> Inadequate dorsiflexion assist
  ¤ Foot slap
  ¤ Toe contact
  ¤ Toe drag/drop foot
  ¤ Steppage
  ¤ Hip hiking
  ¤ Circumduction
  ¤ Vaulting
> Inadequate plantar flexion stop
  ¤ Foot slap
  ¤ Toe contact
  ¤ Toe drag/drop foot
  ¤ Steppage
  ¤ Hip hiking
  ¤ Circumduction
  ¤ Vaulting
> Malalignment of uprights or stirrup in leather-metal orthosis
  ¤ Medial or lateral border contact
  ¤ Toe-in, toe-out
> Inadequate heel and sole lift
  ¤ Toe contact
  ¤ Wide walking base
  ¤ Lateral trunk bending
> Inadequate sole traction
  ¤ Flat foot contact
> KAFO knee lock
  ¤ Hip hiking
  ¤ Circumduction
  ¤ Vaulting
  ¤ Posterior trunk bending

> KAFO high medial upright
  ¤ Wide walking base
  ¤ Lateral trunk bending/waddling
> KAFO inadequate knee lock
  ¤ Excessive knee flexion
  ¤ Hyperextended knee
  ¤ Anterior trunk bending
> KAFO excessively concave bands
  ¤ Hyperextended knee
> HKAFO abducted hip joint
  ¤ Wide walking base
  ¤ Lateral trunk bending
> HKAFO inadequate hip lock
  ¤ Posterior trunk bending

OTHER GAIT ABNORMALITIES

> Cerebrovascular accident[12-21]
  ¤ Usually extensor synergy in lower limb
  ¤ Asymmetrical step length: longer paretic step[11,12,16,17]
  ¤ Slower velocity[14-17,21]
  ¤ Greater oxygen consumption per distance[21]
> Cerebral palsy diplegic gait[22-24]
  ¤ Usually crouching (hip and knee flexion, plantar flexion)
  ¤ May exhibit scissoring (hip adduction)
> Parkinsonian gait[11,25]
  ¤ Difficulty initiating gait
  ¤ Short steps (festination)
  ¤ Tendency to lean and walk backward (retropulsion)
  ¤ Difficulty turning corners
> Ataxia
  ¤ Poor balance
  ¤ Wide base
  ¤ Erratic movement
  ¤ Increased trunk torsion
> Antalgia[3]
  ¤ Decreased stance duration on affected leg
  ¤ Prolonged swing of affected leg
  ¤ Longer step with affected leg
  ¤ Trunk lean, usually toward affected leg
> Normal pressure hydrocephalus
  ¤ Difficulty advancing lower limbs (magnetic, sticky gait)

References

1. Perry J, Burnfield J. *Gait Analysis: Normal and Pathological Function*. 2nd ed. Thorofare, NJ: SLACK Incorporated; 2010.

2. Perry J. Normal and pathological gait. In: Hsu JD, Michael JW, Fisk JR, eds. *AAOS Atlas of Orthoses and Assistive Devices*. 4th ed. Philadelphia, PA: Mosby Elsevier; 2008:71-80.

3. Ayyappa E, Mohamed O. Clinical assessment of pathological gait. In: Lusardi MM, Nielsen CC, eds. *Orthotics and Prosthetics in Rehabilitation*. 2nd ed. St. Louis, MO: Elsevier; 2007:41-68.

4. Whittle MW. *Gait Analysis: An Introduction*. 4th ed. Edinburgh, UK: Butterworth Heinemann; 2007.

5. Hurmuzlu Y, Basdogan C, Stoianovici D. Kinematics and dynamic stability of the locomotion of post-polio patients. *J Biomech Eng*. 1996;118:405-411.

6. Hubley-Kozey CL, Hill NA, Rutherford DJ, et al. Co-activation differences in lower limb muscles between asymptomatic controls and those with varying degrees of knee osteoarthritis during walking. *Clin Biomech (Bristol, Avon)*. 2009;24:407-414.

7. Hubley-Kozey C, Deluzio K, Dunbar M. Muscle co-activation patterns during walking in those with severe knee osteoarthritis. *Clin Biomech (Bristol, Avon)*. 2008;23:71-80.

8. Astephen JL, Deluzio KJ, Caldwell GE, et al. Gait and neuromuscular pattern changes are associated with differences in knee osteoarthritis severity levels. *J Biomech*. 2008;41:868-876.

9. Zeni JA Jr, Higginson JS. Differences in gait parameters between healthy subjects and persons with moderate and severe knee osteoarthritis: a result of altered walking speed? *Clin Biomech (Bristol, Avon)*. 2009;24:372-378.

10. Andriacchi TP, Koo S, Scanlan SF. Gait mechanics influence healthy cartilage morphology and osteoarthritis of the knee. *J Bone Joint Surg Am*. 2009;91(suppl 1):95-101.

11. Boonstra TA, van der Kooij H, Munneke M, Bloem BR. Gait disorders and balance disturbances in Parkinson's disease: clinical update and pathophysiology. *Curr Opin Neurol*. 2008;21:461-471.

12. Kahn JH, Hornby TG. Rapid and long-term adaptations in gain symmetry following unilateral step training in people with hemiparesis. *Phys Ther*. 2009;89:474-483.

13. Balasubramanian CK, Bowden MG, Neptune RR, Kautz SA. Relationship between step length asymmetry and walking performance in subjects with chronic hemiparesis. *Arch Phys Med Rehabil*. 2007;88:43-49.

14. Lin PY, Yang YR, Cheng SJ, Wang RY. The relation between ankle impairments and gait velocity and symmetry in people with stroke. *Arch Phys Med Rehabil*. 2006;87:562-568.

15. Chen G, Patten C, Kothari D, Zajac F. Gait differences between individuals with poststroke hemiparesis and non-disabled controls at matched speeds. *Gait Posture*. 2005;22:51-56.

16. Hsu A, Tang P, Jan M. Analysis of impairments influencing gait velocity and asymmetry of hemiplegic patients after mild to moderate stroke. *Arch Phys Med Rehabil*. 2003;84:1185-1193.

17. Roth EJ, Merbitz C, Mroczek K, et al. Hemiplegic gait: relationships between walking speed and other temporal parameters. *Am J Phys Med Rehabil*. 1997;76:129-133.

18. Olney SJ, Richards C. Hemiparetic gait following stroke. Part I: characteristics. *Gait Posture*. 1996;4:136-148.

19. Ekaterina B, Titianova E, Tarkka I. Asymmetry of walking performance and postural sway in patients with chronic unilateral cerebral infarction. *J Rehabil Res Dev*. 1995;32:236-244.

20. von Shroeder H, Coutts R, Lyden P, et al. Gait parameters following stroke: a practical assessment. *J Rehabil Res Dev*. 1995;32:583-587.

21. Detrembleur C, Dierick F, Stoquart G, et al. Energy cost, mechanical work, and efficiency of hemiparetic walking. *Gait Posture*. 2003;18:47-55.

22. van der Krogt MM, Doorenbosch CA, Becher JG, Harlaar J. Walking speed modifies spasticity effects in gastrocnemius and soleus in cerebral palsy gait. *Clin Biomech (Bristol, Avon)*. 2009;24:422-428.

23. van der Krogt MM, Doorenbosch CA, Harlaar J. The effect of walking speed on hamstrings length and lengthening velocity in children with spastic cerebral palsy. *Gait Posture*. 2009;29:640-644.

24. Crenna P. Spasticity and "spastic" gait in children with cerebral palsy. *Neurosci Biobehav Rev*. 1998;22:571-578.

25. Yang YR, Lee YY, Cheng SJ, et al. Relationships between gait and dynamic balance in early Parkinson's disease. *Gait Posture*. 2008;27:611-615.

Chapter 24

Orthotic Functional Outcomes

Walking in the presence of weakness, with or without sensory alteration, compromises both efficiency and velocity, even if the patient wears orthoses. The clinical decision regarding orthotic prescription concerns whether the added metabolic effort has sufficient physical and emotional benefits to override the anatomic deficits.

ENERGY CONSUMPTION

The metabolic demands of walking with lower-limb orthoses reflect the underlying pathomechanics as well as the weight and restriction or assistance imposed by the orthosis. An abundance of research probes the oxygen consumption of people with amputations. In contrast, much less has been published about the demands of orthotic use, in spite of the much larger number of those who wear orthoses.

ANKLE-FOOT ORTHOSES

Orthotic use appears to reduce oxygen cost for non-disabled men, compared with walking with the feet held in plantar flexion or walking with shoes alone; the benefit occurred regardless of the type of ankle hinge on the ankle-foot orthosis (AFO).[1] Patients with hemiparesis walked 20% faster with a 12% decrease in oxygen consumption when wearing carbon composite AFOs, compared to walking without an orthosis.[2] Other investigators confirmed that patients walked considerably faster at a lower energy cost per meter with the orthosis.[3]

AFOs also improved the performance of children with spastic cerebral palsy. Compared with barefoot gait, use of an AFO was associated with a 9% faster velocity overall. Energy cost declined 6% for those with tetraplegia who walked with an AFO, probably because the orthoses reduced the crouched posture.

Children with hemiplegia and diplegia did not demonstrate greater efficiency when wearing orthoses.[4] Earlier research contradicted these results showing that, on average, children with spasticity walking with flexible plastic AFOs used more energy.[5]

Children with spina bifida at various lumbar levels also performed better when walking with AFOs. Gait velocity improved 14%, stride length increased, and energy demand reduced by one-third.[6]

KNEE-ANKLE-FOOT ORTHOSES

The benefits noted for carbon fiber AFOs also accrue to carbon knee-ankle-foot orthoses (KAFOs). Middle-aged adults who contracted poliomyelitis many years earlier achieved an energy reduction averaging 8% when walking with carbon fiber KAFOs compared to using their previous plastic-metal or leather-metal KAFOs. Walking speed, however, was unchanged.[7] Another study of poliomyelitis survivors confirmed the superiority of carbon fiber KAFOs. Subjects were able to increase step length and speed and consumed significantly less oxygen when walking with the new orthoses.[8] The same research team reported that carbon fiber KAFOs were 28% lighter than the subjects' previous orthoses and remained undamaged for at least 2 years; gait kinematics, however, were not changed by the new orthoses.[9]

TRUNK-HIP-KNEE-ANKLE-FOOT ORTHOSES

Several investigators have reported the metabolic cost of walking for adults with spinal cord injury fitted with a reciprocating gait orthosis (RGO) compared to bilateral KAFOs.[10] Subjects with T_{12} and L_1 lesions wearing a RGO achieved much faster gait at a significantly lower energy demand.[11] Another investigation

Edelstein JE, Muroz A.
Lower-Limb Prosthetics and Orthotics: Clinical Concepts (pp 169-172).
© 2011 Taylor & Francis Group.

on the effects of reciprocating gait orthoses on men with thoracic spinal cord injury revealed that standing in the orthosis caused the heart rate and respiratory rate to increase markedly. Walking a short distance with the orthosis results in unsustainable fatigue.[12] A third comparison of the RGO with another orthosis (medially linked KAFOs) confirmed that subjects with paraplegia walk twice as fast with the RGO and use approximately half as much oxygen.[13] Some clinicians use functional electrical stimulation in combination with a RGO worn by patients with paraplegia. Stimulation reduced heart rate but did not change oxygen consumption. With the orthosis, walking speed was much slower than that of able-bodied people or wheelchair users.[14] The performance of adults with spinal cord injury who wore a RGO was compared with those fitted with a ParaWalker (trunk-hip-knee-ankle-foot orthosis [THKAFO] with hip joints allowing a limited excursion; Orthotic Research and Locomotor Assessment Unit, The Robert Jones and Agnes Hunt Orthopaedic Hospital, Oswestry, England). Subjects were also tested while maneuvering in a wheelchair. Physiologic response was better in the wheelchair than in either type of orthosis.[15] Two analyses at the same clinic concerned children with spina bifida who used the RGO. The results differed somewhat. The later study indicated that walking was faster and the oxygen cost was similar to that with HKAFOs; nevertheless, wheelchair mobility was speedier than walking.[16] Earlier, the investigators reported that HKAFO use required a significantly higher energy consumption rate than did the RGO. Youngsters who perform the swing-through gait in an HKAFO have a significantly faster velocity than those who ambulate with the RGO; altogether, the report concluded that HKAFOs are more energy efficient.[17]

CRUTCH AND WHEELCHAIR USE

Walking with crutches alters the usual arm movement and demands lifting the body with major shoulder and trunk muscle effort in order to advance the legs. Adolescents with spina bifida who walked with crutches used more oxygen per meter than did those who used wheelchairs.[18] Men with incomplete spinal cord injury ranging from C_6 to L_2 walked less efficiently and more slowly, particularly with a walker rather than crutches.[19] In another study comparing adults with incomplete injury to able-bodied people, only one-third of the patients could walk fast enough to cross a street safely. They walked at half the velocity of control subjects with a 26% greater oxygen uptake.[20]

Among unimpaired adults performing the 3-point gait, longer or shorter forearm crutch length, within 1 inch (2.5 cm), affected energy consumption.[21] The swing-through gait with forearm crutches required 2 to 3 times more energy than needed for able-bodied

walking.[22] Able-bodied women used the least oxygen with axillary crutches and had the fastest speed, compared to walkers, when executing the 3-point gait pattern.[23]

With regard to wheelchair use by adults with spinal cord injury, peak oxygen uptake was almost the same for those with tetraplegia and paraplegia, although the latter group had greater power output.[24] Other research into the energy consumption of adults with paraplegia indicates that propelling an ultra light wheelchair was faster and more efficient.[25] One way to diminish energy consumption is by providing patients with powered wheelchairs. They also enabled people with spinal cord injury to increase the distance traveled.[26] Modifying a manually propelled wheelchair also reduced oxygen consumption and heart rate among adults with hemiparesis.[27]

SUBJECTIVE RESPONSE

Functional outcome is also influenced by factors besides the individual's motor and sensory status and the type of orthosis, crutch, or wheelchair the person uses. A survey of consumer satisfaction with orthotic services suggested that though patients are generally quite pleased with service at prosthetics and orthotics facilities, a few complained about slow delivery time and a lack of information about the components of the orthosis or prosthesis.[28,29]

REFERENCES

1. Herndon SK, Bennett BC, Wolovick A, et al. Center of mass motion and the effects of ankle bracing on metabolic cost during submaximal walking trials. *J Orthop Res.* 2006;24:2170-2175.

2. Danielsson A, Sunnerhagen KS. Energy expenditure in stroke subjects walking with a carbon composite ankle foot orthosis. *J Rehabil Med.* 2004;36:165-168.

3. Franceschini M, Massucci M, Ferrari L, et al. Effects of an ankle-foot orthosis on spatiotemporal parameters and energy cost of hemiparetic gait. *Clin Rehabil.* 2003;17:368-372.

4. Brehm MA, Harlaar J, Schwartz M. Effect of ankle-foot orthoses on walking efficiency and gait in children with cerebral palsy. *J Rehabil Med.* 2008;40:529-534.

5. Suzuki N, Shinohara T, Kimizuka M, et al. Energy expenditure of diplegic ambulation using flexible plastic ankle foot orthoses. *Bull Hosp Jt Dis.* 2000;59:76-80.

6. Duffy CM, Graham HK, Cosgrove AP. The influence of ankle-foot orthoses on gait and energy expenditure in spina bifida. *J Pediatr Orthop.* 2000;20:356-361.

7. Brehm MA, Beelen A, Doorenbosch CA, et al. Effect of carbon-composite knee-ankle-foot orthoses on walking efficiency and gait in former polio patients. *J Rehabil Med.* 2007;39:651-657.

8. Hachisuka K, Makino K, Wada F, et al. Oxygen consumption, oxygen cost and physiological cost index in polio survivors: a comparison of walking without orthosis, with an ordinary or a carbon-fibre reinforced plastic knee-ankle-foot orthosis. *J Rehabil Med.* 2007;39:646-650.

9. Hachisuka K, Makino K, Wada F, et al. Clinical application of carbon fibre reinforced plastic leg orthosis for polio survivors and its advantages and disadvantages. *Prosthet Orthot Int.* 2006;30:129-135.

10. Kawashima N, Taguchi D, Nakazawa K, Akai M. Effect of lesion level on the orthotic gait performance in individuals with complete paraplegia. *Spinal Cord.* 2006;44: 487-494.

11. Leung AK, Wong AF, Wong EC, Hutchins SW. The Physiological Cost Index of walking with an isocentric RGO among patients with T(12)-L(1) spinal cord injury. *Prosthet Orthot Int.* 2009;33:61-68.

12. Massucci M, Brunetti G, Piperno R, et al. Walking with the advanced RGO (ARGO) in thoracic paraplegic patients: energy expenditure and cardiorespiratory performance. *Spinal Cord.* 1998;36:223-227.

13. Harvey LA, Davis GM, Smith MB, Engel S. Energy expenditure during gait using the Walkabout and isocentric reciprocal gait orthoses in persons with paraplegia. *Arch Phys Med Rehabil.* 1998;79:945-949.

14. Beillot J, Carré F, Le Claire G, et al. Energy consumption of paraplegic locomotion using RGO. *Eur J Appl Physiol Occup Physiol.* 1996;73:376-381.

15. Merati G, Sarchi P, Ferrarin M, et al. Paraplegic adaptation to assisted-walking: energy expenditure during wheelchair versus orthosis use. *Spinal Cord.* 2000;38:37-44.

16. Thomas SS, Buckon CE, Melchionni J, et al. Longitudinal assessment of oxygen cost and velocity in children with myelomeningocele: comparison of the hip-knee-ankle-foot orthosis and the RGO. *J Pediatr Orthop.* 2001;21: 798-803.

17. Cuddeford TJ, Freeling RP, Thomas SS, et al. Energy consumption in children with myelomeningocele: a comparison between RGO and hip-knee-ankle-foot orthosis ambulators. *Dev Med Child Neurol.* 1997;39:239-242.

18. Bruinings AL, van den Berg-Emons HJ, Buffart LM, et al. Energy cost and physical strain of daily activities in adolescents and young adults with myelomeningocele. *Dev Med Child Neurol.* 2007;49:672-677.

19. Ulkar B, Yavuzer G, Guner R, Ergin S. Energy expenditure of the paraplegic gait: comparison between different walking aids and normal subjects. *Int J Rehabil Res.* 2003;26:213-217.

20. Lapointe R, Lajoie Y, Serresse O, Barbeau H. Functional community ambulation requirements in incomplete spinal cord injured subjects. *Spinal Cord.* 2001;39:327-335.

21. Mullis R, Dent RM. Crutch length: effect on energy cost and activity intensity in non-weight-bearing ambulation. *Arch Phys Med Rehabil.* 2000;81:569-572.

22. Thys H, Willems PA, Saels P. Energy cost, mechanical work and muscular efficiency in swing-through gait with elbow crutches. *J Biomech.* 1996;29:1473-1482.

23. Holder CG, Haskvitz EM, Weltman A. The effects of assistive devices on the oxygen cost, cardiovascular stress, and perception of nonweight-bearing ambulation. *J Orthop Sports Phys Ther.* 1993;18:537-542.

24. Haisma JA, van der Woude LH, Stam HJ, et al. Physical capacity in wheelchair-dependent persons with a spinal cord injury: a critical review of the literature. *Spinal Cord.* 2006;44:642-652.

25. Beekman CE, Miller-Porter L, Schoneberger M. Energy cost of propulsion in standard and ultralight wheelchairs in people with spinal cord injuries. *Phys Ther.* 1999;79: 146-158.

26. Nash MS, Koppens D, van Haaren M, et al. Power-assisted wheels ease energy costs and perceptual responses to wheelchair propulsion in persons with shoulder pain and spinal cord injury. *Arch Phys Med Rehabil.* 2008;89: 2080-2085.

27. Mandy A, Lesley S. Measures of energy expenditure and comfort in an ESP wheelchair: a controlled trial using hemiplegic users. *Disabil Rehabil Assist Technol.* 2009;4:137-142.

28. Bosmans J, Geertzen J, Dijkstra PU. Consumer satisfaction with the services of prosthetics and orthotics facilities. *Prosthet Orthot Int.* 2009;33:69-77.

29. Phillips B, Zhao H. Predictors of assistive technology abandonment. *Assist Technol.* 1993;5:36-45.

Chapter 25

Orthotics in Management of Musculoskeletal and Neuromuscular Disorders

Orthotic management is part of comprehensive clinical care for some patients with musculoskeletal or neuromuscular disorders. As with any prescription decision, selecting a particular device for a patient depends on a thorough history, careful physical examination, detailed review of laboratory and functional tests, and in-depth discussion with the patient, family, and rehabilitation team members regarding feasible goals.

Orthoses are presented in order of preference, with the most practical option first. In all instances, the orthosis should be worn with a low-heeled shoe. Assistive devices (eg, canes, walkers, and crutches) may be used with or instead of orthoses.

FOOT DEFORMITIES

Heel Spur

Also known as *infracalcaneal exostosis*, the spur interferes with comfortable heel contact at the start of the gait cycle. The goal of orthotic intervention is to reduce pressure at the painful site.

> - Heel insert: The simplest approach; the insert should have a wall extending from the distomedial edge to the posterior edge to the distolateral edge. The wall reduces the likelihood that the anatomic heel will slide inside the shoe. The insert is gently sloped forward, transferring some weight anteriorly away from the spur. Beneath the spur, the insert should have a concavity that increases the contact area, thereby reducing pressure. Heel inserts vary in resilience, durability, and cost.

Pes Planovalgus

Pes planovalgus (flat foot) occurs when the subtalar joint subluxes. Consequently, the orthosis should apply upward and laterally directed force on the medial aspect of the rear foot and, ideally, medially directed force on the heel.

> - Medial heel wedge: Shifts weight away from the medial border. Effective only if the posterior portion of the shoe fits the anatomic heel snugly.

> - Arch support[1]: Applies upward force over a broad area of the foot with the apex of the arch in the vicinity of the sustentaculum tali of the calcaneus. May be built into the shoe at the time of its manufacture or added later as an internal modification. Made in a wide range of materials. Extent of convexity at the apex of the arch varies.

> - University of California Biomechanics Laboratory (UCBL) insert: Three-quarter insert custom-made over a plaster cast of the foot positioned in maximum supination, with the leg externally rotated. Encompasses all of the intertarsal joints, maintaining the mid- and rearfoot in the corrected position. When the orthosis is removed, the foot returns to its planovalgus posture.

> - Solid ankle-foot orthosis (AFO)

> - Limited motion AFO with stirrup, bilateral metal upright(s), and valgus correction strap

Pes Varus

Foot bears excessive weight on the lateral border.

> - Lateral outsole or insole wedge: For flexible pes varus. Reduces the deformity. Height of the wedge depends on the extent of foot deformity and the patient's comfort and function.

> - Medial outsole or insole wedge: For rigid pes varus. Increases the bearing area.

> - Solid ankle AFO

> - Hemispiral AFO

> - Limited motion AFO with stirrup, bilateral metal upright(s), and varus correction strap

Edelstein JE, Muroz A.
Lower-Limb Prosthetics and Orthotics: Clinical Concepts (pp 173-182).
© 2011 Taylor & Francis Group.

Pes Cavus

Pes cavus is often accompanied by pes varus. The cavovarus foot usually lacks joint mobility.

> ➤ Insert with convexity under the mid-foot[2]: Broadens the weight-bearing surface to reduce unit pressure.

> ➤ Resilient insole or outsole: Aids shock absorption during the stance phase of walking.

Pes Equinus

Plantar flexed foot overloads forefoot and prevents heel contact at the beginning of stance phase.

> ➤ Heel lift: For fixed deformity. Enables the patient to stand with equal weight on the rear foot and the forefoot. The lift also improves balance and weight transition from early through late stance.

> ➤ Heel and sole lift on contralateral shoe: For unilateral pes equinus if the pelvis is tilted. Equalizes leg length.

Metatarsal Subluxation

Women who have worn high-heeled shoes for a long time may develop pain in both forefeet. The higher the heel, the greater the load borne by the forefoot. Typically, the patient will have limited ankle and metatarsophalangeal excursion, interfering with heel contact, as well as late stance propulsion. The plantar surface often has callus beneath the metatarsal heads.

> ➤ Shoe selection: Because it is unrealistic to expect the patient to abandon high-heeled shoes, a more feasible approach involves selecting shoes with slightly lower heels. Such footwear will still be stylish and will subject the Achilles tendon to a slight stretch throughout the day. After several months of wearing the new shoes, the person should obtain shoes with heels lower than now worn. The process of gradually decreasing heel height enables the individual to accommodate the aesthetics of lower heels and to adjust to the lengthening of the Achilles tendon.

> ➤ Three-quarter or full length insert with metatarsal pad: Shift load from the sensitive metatarsophalangeal joints to the metatarsal shafts, which are relatively insensitive. The pad should lie proximal to the metatarsal heads, between the first and the fifth metatarsals.

> ➤ Metatarsal bar: External sole modification shifts weight bearing posterior to the metatarsophalangeal joints and reduces irritative forefoot motion. The metatarsal bar is ordinarily placed on the sole of a low-heeled shoe.

Hallux Valgus

Angulation of the first toe may be accompanied by lateral displacement of the sesamoid bones as well as medial angulation of the fifth toe (bunionette). Severe hallux valgus displays overlapping of the second toe. The patient is likely to experience pain during late stance.

> ➤ Shoe selection: Ample width for the forefoot. If toes overlap, the upper must provide sufficient vertical space to avoid irritating the dorsum of the displaced toe.

> ➤ Bunion patch in the upper: Material is removed from the upper overlying the bunion. A leather patch over the resulting hole provides extra room for the medial aspect of the forefoot.

> ➤ Rocker bar: Aids propulsion during late stance.

Hammer and Claw Toes

Both hammer and claw toe deformities affect the middle toes, typically the second or third toes, which are hyperextended at the metatarsophalangeal joint and flexed at the proximal interphalangeal joint. The distal interphalangeal joint is in neutral position in hammer toe and is flexed in claw toe. Angulation of one or more toes can make shoe wear painful. The deformities result either from shoes that constrict the toes or imbalance between intrinsic and extrinsic toe muscles. Calluses eventually form on the dorsum of the head of the proximal phalanx of the affected toe.

> ➤ Shoe selection: Moccasin toe shoes provide more room for the toes than do other upper designs. Thermomold shoes are another option; the leather is specially treated in the factory. Subsequently, the clinician can remove the shoe from the foot, spot heat the leather over the tender toes, and stretch the material to provide more toe space. Upon cooling, the leather retains the stretched contour.

> ➤ Toe crest: A convex pad under the toes increases the area that sustains the force of weight bearing.

Foot Size Inequality

Whether size inequality is congenital or results from surgery or asymmetrical growth following childhood disease, each foot should be fitted properly, as described in Chapter 18. Depending on the extent of size inequality, some patients simply stuff cotton or similar material in the shoe intended for the smaller foot. The drawback of this approach is that the shoe on the smaller foot may not provide adequate support during stance phase.

> ➤ Custom insert in shoe for smaller foot: The patient can purchase one pair of shoes and transfer the insert into the new shoe for the smaller foot.

➢ Two pairs of shoes, one size for the larger foot and another for the smaller foot: Discard the unneeded shoes. This method will enable a good fit for both feet and enables the widest shoe selection but doubles the cost of shoes.

➢ Split size (mismatched) shoes: Available from orthotists and pedorthists. Each foot will be properly fitted; however, the styles and colors are limited and the cost is appreciable because wholesalers must stock many shoes to meet the requirements of particular customers.

Leg Length Inequality

Although the feet are usually unimpaired in the presence of leg length inequality, conservative management involves modifying the shoe on the side of the shorter limb.

➢ Sole and heel lift on the shoe on the shorter side: Measure the extent of inequality by placing boards under the shorter limb until the pelvis is level. Subtract 0.5-inch (6 mm) from the height of boards to provide adequate clearance during swing phase. A low quarter shoe on the shorter side can accommodate a 0.5-inch internal heel lift, with the remaining lift on the exterior of the heel and sole. Sole lift should be beveled to create a rocker sole to facilitate late stance.

Knee Deformities

Knee Flexion Contracture

➢ Knee-ankle-foot orthosis (KAFO) with bilateral uprights and fan lock, serrated lock, or ratchet lock: Adjust the fan or serrated lock to accommodate the contracture or apply a slight stretch to the knee. The ratchet lock accommodates the contracture.

Genu Recurvatum

➢ KAFO with bilateral uprights, knee lock, and shallow calf and distal thigh bands: Shallow (less concave) bands provide anteriorly directed force at posterior knee.

Genu Valgum

➢ AFO with plastic calf band with proximally extended medial side: Medial extension applies laterally directed force at the knee.

➢ KAFO with bilateral (or lateral) uprights with plastic calf band having proximal medial extension: KAFO exerts greater leverage than the AFO.

➢ KAFO with bilateral uprights with 5-strap leather knee pad or padded disc on the medial upright near the orthotic knee joint

Genu Varum

➢ AFO with plastic calf band with proximally extended lateral side: Lateral extension applies medially directed force at the knee.

➢ KAFO with bilateral (or lateral) uprights with plastic calf band having proximal lateral extension

➢ KAFO with bilateral uprights with 5-strap leather knee pad or padded disc on the lateral upright near the orthotic knee joint

Nonunited Femoral Fracture

Patient is unable to bear weight through the affected limb.

➢ KAFO with locked knee, ischial weight-bearing brim, and patten bottom, plus contralateral shoe lift: Weight transmitted from pelvis to brim, through uprights to patten bottom. Shoe does not touch the floor. Walking aid is often required.

Diabetes

Diabetic foot disorders are multiple. Peripheral neuropathy can cause intrinsic muscle imbalance, leading to hammer and claw toes. Neuropathy also affects sensation, typically with diminished awareness of light touch on the dorsum and sole of the feet. Autonomic consequences include reduced perspiration, which may cause drying of the skin, with fissures that can become infected. Advanced diabetic neuropathy can manifest itself by decubitus ulcers, Charcot neuropathic joints, or both. Nephropathy may be evident by fluctuating foot volume, and retinopathy may complicate inspecting the feet and fastening the shoes.

In addition to an educational program emphasizing meticulous foot and shoe inspection, hygiene, and medical and dietary control, the patient is likely to benefit from specific shoes and foot orthoses.

➢ Shoe selection[3-13]

¤ Blucher upper for maximum adjustability, particularly when the foot is edematous

¤ Supple upper, such as kid or deerskin

¤ Extra depth shoe provides maximum room for deformities and wound dressings

¤ Toe box high enough to encompass any hammer or claw toes that may be present

¤ Hook and pile straps, rather than laces, if vision is poor

- ¤ Resilient insole and outsole[14]
- ¤ Proper shoe fit is essential to avoid pressure concentration or abrasion of hypesthetic skin or abrasion
- ¤ Healing shoe, intended to be worn while ulcers are healing, has a thermoplastic foam upper
- ➢ Metatarsal pad[14]
- ➢ AFO with solid ankle[15]: May improve balance in the presence of sensory loss.

ARTHRITIS

Osteoarthritis (degenerative, traumatic arthritis), as well as gout and rheumatoid arthritis, can cause pain, deformity, and limitation of joint movement, which lead to restriction of overall function. Orthoses, in combination with other interventions, can absorb shock, reduce painful motion, and redirect stress from damaged joint surfaces.

Ankle and Foot Arthritis

- ➢ Shoe selection
  - ¤ Resilient insole and outsole[16-20]
  - ¤ Supple upper
  - ¤ Hook and pile straps, rather than laces, if manual dexterity is poor
- ➢ AFO with ankle hinge[21,22]

Knee Arthritis

- ➢ Medial sole wedge in the presence of medial compartment disease[23-34]
- ➢ Lateral sole wedge in the presence of genu valgum[35]
- ➢ Knee orthoses: Over-the-counter orthoses, custom-fitted, restrict mediolateral and rotation movement and provide sensory cues to accustom the wearer to avoid abrupt movement.

POLIOMYELITIS, PERIPHERAL NEUROPATHIES, AND GUILLAIN-BARRÉ DISEASE

In North and South America, Europe, and Australia, poliomyelitis is exceedingly uncommon, given widespread inoculation in childhood. Consequently, most patients present a history of poliomyelitis contracted many years earlier. Paralysis is thus complicated by age-related changes and whatever maneuvers the individual has come to rely upon. A typical adaptation results in genu recurvatum with pain caused by tension in the cruciate and collateral ligaments of the knee. Sensation usually remains intact.

Peripheral neuropathy may result from disease, such as diabetes, trauma, or tumor. Usually the patient presents both motor and sensory loss. The person is thus vulnerable to decubitus ulceration caused by an ill-fitting orthosis or other irritants that press excessively or continually rub against the skin.

Guillain-Barré disease, an infectious peripheral neuropathy, usually starts as ascending paralysis progressing from the legs to the upper limbs. Although the disease is generally self-limiting, rehabilitation during the 6 to 12 months of illness is important to prevent complications. Sensory changes usually include dysesthesias, loss of proprioception, areflexia, loss of temperature sensation, and an aching pain in the weakened muscles.

For these diverse etiologies, functional deficits and orthoses are similar, associated with the particular muscles that are paralyzed.[36]

Dorsiflexor Paralysis

Injury to the common peroneal (fibular) nerve often occurs at the head of the fibula where the nerve is superficial. More distal lesions to the deep peroneal nerve are generally caused by tibial, fibular, or tarsal fracture or penetrating wounds. The most serious consequence is paralysis of the anterior tibialis, usually associated with extensor hallucis longus and extensor digitorum longus paralysis. Proximal lesions also weaken or paralyze the peroneal (fibular) muscles. Sensory loss is located along the dorsum of the foot and anterior leg.

- ➢ Functional deficits
  - ¤ Toe drag in swing phase which is likely to cause tripping. Some patients compensate by exaggerated hip flexion (steppage gait), excessive contralateral plantar flexion (vaulting), or circumduction.
  - ¤ Foot slap in early stance phase
  - ¤ Pes equinus if paralysis is not compensated
  - ¤ Pes valgus may occur in the presence of pes equinus
  - ¤ Pes varus caused by severance of the superficial peroneal nerve may jeopardize ankle stability in early stance phase
- ➢ Orthoses
  - ¤ A 0.5-inch (6 mm) heel and sole lift on contralateral shoe if paralysis is unilateral
  - ¤ Heel elevation in the presence of fixed pes equinus
  - ¤ Medial heel and sole wedge in the presence of fixed pes valgus
  - ¤ Lateral heel and sole wedge in the presence of fixed pes varus
  - ¤ Plastic or carbon fiber posterior leaf spring AFO[37,38]

- ¤ Carbon fiber AFO with anterior upright
- ¤ Solid ankle AFO
- ¤ AFO with stirrup foundation, bilateral or unilateral uprights, and dorsiflexion spring assist; valgus or varus correction strap may be added
- ¤ AFO with stirrup foundation, bilateral or unilateral uprights, and posterior stop with optional valgus or varus correction strap
- ¤ Spiral AFO
- ¤ Hemispiral AFO

Plantar Flexor Paralysis

After passing through the popliteal fossa, the tibial nerve lies deep within the calf. Thus, injury to the tibial nerve is relatively rare, although tibial or fibular fracture or penetrating wounds may damage the nerve. The most serious consequence is paralysis of the triceps surae, associated with flexor hallucis longus, flexor digitorum longus, and posterior tibialis paralysis. Sensory loss is on the plantar surface of the foot.

- ➤ Functional deficits
  - ¤ Insufficient propulsion in late stance
  - ¤ Pes calcaneus
  - ¤ Pes valgus if posterior tibialis is paralyzed
  - ¤ Pes cavus if dorsiflexors overpower paralyzed plantar flexors
- ➤ Orthoses
  - ¤ Shoe with rocker bar on the sole and insert to accommodate pes calcaneus and pes cavus
  - ¤ Solid ankle AFO
  - ¤ AFO with hinged shell
  - ¤ AFO with stirrup foundation, bilateral or unilateral uprights, and limited motion ankle joint. bichannel adjustable ankle locking (BiCAAL; Kingsley, Costa Mesa, California; Becker Orthopedic, Troy, Michigan; Fillauer, Chattanooga, Tennessee) joint may be substituted for limited motion joint. Valgus correction strap may be added.

Dorsiflexor and Plantar Flexor Paralysis

- ➤ Orthoses[39-43]
  - ¤ Solid ankle AFO
  - ¤ Hinged AFO
  - ¤ Limited motion AFO with stirrup and bilateral metal upright(s)
  - ¤ BiCAAL AFO with stirrup and bilateral metal uprights
  - ¤ Weight-reducing brim with bilateral metal uprights, BiCAAL ankle joints with bilateral metal uprights

Quadriceps Paralysis

Injury to the femoral nerve may result from pelvic fracture or penetrating injury to the anterior thigh. Severance within the pelvis can interrupt innervation of the rectus femoris. Sensory loss is confined to the anterior thigh.

- ➤ Functional deficits
  - ¤ Inability to extend the knee, such as when rising from a chair, ascending stairs, and maintaining stability during the early stance phase of gait
  - ¤ Knee extensor paralysis also interferes with controlled knee flexion during stair descent and lowering oneself to a chair
  - ¤ Knee flexion contracture if patient remains seated
  - ¤ Genu recurvatum results eventually if patient persistently compensates by forcing the knee into hyperextension by leaning forward with or without pressing the anterior thigh
- ➤ Orthoses
  - ¤ AFO with solid ankle and anterior band
  - ¤ KAFO with stance control knee joint[44-46]
  - ¤ KAFO with bilateral (or unilateral) uprights and drop ring lock; thigh release may be added
  - ¤ KAFO with bilateral uprights and pawl lock with bail or lever release
  - ¤ AFO with stirrup, BiCAAL ankle joints, bilateral metal uprights with anterior band
  - ¤ KAFO with ratchet joint
  - ¤ KAFO with fan, serrated, or ratchet knee joint in the presence of flexion contracture
  - ¤ KAFO with relatively shallow calf and distal thigh bands and knee lock in the presence of genu recurvatum

Hamstring Paralysis

Pelvic fracture may damage the sciatic nerve, paralyzing the hamstrings, plantar flexors, and dorsiflexors often resulting in referred pain along the posterior thigh. Functional deficits and orthoses are those associated with dorsiflexor and plantar flexor paralysis.

CHARCOT-MARIE-TOOTH DISEASE (PERONEAL MUSCULAR ATROPHY)

The relatively common inherited neuropathy features bilateral weakness, atrophy, and anesthesia, particularly in the feet and legs along the distribution of the peroneal nerve. Atrophy of the legs is known as *stork leg* or *champagne bottle* appearance. Other involvements include hammer toes, malformed acetabula, and hand and forearm atrophy. Functional deficits and orthoses are those associated with dorsiflexor and evertor paralysis.[47-51]

CEREBROVASCULAR ACCIDENT

Because cerebrovascular accident (CVA), neoplasm, and traumatic brain injury present similar disabilities, orthotic management is comparable, although the clinical course and associated disorders differ. Hypertonic reflexes usually appear after the initial flaccidity. Extensor synergy in the affected lower limb and flexor synergy in the upper limb is most common, particularly with CVA. Most patients achieved better gait and balance with orthoses.[52]

> Typical functional deficits
  ¤ Hip is extended, adducted, internally rotated
  ¤ Knee is extended
  ¤ Ankle is plantar flexed
  ¤ Foot is inverted
  ¤ Toes are frequently flexed
  ¤ Early stance, floor contact with the forefoot
  ¤ Mid-stance on the paretic limb, the patient tends to flex the hip over the extended knee, increasing the knee extension moment of force
  ¤ Late stance propulsion is poor
  ¤ Swing phase, foot drop is likely making the patient vulnerable to tripping
  ¤ Patients often compensate by elevating the pelvis with or without circumduction to clear the foot during swing phase
  ¤ Flexor synergy in the upper limb deprives the patient of the propulsive effect normally provided by the arms
> Orthoses
  ¤ Minimal spasticity
    » A 0.5-inch (6 mm) heel and sole lift on the contra-lateral shoe[53]
    » Pick-up strap from ankle to distal shoe lace
    » Posterior leaf spring AFO[54-60]
    » Functional electrical stimulation[61-72]
    » Several commercial systems include an upper leg cuff holding a skin electrode over the peroneal nerve
    » AFO with stirrup foundation or full length foot plate,[73] bilateral or unilateral uprights, and posterior stop. Valgus correction strap may be added

¤ Moderate spasticity
  » Spiral AFO
  » Hemispiral AFO
  » Solid ankle AFO
  » AFO with anterior hinged shell[74]
  » AFO with stirrup foundation, bilateral or unilateral uprights, and limited motion ankle joint. Valgus correction strap may be added
¤ Severe spasticity
  » Solid ankle AFO
  » AFO with stirrup foundation, bilateral uprights, and limited motion ankle joint. Valgus correction strap may be added.
  » KAFO with stance control and limited motion ankle joint
  » KAFO with limited motion ankle joint and locked knee joint, only for in-patient use on limited basis[75]

SPINAL CORD INJURY

Orthoses may address impairment of standing and walking among the many, often life-threatening, disorders confronting the patient with spinal cord injury. The extent of motor and sensory loss depends on the site of the lesion, whether traumatic, neoplastic, or disease related. In addition, body weight, general health, absence of contractures and decubiti, and motivation are major determinants of orthotic use. Although traumatic lesions are seldom clear-cut, for the sake of clarity, the following discussion assumes straight, horizontal damage with the terminology approved by the American Spinal Injury Association in which the level indicates the most distal functioning level.

CERVICAL AND HIGH THORACIC LESIONS

Unilateral Paralysis
> Hip-knee-ankle-foot orthosis (HKAFO) with unilateral pelvic band, unlocked or locked hip joint, locked knee joint; solid ankle, BiCAAL ankle joint, or posterior ankle stop

Bilateral Paralysis
> HKAFO with bilateral pelvic band, unlocked or locked hip joints, locked knee joints; solid ankles, BiCAAL ankle joints, or posterior ankle stops; may have spreader bar if adductor spasticity is severe[76]

THORACOLUMBAR AND LUMBAR LESIONS

➤ Trunk-hip-knee-ankle orthosis (THKAFO) with locked hip joints, locked knee joints; solid ankles, BiCAAL ankle joints, or posterior ankle stops: Because donning a THKAFO is relatively time consuming and gait velocity is slow, orthosis is used primarily for the physiological benefits of standing.[77]

➤ KAFOs with medial linkage[78]

➤ Reciprocating gait orthoses[79,80]

➤ Wheelchair, powered or manual, for most mobility needs

➤ Standing frame, standing table or standing wheelchair, rather than THKAFOs

T_{12} Paraplegia

➤ Functional deficits
  ¤ Paralysis and anesthesia of the hips and distal parts compels reliance on a wheelchair for practical travel; however, many patients will wear lower-limb orthoses for therapeutic weight bearing

➤ Orthoses
  ¤ Pair of stabilizing boots, AFOs with solid ankles, plantar-flexed ankles, and anterior strap at the proximal portion of the orthoses; a pair of crutches or a walker for ambulation
  ¤ Pair of KAFOs with solid ankles, locked knee joints permits standing with hips extended, relying on tension in the iliofemoral ligaments; crutches for ambulation
  ¤ Functional electrical stimulation to hip and knee extensors[81-84]

L_1-L_3 Paraplegia

➤ Functional deficits
  ¤ Paralysis and anesthesia, except for voluntary hip flexor control with some adductor strength

➤ Orthoses
  ¤ Same options as for T_{12} paraplegia

L_4 Paraplegia

➤ Functional deficits
  ¤ Presence of quadriceps strength, together with some power in the hip extensors and abductors, facilitates transferring from chair to standing if the ankles are stabilized and walking short distances with the aid of assistive devices

➤ Orthoses
  ¤ Same options as for T_{12} paraplegia

L_5 Paraplegia

➤ Functional deficits
  ¤ Imbalance between functioning dorsiflexors and paralyzed plantar flexors causes pes calcaneus

➤ Orthoses
  ¤ Pair of solid ankle AFOs with heel lifts to compensate for pes calcaneus

MULTIPLE SCLEROSIS

Autoimmune disorder is characterized by patchy demyelination of virtually any portion of the central and peripheral nervous systems, interfering with conducting impulses. Each patient presents a different complex of weakness and sensory loss, particularly hypoesthesias and paresthesias. Disease course is characterized by exacerbations and remissions, with gradual deterioration. Visual and cerebellar disorders compound the difficulty of walking.

Because of the progressive nature of the disease, periodic revision of the orthotic prescription is usually necessary. Functional deficits and orthoses depend on the particular weaknesses.[85]

REFERENCES

1. Mulford D, Taggart HM, Nivens A, Payrie C. Arch support use for improving balance and reducing pain in older adults. *Appl Nurs Res.* 2008;21:153-158.

2. Burns J, Landorf KB, Ryan MM, et al. Interventions for the prevention and treatment of pes cavus [serial on CD-ROM]. *Cochrane Database Syst Rev.* 2007;4:CD006154.

3. Reiber GE, Smith DG, Wallace CM, et al. Footwear used by individuals with diabetes and a history of foot ulcer. *J Rehabil Res Dev.* 2002;39:615-622.

4. Bus SA. Foot structure and footwear prescription in diabetes mellitus. *Diabetes Metab Res Rev.* 2008;24(suppl 1): S90-S95.

5. Lobmann R, Kayser R, Kasten G, et al. Effects of preventative footwear on foot pressure as determined by pedobarography in diabetic patients: a prospective study. *Diabet Med.* 2001;18:314-319.

6. Hijmans JM, Geertzen JH, Dijkstra PU, Postema K. A systematic review of the effects of shoes and other ankle or foot appliances on balance in older people and people with peripheral nervous system disorders. *Gait Posture.* 2007;25:316-323.

7. Lott DJ, Hastings MK, Commean PK, et al. Effect of footwear and orthotic devices on stress reduction and soft tissue strain of the neuropathic foot. *Clin Biomech (Bristol, Avon).* 2007;22:352-359.

8. Lavery LA, Peters EJ, Armstrong DG. What are the most effective interventions in preventing diabetic foot ulcers? *Int Wound J*. 2008;5:425-433.

9. Charanya G, Patil KM, Narayanamurthy VB, et al. Effect of foot sole hardness, thickness and footwear on foot pressure distribution parameters in diabetic neuropathy. *Proc Inst Mech Eng H*. 2004;218:431-443.

10. Burns J, Begg L, Vicaretti M. Comparison of orthotic materials on foot pain, comfort, and plantar pressure in the neuroischemic diabetic foot: a case report. *J Am Podiatr Med Assoc*. 2008;98:143-148.

11. Zequera M, Stephan S, Paul J. Effectiveness of moulded insoles in reducing plantar pressure in diabetic patients. *Conf Proc IEEE Eng Med Biol Soc*. 2007;2007:4671-4674.

12. Bus SA, Valk GD, van Deursen RW, et al. The effectiveness of footwear and offloading interventions to prevent and heal foot ulcers and reduce plantar pressure in diabetes: a systematic review. *Diabetes Metab Res Rev*. 2008;24(suppl 1): S162-S180.

13. Hastings MK, Mueller MJ, Pilgram TK, et al. Effect of metatarsal pad placement on plantar pressure in people with diabetes mellitus and peripheral neuropathy. *Foot Ankle Int*. 2007;28:84-88.

14. Mueller MJ, Lott DJ, Hastings MK, et al. Efficacy and mechanism of orthotic devices to unload metatarsal heads in people with diabetes and a history of plantar ulcers. *Phys Ther*. 2006;86:833-842.

15. Rao N, Aruin AS. Automatic postural responses in individuals with peripheral neuropathy and ankle-foot orthoses. *Diabetes Res Clin Pract*. 2006;74:48-56.

16. Hawke F, Burns J, Radford JA, du Toit V. Custom-made foot orthoses for the treatment of foot pain [serial on CD-ROM]. *Cochrane Database Syst Rev*. 2008;3:CD006801.

17. Trotter LC, Pierrynowski MR. Changes in gait economy between full-control custom-made foot orthoses and prefabricated inserts in patients with musculoskeletal pain: a randomized clinical trial. *J Am Podiatr Med Assoc*. 2008;98:429-435.

18. Hinman RS, Bennell KL. Advances in insoles and shoes for knee osteoarthritis. *Curr Opin Rheumatol*. 2009;21: 164-170.

19. Egan M, Brosseau L, Farmer M, et al. Splints/orthoses in the treatment of rheumatoid arthritis [serial on CD-ROM]. *Cochrane Database Syst Rev*. 2003;1:CD004018.

20. Novak P, Burger H, Tomsic M, et al. Influence of foot orthoses on plantar pressures, foot pain and walking ability of rheumatoid arthritis patients: a randomized controlled study. *Disabil Rehabil*. 2008;21:1-8.

21. Huang YC, Harbst K, Kotajarvi B, et al. Effects of ankle-foot orthoses on ankle and foot kinematics in patients with subtalar osteoarthritis. *Arch Phys Med Rehabil*. 2006;87:1131-1136.

22. Huang YC, Harbst K, Kotajarvi B, et al. Effects of ankle-foot orthoses on ankle and foot kinematics in patients with ankle osteoarthritis. *Arch Phys Med Rehabil*. 2006;87:710-716.

23. Zhang W, Moskowitz RW, Nuki G, et al. OARSI recommendations for the management of hip and knee osteoarthritis, part II OARSI evidence-based, expert consensus guidelines. *Osteoarthritis Cartilage*. 2008;16:137-162.

24. Gelis A, Coudevre E, Hudry C, et al. Is there an evidence-based efficacy for the use of foot orthotics in knee and hip osteoarthritis? Elaboration of French clinical practice guidelines. *Joint Bone Spine*. 2008;75:714-720.

25. Kakihana W, Akai M, Nakazawa K, et al. Inconsistent knee varus moment reduction caused by a lateral wedge in knee osteoarthritis. *Am J Phys Med Rehabil*. 2007;86: 446-454.

26. Kakihana W, Akai M, Nakazawa K, et al. Effects of laterally wedged insoles on knee and subtalar joint moments. *Arch Phys Med Rehabil*. 2005;86:1465-1471.

27. Reilly KA, Barker KL, Shamley D. A systematic review of lateral wedge orthotics—how useful are they in the management of medial compartment osteoarthritis? *Knee*. 2006;13:177-183.

28. Krohn K. Footwear alterations and bracing as treatments for knee osteoarthritis. *Curr Opin Rheumatol*. 2005;17: 653-656.

29. Barrios JA, Crenshaw JR, Royer TD, Davis IS. Walking shoes and laterally wedged orthoses in the clinical management of medial tibiofemoral osteoarthritis: a one-year prospective controlled trial. *Knee*. 2009;16:136-142.

30. Maillefert JF, Hudry C, Baron G, et al. Laterally elevated wedged insoles in the treatment of medial knee osteoarthritis: a prospective randomized controlled study. *Osteoarthritis Cartilage*. 2001;9:739-745.

31. Pham T, Maillefert JF, Hudry C, et al. Laterally elevated wedged insoles in the treatment of medial knee osteoarthritis: a two-year prospective randomized controlled study. *Osteoarthritis Cartilage*. 2004;12:46-55.

32. Kerrigan DC, Lelas JL, Goggins J, et al. Effectiveness of a lateral-wedge insole on knee varus torque in patients with knee osteoarthritis. *Arch Phys Med Rehabil*. 2002;83: 889-893.

33. Butler RJ, Barrios JA, Royer T, Davis IS. Effect of laterally wedged foot orthoses on rearfoot and hip mechanics in patients with medial knee osteoarthritis. *Prosthet Orthot Int*. 2009;33:107-116.

34. Nakajima K, Kakihana W, Nakagawa T, et al. Addition of an arch support improves the biomechanical effect of a laterally wedged insole. *Gait Posture*. 2009;29:208-213.

35. Rodrigues PT, Ferreira AF, Pereira RM, et al. Effectiveness of medial-wedge insole treatment for valgus knee osteoarthritis. *Arthritis Rheum*. 2008;59:603-608.

36. Hijmans JM, Geertzen JHB. Development of guidelines for the prescription of orthoses in patients with neurological disorders in the Netherlands. *Prosthet Orthot Int*. 2006;30:35-43.

37. Steinfeldt F, Seifert W, Günther KP. Modern carbon fibre orthoses in the management of polio patients—a critical evaluation of the functional aspects. *Z Orthop Ihre Grenzgeb*. 2003;141:357-361.

38. Hachisuka K, Makino K, Wada F, et al. Clinical application of carbon fibre reinforced plastic leg orthosis for polio survivors and its advantages and disadvantages. *Prosthet Orthot Int.* 2006;30:129-135.

39. Lin SS, Sabharwal S, Bibbo C. Orthotic and bracing principles in neuromuscular foot and ankle problems. *Foot Ankle Clin.* 2000;5:235-264.

40. Sackley C, Disler PB, Turner-Stokes L, et al. Rehabilitation interventions for foot drop in neuromuscular disease [serial on CD-ROM]. *Cochrane Database Syst Rev.* 2009;3: CD003908.

41. Geboers JF, Drost MR, Spaans F, et al. Immediate and long-term effects of ankle-foot orthosis on muscle activity during walking: a randomized study of patients with unilateral foot drop. *Arch Phys Med Rehabil.* 2002;83:240-245.

42. Geboers JF, Janssen-Potten YJ, Seelen HA, et al. Evaluation of effect of ankle-foot orthosis use on strength restoration of paretic dorsiflexors. *Arch Phys Med Rehabil.* 2001;82: 856-860.

43. Farmer SE, Pearce G, Whittall J, et al. The use of stock orthoses to assist gait in neuromuscular disorders: a pilot study. *Prosthet Orthot Int.* 2006;30:145-154.

44. Hebert JS, Liggins AB. Gait evaluation of an automatic stance-phase control knee orthosis in a patient with post-poliomyelitis. *Arch Phys Med Rehabil.* 2005;86:1976-1979.

45. Hebert JS, Liggins AB. Gait evaluation of an automatic stance-control knee orthosis in a patient with postpoliomyelitis. *Arch Phys Med Rehabil.* 2005;86:1676-1680.

46. Huang S, Kang S, Cho K, Kim Y. Biomechanical effect of electromechanical knee-ankle-foot-orthosis on knee joint control in patients with poliomyelitis. *Med Biol Eng Comput.* 2008;46:541-549.

47. Don R, Serrao M, Vinci P, et al. Foot drop and plantar flexion failure determine different gait strategies in Charcot-Marie-Tooth patients. *Clin Biomech (Bristol, Avon).* 2007;22:905-916.

48. Newman CJ, Walsh M, O'Sullivan R, et al. The characteristics of gait in Charcot-Marie-Tooth disease types I and II. *Gait Posture.* 2007;26:120-127.

49. Young P, De Jonghe P, Stögbauer F, Butterfass-Bahloul T. Treatment for Charcot-Marie-Tooth disease [serial on CD-ROM]. *Cochrane Database Syst Rev.* 2008;1:CD006052.

50. Bean J, Walsh A, Frontera W. Brace modification improves aerobic performance in Charcot-Marie-Tooth disease: a single-subject design. *Am J Phys Med Rehabil.* 2001;80:578-582.

51. Vinci P, Gargiulo P. Poor compliance with ankle-foot orthoses in Charcot-Marie-Tooth disease. *Eur J Phys Rehabil Med.* 2008;44:27-31.

52. Tyson SF, Kent RM. Orthotic devices after stroke and other non-progressive brain lesions [serial on CD-ROM]. *Cochrane Database Syst Rev.* 2009;1:CD003694.

53. Kitisomprayoonkul W, Cheawchanwattana S, Janchai S, E-Sepradit P. Effects of shoe lift on weight bearing in stroke patients. *J Med Assoc Thai.* 2005;88:S79-S84.

54. Wang RY, Lin PT, Lee CC, Yang YR. Gait and balance performance improvements attributable to ankle-foot orthosis in subjects with hemiparesis. *Am J Phys Med Rehabil.* 2007;86:556-562.

55. Teasell RW, McRae MP, Foley N, Bhardwaj A. Physical and functional correlations of ankle-foot orthosis use in the rehabilitation of stroke patients. *Arch Phys Med Rehabil.* 2001;82:1047-1049.

56. Gok H, Kucukdeveci A, Altinkaynak H, et al. Effects of ankle-foot orthoses on hemiparetic gait. *Clin Rehabil.* 2003;17:137-139.

57. de Wit DC, Buurke JH, Nijlant JM, et al. The effect of an ankle-foot orthosis on walking ability in chronic stroke patients: a randomized controlled trial. *Clin Rehabil.* 2004;18:550-557.

58. Wang RY, Yen L, Lee CC, et al. Effects of an ankle-foot orthosis on balance performance in patients with hemiparesis of different durations. *Clin Rehabil.* 2005;19:37-44.

59. Hesse S, Werner C, Matthias K, et al. Non-velocity-related effects of a rigid double-stopped ankle-foot orthosis on gait and lower limb muscle activity of hemiparetic subjects with an equinovarus deformity. *Stroke.* 1999;30:1855-1861.

60. Chen CK, Hong WH, Chu NK, et al. Effects of an anterior ankle-foot orthosis on postural stability in stroke patients with hemiplegia. *Am J Phys Med Rehabil.* 2008;87:815-820.

61. Stein RB, Chong SL, Everaert D, et al. A multicenter trial of a foot drop stimulator controlled by a tilt sensor. *Neurorehabil Neural Repair.* 2006;20:317-379.

62. Yan T, Hui-Chan CWY, Li LSW. Functional electrical stimulation improves motor recovery of the lower extremity and walking ability of subjects with first acute stroke: a randomized placebo-controlled trial. *Stroke.* 2005;36:80-85.

63. Dunning K, Black K, Harrison A, et al. Neuroprosthesis peroneal functional electrical stimulation in the acute inpatient rehabilitation setting: a case series. *Phys Ther.* 2009;89:499-506.

64. Burridge JH, Taylor PN, Hagan SA, et al. The effects of common peroneal stimulation on the effort and speed of walking: a randomized control trial with chronic hemiplegic patients. *Clin Rehabil.* 1997;11:201-210.

65. Ring H, Rosenthal N. Controlled study of neuroprosthetic functional electrical stimulation in sub-acute post-stroke rehabilitation. *J Rehabil Med.* 2005;37:32-36.

66. Daly JJ, Roenig K, Holcomb J, et al. A randomized controlled trial of functional neuromuscular stimulation in chronic stroke subjects. *Stroke.* 2006;37:172-178.

67. Sheffler LR, Hennessey MT, Naples GG, Chae J. Peroneal nerve stimulation versus an ankle foot orthosis for correction of foot drop in stroke: impact on functional ambulation. *Neurorehabil Neural Repair.* 2006;20:355-360.

68. Thompson AK, Doran B, Stein RB. Short-term effects of functional electrical stimulation on spinal excitatory and inhibitory reflexes in ankle extensor and flexor muscles. *Exp Brain Res.* 2006;170:216-226.

69. Robbins SM, Houghton PE, Woodbury MG, Brown JL. The therapeutic effect of functional and transcutaneous electric stimulation on improving gait speed in stroke patients: a meta-analysis. *Arch Phys Med Rehabil.* 2006;87:853-859.

70. Kottink AI, Hermens HJ, Nene AV, et al. Therapeutic effect of an implantable peroneal nerve stimulator in subjects with chronic stroke and footdrop: a randomized controlled trial. *Phys Ther.* 2008;88:437-448.

71. Lindquist A, Prado CL, Barros RML, et al. Gait training combining partial body-weight support, a treadmill, and functional electrical stimulation: effects on poststroke gait. *Phys Ther.* 2007;87:1144-1154.

72. Ng MF, Tong RK, Li LS. A pilot study of randomized clinical controlled trial of gait training in subacute stroke patients with partial body-weight support electromagnetic gait trainer and functional electrical stimulation: a six month follow-up. *Stroke.* 2008;39:154-160.

73. Fatone S, Gard SA, Malas BS. Effect of ankle-foot orthosis alignment and foot-plate length on the gait of adults with poststroke hemiplegia. *Arch Phys Med Rehabil.* 2009;90: 810-818.

74. Park JH, Chun MH, Ahn JS, et al. Comparison of gait analysis between anterior and posterior ankle foot orthosis in hemiplegic patients. *Am J Phys Med Rehabil.* 2009;88: 630-634.

75. Hurley EA. Use of KAFOs for patients with cerebral vascular accident, traumatic brain injury, and spinal cord injury. *Proc Amer Acad Orthot Prosthet.* 2006;7:P199-P201.

76. Kaplan LK, Grynbaum BB, Rusk HA, et al. A reappraisal of braces and other mechanical aids in patients with spinal cord dysfunction: results of a follow-up study. *Arch Phys Med Rehabil.* 1996;77:393-405.

77. Plassat R, Perrouin-Verbe B, Stéphan A, et al. Gait orthosis in patients with complete thoracic paraplegia: review of 43 patients. *Ann Readapt Med Phys.* 2005;48:240-247.

78. Suzuki T, Sonoda S, Saitoh E, et al. Prediction of gait outcome with the knee-ankle-foot orthosis with medial hip joint in patients with spinal cord injuries: a study using recursive partitioning analysis. *Spinal Cord.* 2007;45: 57-63.

79. Franceschini M, Baratta S, Zampolini M, et al. Reciprocating gait orthoses: a multicenter study of their use by spinal cord injured patients. *Arch Phys Med Rehabil.* 1997;78:582-586.

80. Scivoletto G, Petrelli A, Lucente LD, et al. One year follow up of spinal cord injury patients using a reciprocating gait orthosis: preliminary report. *Spinal Cord.* 2000;38: 555-558.

81. Field-Fote EC. Combined use of body weight support, functional electric stimulation, and treadmill training to improve walking ability in individuals with chronic incomplete spinal cord injury. *Arch Phys Med Rehabil.* 2001;82:818-824.

82. Ladouceur M, Barbeau H. Functional electrical stimulation-assisted walking for persons with incomplete spinal injuries: longitudinal changes in maximal overground walking speed. *Scand J Rehabil Med.* 2000;32:28-36.

83. Nightingale EJ, Raymond J, Middleton JW, et al. Benefits of FES gait in a spinal cord injured population. *Spinal Cord.* 2007;45:646-657.

84. Kim CM, Eng JJ, Whittaker MW. Effects of a simple functional electrical system and/or hinged ankle-foot orthosis on walking in persons with incomplete spinal cord injury. *Arch Phys Med Rehabil.* 2004;85:1718-1723.

85. Sheffler LR, Hennessey MT, Knutson JS, et al. Functional effect of an ankle foot orthosis on gait in multiple sclerosis: a pilot study. *Am J Phys Med Rehabil.* 2008;87:26-32.

Chapter 26

Pediatric Prosthetics and Orthotics

Joan T. Gold, MD and Joan E. Edelstein, MA, PT, FISPO, CPed

Children who require orthoses or prostheses differ from adult patients. Consequently, implementing juvenile habilitation or rehabilitation presents distinctive prescription considerations. Developmental concerns extend to the complexity of the device and the timing with which one is prescribed. For the child with an acquired disorder, issues relate to the age of the patient when the disorder occurred and the grief about the lost function expressed by both the child and the child's family. Most importantly, prescription of orthoses and prostheses, or their revision, does not constitute complete medical treatment. Underlying changes in the patient's medical diagnosis or potential complications should be addressed concurrently.

DIFFERENCES BETWEEN CHILDREN AND ADULTS

➢ Size: Fewer prosthetic and orthotic components are manufactured in children's sizes.

➢ Growth: Appliances should have provision for enlarging length and girth, as well as accommodating larger shoes as the child grows.

➢ Development: The complexity of orthoses and prostheses should keep pace with the child's development. Young children need relatively simple components that they can manage. The developmental age of the child, rather than just the chronological age, should be considered, especially in patients with cerebral palsy and spina bifida. Adolescents place more force on devices; thus, sturdier components and stronger construction are required. Cosmetic concerns, a major anxiety among teenagers, can be addressed by streamlined appliances, possibly in bright colors. At all ages, the device should allow the wearer to engage in the full range of activities for which the person is physically capable.

➢ Diagnoses: Pediatric practice focuses on cerebral palsy, congenital limb deficiency, muscular dystrophy, and other disorders that are either unique to childhood or more common among young patients.

➢ Parental role: Parents or guardians are ultimately responsible for their children, especially with regard to financial and legal considerations. Successful care of children, especially the very young, involves constant parental participation. It is important to have social services at hand to assist with potential strategies for addressing these issues.

COMPREHENSIVE TREATMENT

The broad goal of treatment is to prepare children for a lifetime of function. To achieve this goal, every patient deserves good overall medical care. Children with musculoskeletal and neurologic disorders should have a thorough examination seeking to identify the cause of abnormal movement. Cerebral palsy, rapidly progressive muscular dystrophy, and spinal cord tumors, among other causes, can all present similar signs yet have vastly different prognoses and interventions. Identification of the cause of a patient's gross motor deficits and motor planning issues permits the most effective orthotic, prosthetic, pharmacological, surgical, and exercise management. Active treatment may continue for the lifetime of the patient.

Edelstein JE, Muroz A.
Lower-Limb Prosthetics and Orthotics: Clinical Concepts (pp 183-196).
© 2011 Taylor & Francis Group.

GOALS OF ORTHOTIC AND PROSTHETIC MANAGEMENT

➤ Sitting stability: Head, neck, and trunk control is essential for swallowing, speech, sitting, and walking and contributes substantially to the patient's intellectual and emotional development. Sitting stability also frees the child's hands to perform self-care, graphomotor, and other essential functions.

➤ Upright posture: Among the many benefits of standing are reduction in osteopenia, contractures, and the risk of skin ulceration; stress on the skeleton encourages bony growth, improves respiration and urinary function, and facilitates muscle re-education, sensory stimulation, tone modulation, and self-esteem. Vertical orientation may reduce perceptual motor issues concurrent with the underlying diagnosis.

➤ Interaction with the environment: Children who stand and walk have more opportunities to interact with people and objects in their environment, at home, school, and elsewhere.

ORTHOTIC AND PROSTHETIC PRESCRIPTION CONSIDERATIONS

➤ Other medical issues: Designs may need to be modified to bypass any tubes, shunts, or other equipment on the child. Some children present a severe gibbus or other deformity that must be accommodated by the appliance. Sensory deficits also must be compensated by the device.

➤ Facilitating age-appropriate function: The device should facilitate the child's function; for example, water-resistant materials may enable the child to frolic under a playground sprinkler. Such materials also permit cleansing of the device in the presence of urinary or fecal incontinence, to avoid socially unacceptable malodor. Conversely, restricting ankle motion can hamper attempts at rising from a chair and climbing stairs. School-aged children should be able to don and doff the appliance easily for purposes of dressing and using a toilet with minimal assistance.

➤ Weight: The device should be as lightweight as feasible, particularly for children with muscular deficiency. The prescription should also address the force that the individual (eg, an obese adolescent or a rambunctious 10-year-old) is likely to apply.

➤ Easy repair and adjustment: In the absence of conditions causing the failure to thrive, children grow in height, girth, and foot size. The orthosis should be designed to minimize the time needed for adjustments and repairs so that the child can achieve the maximum benefit from using it. Expandable uprights and removable liners extend the duration during which the device can be worn. Patients who have fluctuating edema need to have a device that they, or their caregivers, can adjust throughout the day.

➤ Cosmetic acceptability: Most people prefer streamlined devices, usually made of thermoplastics, polymeric resins, or carbon fiber. They are unobtrusive, especially if worn under clothing. By providing intimate skin contact, they offer better control of the limb. Plastic orthoses enable the patient to wear a wide range of shoes of similar heel height. Plastic is more easily cleaned than leather, improving the hygienic and esthetic qualities of the appliance. Bright colors or cartoon characters on the prostheses or orthoses may foster the child's pride in using the appliance.

➤ Cost: Prescription must address the cost of the device in light of the financial resources of the child's parents or other paying agency. A reasonable cost for children's appliances is especially important, because replacement is needed every 1 to 2 years until growth has ceased. Replacement is also likely following orthopedic revision of deformities.

➤ Comprehensive prescription: Essential elements of the orthotic or prosthetic prescription include the following:
   ¤ Detailed description of the device
   ¤ Diagnosis and disability
   ¤ Any sensory loss
   ¤ Any allergy to particular materials, especially latex
   ¤ Anticipated length of use during the day and the number of weeks or months of likely usage, as well as conditions during which the device should or should not be used

GAIT DEVELOPMENT

Young children walk differently from the adult pattern as described in Chapter 1. Concurrent perceptual motor and upper motor neuron disorder, perceptual motor limitations, visual and cognitive impairments, and upper limb dysfunction may interfere with the acquisition of ambulation, as may any pain associated with the condition.

CEREBRAL PALSY

Cerebral palsy is a static encephalopathy with onset in the pre-, peri-, or postnatal period presenting abnormalities of posture, muscular control, and tone; spasticity is the most common. Although the cerebral lesion does not progress, tone may be amplified with maturation of the nervous system and concurrent myelination. Contractures may progress, and increased weight and height result in an ascending center of gravity, increasing balance difficulties. Patients most commonly are diplegic (ie, all limbs and trunk involved, with greatest abnormality in the lower limbs) or hemiplegic (ie, ipsilateral upper and lower limb involved). Prognoses for ambulation and deformities depend, in part, on the type of motor disturbance and the extent to which positive primitive reflexes persist. Ambulation is most likely with children with hemiplegia and diplegia, and poorest in those with hypotonic tetraplegia.

Clinical assessment should include assessment of leg length discrepancy, evaluation of hip and knee contractures, and determining whether cospasticity is present. Evaluation of upper limb function determines whether the child will be able to use an assistive device for ambulation. Computerized gait analysis, although not readily available in most clinical practices, is an adjunct that may assist when clinical decisions are complex and when surgery is contemplated. The Gross Motor Function test[1] objectifies the effect of clinical interventions, especially where gait analysis and pathologic studies are unavailable. The test is sensitive to changes under various ambulatory conditions, such as walking with and without orthoses and with various ambulatory aids. The most typical gait patterns feature crouching, with hips and knees flexed and ankles dorsiflexed; toe walking; and scissoring, with marked hip adduction. These manners of walking are unstable and fatiguing.[2-6]

Orthoses often result in better balance, longer strides, and improved cadence.[7,8] Most children with hemiplegia walk, as do one-half to three-quarters of those with diplegia. Function may be improved with multilevel orthopedic and neurologic surgery. The use of Botox and intrathecal baclofen may provide limited, rather than sustained, benefits.

In infancy and early childhood, prior to developing steady standing balance, bracing can control foot deformities and prevent their progression. Equinus with pronation is typical for those with diplegia, whereas equinus with supination prevails among children with hemiplegia. Muscles demonstrate an intrinsic change in resistance to passive stretch (or easier elongation) in children who wear orthoses for at least 6 hours a day. Improvement may be associated with increased numbers of sarcomeres in sequence, reflecting an influence in muscle growth, change in muscle protein, and

optimal overlap of actin and myosin to maximize evoked muscle tension that the muscle can generate. Unilateral ankle-foot orthoses (AFOs) with a full-length foot plate can decrease the need for Achilles tendon lengthening in hemiplegic children; improvement may reflect a dynamic advantage, rather than the orthosis used solely to establish a stable base of support.

Solid ankle AFOs in patients with spastic diplegia control ankle excursion, improve heel contact and swing phase clearance, and allow faster velocity and longer strides; single-limb support time increases in comparison to barefoot ambulation. Similar results can be achieved with hinged AFOs and posterior leaf spring AFOs.[9-14] Children tend to prefer hinged AFOs or ones with a posterior leaf spring.[10] Hinges may have adjustable excursion or the orthosis may have a posterior strap to increase ankle range gradually without losing proximal control. With the rare exception of hemiplegic patients with true flaccid drop foot, spring-loaded joints are rarely utilized to assist dorsiflexion because spring tension may provoke a fast stretch to the already spastic gastrocnemius-soleus complex, exacerbating abnormal tone. During late stance, hinged AFOs, in contrast to solid ankle AFOs, enable more normal dorsiflexion and increase ankle power. Hinged AFOs also facilitate sit-to-stand transfers[15] and make stair climbing somewhat easier.[16]

The contour and trim lines of the AFOs vary. Full-length foot plates are customary to prevent spastic toe flexors from interfering with donning shoes but may have a reflex effect, reducing spasticity in proximal portions of the limb. Foot plates can be modified with a toe crest to keep toes extended. Intrinsic tonic reflexes are associated with toe extension past the level of the metatarsal heads, thus reducing the extension synergy proximally and improving gait. It is more difficult for the child to walk on the toes when the feet are kept in neutral position, thus fostering better swing phase clearance. AFOs can control the subtalar and midtarsal joints with flexible medial and lateral walls and can support the transmetatarsal arch.

Postrhizotomy patients with residual proximal weakness, with or without dynamic internal rotation, often benefit from hinged AFOs attached to single lateral uprights with unlocked hip and knee joints and a pelvic band. The pelvic band may be jointed when isolated hip abduction is possible. Total contact orthoses and serial casting can help these patients achieve tone reduction. Skin pressure may modulate tone through the servomechanism in the muscle spindle, resulting in physiologic responses to tone and histological changes including alterations in the cross-bridge attachments, numbers of sarcomeres, and amount of connective tissue in a muscle. Improvement correlates with resistance to passive torque and greater muscle length and joint range.

If the child has adequate swing clearance, supra-malleolar AFOs may be sufficient to control residual pes valgus or varus. The orthosis should stabilize the calcaneus.

Recurvatum is likely if there is cospasticity of the quadriceps with insufficient foot clearance. An AFO with the ankle set in 5 degrees of dorsiflexion may avoid the use of a knee-ankle-foot orthosis (KAFO). Conversely, for a progressive crouch gait with excessive dorsiflexion, an AFO with solid ankle and anterior band, also known as a *floor-reaction orthosis*, can provide knee extension.

Limited experience with TheraTogs (TheraTogs, Telluride, Colorado), a garment with strategically placed elastic webbing, suggests that some children with cerebral palsy may improve their gait when wearing it.[17]

SPINA BIFIDA AND ACQUIRED SPINAL CORD INJURIES

Interdisciplinary treatment of the child with myelomeningocele represents a paradigm for advocacy of virtually any child with a physical disability. Survival has increased dramatically following closure of the spinal defect at birth, early shunting of hydrocephalus associated with a Chiari II malformation, and strict attention to the management of a neurogenic bowel and bladder.

Most children with spina bifida are able to ambulate with or without orthoses[18-20]; however, walking is slower and the energy cost is higher than that of able-bodied youngsters.[21-31] Reciprocal gait is more strenuous than swing-through gait.[21] Muscular and respiratory deconditioning appear to account for the high metabolic demand.[25] Generalizations regarding functional prognosis made on the basis of neurological level must be qualified by the presence of any asymmetrical innervation and concurrent spasticity. Other factors that influence the achievement of ambulation include scoliosis with or without gibbus deformity, hip dislocation associated with pain and range limitation, hip and knee flexion contractures in excess of 35 degrees, inability to achieve a plantigrade foot, upper limb dysfunction, impaired cognition, lack of motivation, excessive body weight, and spasticity, which may indicate a tethered spinal cord. Parents are a major influence on the child's performance.

Although children with thoracic-level lesions are usually fitted with trunk-hip-knee-ankle-foot orthoses (THKAFOs), they are unlikely to remain ambulators throughout their lifetime. Patients with upper lumbar lesions also need THKAFOs and are likely be therapeutic and household ambulators. Those with lower lumbar and more distal lesions require less extensive bracing and will usually be lifelong community ambulators. Patients with lesions that primarily involve the cauda equina have flaccid, partially insensate limbs at risk for

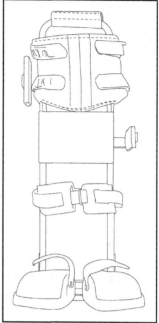

Figure 26-1. Standing frame.

skin breakdown and pathological fracture. Functional ambulation depends primarily upon the strength of the hip abductors, flexors, and knee extensor muscles. Habilitation should focus on bladder and bowel management.[26]

Infants

Solid ankle AFOs that have non-latex padding with a removable abduction bar keeps hips in the neutral position, avoiding excessive external rotation. A trunk orthosis can aid sitting balance, particularly if the child has central hypotonia associated with hydrocephalus and unopposed contraction of the hip flexors, which pulls the child forward. A low cart enhances mobility without the infant crawling on insensate limbs. The child older than 18 months with a high lesion can use a standing frame (Figure 26-1) or a parapodium (Figure 26-2) to acclimate to upright posture and movement.

Young Children—4 or 5 Years of Age

The child with a high lumbar or more proximal lesion can advance to THKAFOs. Other components are knee locks, wide thigh cuffs to reduce pressure concentration, and limited motion ankle joints.

The ParaWalker (Orthotic Research and Locomotor Assessment Unit, The Robert Jones and Agnes Hurt Orthopaedic Hospital, Oswestry, England), also known as the Hip Guidance Orthosis, is an option. Ball bearings in the orthotic hip joints reduce flexion constraint. Lateral rocking on the base permits maneuvering indoors without crutches. Reciprocating gait orthoses are another THKAFO. They allow alternating movements at the hips via 1 or 2 cables or a bar

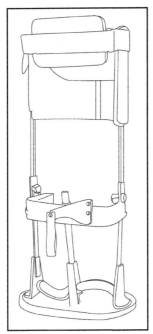

Figure 26-2. Parapodium.

attached posteriorly to both thigh uprights. Although these devices are cumbersome, difficult to don, and facilitate slow, arduous gait, some children wear them for several hours daily for supervised ambulation.

Older Children

Children with lower lesions may have adequate hip and knee strength but often have plantar flexor paralysis. They may benefit from solid ankle AFOs[27] or AFOs with anterior stops with anterior bands or slight plantar flexion alignment with a padded pretibial shell. Excessive pressure must be avoided. Difficulty with ongoing fitting may indicate the desirability of muscle transfer or other procedures to address the underlying neuromuscular deformity. A carbon fiber spring in an AFO may also facilitate energy return and permit more physiologic push-off.[28,29]

Foot deformities predisposing to skin ulceration often exist, depending on the extent of innervation and muscle balance. With an L5 lesion, pes calcaneus due to the unopposed pull of the tibialis anterior is common. Transfer of the tibialis anterior tendon to the plantar aspect of the foot can be considered between 5 and 13 years of age. Calcaneal osteotomy and, less frequently, triple arthrodesis (ie, fusion of subtalar, talonavicular, and calcaneal cuboid joints) may be considered. Patients with sacral lesions may need only minor shoe modifications or shoe inserts to provide optimal foot alignment.

School-age children with full passive knee extension may be able to utilize bilateral KAFOs.[30] Stance-phase locking knee joints can be incorporated in the orthoses if the child is tall enough to meet the size requirements for these components. Some can ambulate with orthoses but without assistive devices. The hips, however, are often weak, causing the patient to walk with a Trendelenburg, lateral trunk bending gait. Excessive valgus force at the knees can progressively deteriorate comfort and joint stability. More extensive bracing, crutches or a cane, or both can limit damaging gait deviations. Reciprocating gait orthoses are another option.[31,32]

Children with acquired spinal cord disorders have similar orthotic options. Ambulation is more likely to be restored in those who are younger age at the time of injury and who have lower lesion levels. Community ambulation is most unlikely to occur in patients with complete cervical and high thoracic-level injuries. Robotic-assisted, body-weight-supported treadmill training may be beneficial in the rehabilitation department, rather than in the community.

MUSCULAR DYSTROPHY AND SIMILAR NEUROMUSCULAR DISORDERS

Duchenne dystrophy (rapidly progressive muscular dystrophy of childhood) is a sex-linked recessive condition affecting boys. Creatine phosphokinase is markedly elevated. The average age of diagnosis is about 4.5 years of age, unless a family history of the disease already exists. Genetic testing can assist with in utero diagnosis and identification of carrier states. Characteristic deformities include lumbar lordosis with a forward shift of the center of gravity in standing, hip abduction and flexion, calf pseudohypertrophy, pes equinus, and calcaneocavovarus, leading to toe walking, slow gait, and loss of balance.[33,34] Proximal weakness increases bilateral lateral displacement, known as *waddling*.

Although no treatment of the histologic abnormality is available, attempts are made to prolong the child's mobility. Most patients require a wheelchair by 12 years of age. Those who can ambulate in adolescence usually have the more slowly progressive Becker myopathy.

Lightweight bilateral orthoses, exercise, and surgical lengthening of the Achilles tendon, posterior tibial transfer with or without release of the iliotibial band, may prolong ambulation for several years. Periods of immobilization after surgery must be strictly limited to avoid marked functional decline.

Orthoses should be as lightweight as possible because of the progressive weakness. AFOs can help to correct foot drop and provide some ankle stability. Orthoses, however, should have some flexibility at the ankle because rigid fixation in the neutral position can exacerbate the tendency toward knee instability and hamper the push-off that plantar flexion ordinarily provides. Air splints are a temporary option to control mediolateral instability without significantly affecting ankle position. Knee stability and prevention of knee contractures can be obtained with KAFOS[30,35-37]; however, these relatively heavy, cumbersome orthoses are not very effective when used for ambulation. An alternative to KAFOs are AFOs with limited motion ankle joints and an anterior band; they are ineffective in the presence of knee flexion contractures. A posterior rolling walker may allow the patient to maintain his compensatory hyperlordotic stance.

Upright posture and a properly fitted wheelchair can retard development of scoliosis and respiratory problems. Lower-limb bracing should not cease when ambulation stops. Progressive deformities interfere with wearing ordinary shoes, make resting the feet on wheelchair footrests uncomfortable, and result in discomfort and problems with bed positioning. These considerations are especially important because advances in respiratory care have begun to extend longevity into the third and even fourth decades of life.

Related disorders include the spinal muscular atrophies (SMA), Werdnig-Hoffmann disease (SMA I), chronic infantile (SMA II), and Kugelberg-Welander disease (SMA III). These are autosomal recessive conditions with anterior horn cell dysfunction usually resulting from absence of the survival motor neuron gene on chromosome #5. They have widely varied presentations. Most patients diagnosed at birth with Werdnig-Hoffman disease are totally dependent and do not attain gross motor milestones. About a quarter of patients are outliers who survive beyond the anticipated life expectancy of about 2 years of age. They are generally alert and cognitively normal; consequently, noninvasive respiratory support and enteral nutrition have resulted in modest but significant improvements in survival of a few years. Gait of patients with SMA II features pelvic rotation to propel the leg forward.[38]

Orthoses should be utilized for support and to prevent painful contractures, rather than acquisition or restitution of function. A few patients may be able to achieve standing but are unlikely to be functional ambulators.

Boys and girls with Kugelberg-Welander disease may present in early childhood with a gait reminiscent of patients with Duchenne dystrophy. Multiple tendon releases and bilateral KAFOs or AFOs may improve standing and ambulation.

DOWN SYNDROME

Down syndrome, the most common cause of mental retardation and malformation, occurs in the newborn because of the presence of 1 of 3 extra chromosomes, known as *Trisomy 21*. In addition to the almond-shaped eyes, round skull with flattened occiput, and broad, flattened nose, children typically present characteristic foot deformities, including pronation and a gap between the hallux and second toes, as well as hyperflexibility and patellar subluxation, leading to clumsy gait with short

strides, wide base, and reduced swing-phase clearance.[39-43] Foot orthoses that stabilize the foot and reduce heel eversion appear to decrease walking speed.[44]

OSTEOGENESIS IMPERFECTA

A less common challenge to the rehabilitation team is osteogenesis imperfecta, a group of autosomal-dominant disorders of connective tissue featuring brittle, fragile bones. In addition to occasional surgery, drugs, and exercise, upper-limb, trunk, and lower-limb orthoses may improve the child's quality of life.[45] Gait is slower than normal with less ankle motion in late stance[46] as well as in-toeing resulting from hip anteversion, internal tibial torsion, and metatarsus adductus. Children risk falling, with subsequent fractures and limb distortion.[47]

Orthotic management of the malaligned, fragile limbs often requires using the smallest components so that children can stand and walk. Some benefit from a standing frame and then use of a parapodium.[48] Those who have the potential for walking may use KAFOs.[30] Nonambulatory children should be fitted with trunk orthoses to minimize development of scoliosis and enable more comfortable, stable sitting.

FOOT PAIN

School-age children may complain of pain, particularly when engaged in sports activities, especially basketball, and less commonly with football, gymnastics, handball, dancing, tennis and combat sports. Pain is usually localized to the medial longitudinal arch. Sometimes knee pain occurs in association with patellofemoral syndrome. Orthotic use generally reduces foot and knee pain. Foot orthoses also address alignment and enable the child to present a more normal appearance.

CLUB FOOT

Talipes equinovarus is the most common congenital foot deformity. Typically the newborn infant is placed in corrective casts. Surgery may be performed when the deformity is unresponsive. Extensive surgery with nonteratologic deformity has been uncommon with the growing popularity of the Ponsetti manipulation of the foot around the talus. The ambulatory child is fitted with outflare lasted shoes to sustain the correction. Without correction, children walk with pes equinus and have difficulty with late-stance propulsion and foot clearance during swing phase. In-toeing is also seen occasionally.[49] Unilateral club foot demonstrates gastrocnemius-soleus atrophy.[50] If the foot is pliable, corrective shoes may enable a more functional gait. In the presence of rigid club foot, the shoe needs to accommodate the deformities.

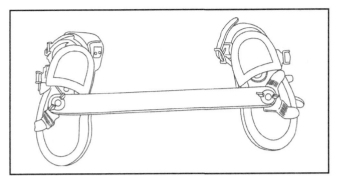

Figure 26-3. Denis-Browne splint.

IN-AND OUT-TOEING

In-toeing may occur as a result of metatarsus adductus (varus), internal tibial torsion, and femoral anteversion. Out-toeing is usually caused by hip external rotation contracture, external femoral torsion, or external tibial torsion. Many of these developmental variants correct spontaneously.[51] Osseous malformations, inflammation, and neurogenic disorders should be excluded.

A common device for the child who is not yet walking is the Denis-Browne splint (Figure 26-3). It has a bar that is as wide as the pelvic brim, to which are fastened open-toed high-top shoes with straight or reverse lasts. The shoes minimize pressure on the feet, and the attachment on the soles permits adjustable foot positioning. If misused, the device may place a valgus stress on the knees. The bar should be bent downward for varus correction and upward for valgus correct. The efficacy of the Denis-Browne splint is unclear. Some developmental deformities correct spontaneously. Plastic AFOs, shoe wedges, gait plates,[52] and torque heels may improve gait but do not necessarily correct the rotational abnormality.

DEVELOPMENTAL HIP DYSPLASIA

Hip anomalies occur in 2 of 1000 births, with a female predominance. Disorders range from acetabular malformation to dislocation. The affected limb is likely to be externally rotated, with foreshortening of the thigh and a clunking sound when the hip is abducted. Ortolani and Barlow signs are positive in newborns. Ortolani sign is produced with the hip and knee flexed 90 degrees; when the thigh is abducted to reduce the dislocation, an audible clunk is heard. Barlow's sign occurs when the hip is adducted and flexed to confirm instability. Ultrasound studies of infants younger than 8 months of age subject the patient to less x-ray exposure. In older infants, the ossified femoral head is displaced laterally and superiorly, with an abnormal center-edge angle and abnormal acetabular indices; ossification may be delayed in comparison to the contralateral side.

Though ambulation can occur in untreated dislocation, the child risks pain, leg length discrepancy, and

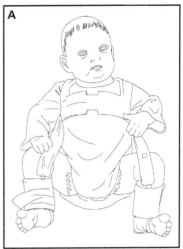
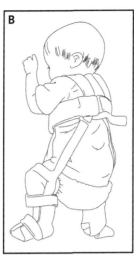

Figure 26-4. Pavlik harness. (A) Anterior. (B) Posterior.

gait disorder. Early onset of osteoarthritis may necessitate total hip replacement in young adults. Effective treatment is necessary in an attempt to prevent these sequelae and is generally quite successful unless the deformity is teratologic.

In infancy, the hips should be kept abducted. Double diapers are ineffective. The most common orthosis is the Pavlik harness (Figure 26-4), which should be applied to infants younger than 6 months but can be used up to 12 months of age.[53] The harness has a chest strap with shoulder straps to provide anchorage. Anterior straps are attached to the feet in order to flex the hips 90 to 110 degrees. Posterior straps prevent hip adduction, with the hips abducted 30 degrees. Efficacy can be demonstrated with serial sonograms or x-rays. Treatment generally lasts from 3 to 10 months. Satisfactory results are achieved in up to 90% of cases. The device is inappropriate for large children or those in which a sense of reduction is not yet appreciated and where internal rotation is required to achieve reduction. If there is no improvement after 4 weeks of application, other interventions should be considered. These include traction, plaster cast, or open reduction with adductor tenotomies and resection of interposed abnormal soft tissue. Complications include parental noncompliance, skin crease dermatitis, feet slipping from the harness, difficulty dressing the child,[54] and inability of the infant to be accommodated in a car seat. More serious complications are the risk of avascular necrosis, medial ligament instability, anterior hip dislocation, and femoral nerve or brachial plexus traction injuries due to misapplication of the straps.[55]

Other less popular devices are the von Rosen splint and the Frejka pillow splint. The von Rosen splint consists of a plastic frame that is shaped to conform to the infant's torso. The Frejka splint is a 9 × 9 × ¾-inch pillow with shoulder straps and chest ties. It may not provide adequate hip positioning.

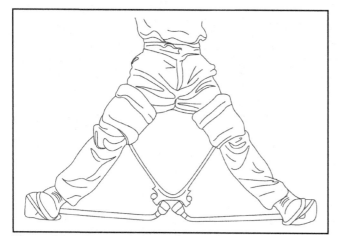

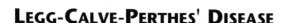

Figure 26-5. Toronto Legg-Calve-Perthes' orthosis.

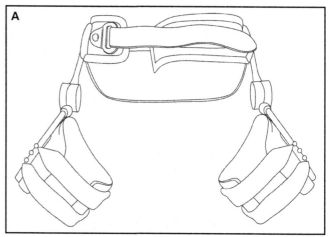

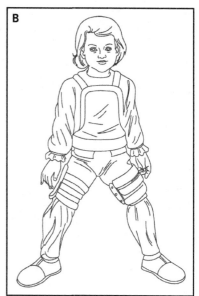

Figure 26-6. Scottish Rite Legg-Calve-Perthes' orthosis. (A) Orthosis. (B) Orthosis on patient.

LEGG-CALVE-PERTHES' DISEASE

Legg-Calve-Perthes' disease occurs primarily in boys 4 to 11 years of age who have idiopathic impairment of the blood supply to the head of the femur. This results in recurrent episodes of synovitis with damage to the ossific nucleus of the femoral head. Patients complain of pain in the knees and thighs and may develop hip flexion contractures, restricted internal rotation, and a positive Trendelenburg sign.[56,57] Radiographic findings include poorly developed osseous nucleus, subchondral radiolucent fracture line, subluxation, sclerosis, and flattening of the femoral head.

Initial treatment includes bed rest, sometimes with traction until spasms and pain abate, and use of anti-inflammatory agents. The period of immobilization is related to radiographic evidence of reconstitution of the femoral head contour.

Bracing to contain the hip so that it remodels properly is most successful with children under the age of 6 years and with Catterall x-ray classification groups I and II, although these groups may do well with limited intervention. Devices include the Toronto (Hugh McMillan Medical Center, Toronto, Ontario, Canada; Figure 26-5), Tachdjian trilateral, and Scottish Rite (Fillauer, Chattanooga, Tennessee; Figure 26-6) orthoses.[57,58]

The Toronto orthosis allows each hip to be maintained in 45 degrees of internal rotation and abduction, allowing hip and knee movement. Bilateral thigh cuffs extend from 2 inches (5 cm) below the perineum to an inch over the patellae. Some children need crutches in order to ambulate. Sitting may cause anterior uncovering of the femoral heads.

The Tachdjian trilateral orthosis is suitable for unilateral disease. The orthosis has a socket attached to a lateral upright attached to the shoe. The upright includes a locked knee joint. The shoe is attached to a wedged sole, preventing the child from placing weight through the orthosis. A lift on the contralateral shoe is necessary.

The Scottish Rite orthosis is most commonly used. It has a pelvic band joined to bilateral thigh cuffs by extra-sturdy abducted hip joints. Knees, ankles, and feet are not braced.

When orthotic treatment is not successful or where there is greater than 50% femoral head necrosis, proximal femoral varus osteotomy should realign the femoral head.

LIMB ABSENCE AND AMPUTATIONS

Because children compose a small fraction of the population having limb loss,[59] the developmental concerns noted at the beginning of this chapter may not be appreciated by inexperienced clinicians. The total population of children with amputations consists primarily of those with lower-limb involvement, with the leading cause being congenital limb absence.[60,61] Amputation in osteogenic sarcoma and other neoplastic diseases is less common than aggressive chemotherapy and limb salvage procedures. Virtually all patients with lower-limb loss walk without canes or other aids.[60]

Congenital Limb Absence

Patterns of deformities need to be recognized as part of syndromes. If a genetic factor is associated with the absence, assessment of other organ systems needs to be performed as well as screening of subsequent pregnancies.

Congenital Absence of the Fibula

Congenital absence of the fibula, formerly termed *fibular hemimelia*,[62] is associated with tibial bowing, talocalcaneal fusion, and lateral ray deficiencies. A few infants have bilateral involvement. Untreated, unilateral deficiency results in a very significant leg length discrepancy progressing to an ultimate difference averaging 10 inches (25 cm). A prosthesis is needed to provide support and equalize leg length for bipedal weight bearing and ambulation. If the foot is relatively stable, the very young patient can often walk without a prosthesis prior to incremental leg length discrepancy.

Some children benefit from surgical resection, particularly ankle disarticulation, to yield an end-bearing amputation limb. The limb is less bulbous than in adults because the immature malleoli are not well formed; a standard transtibial prosthesis is suitable. Limb ablation should be performed prior to 2 years of age when the child is less aware of the surgical changes. Disarticulation preserves the distal epiphyseal plate, making bony overgrowth unlikely.

Other procedures used for unilateral absence include soft tissue releases with Achilles tendon lengthening, posterior capsulotomy, peroneal tendon lengthening, and tibial osteotomy. With growth, medial femoral epiphyseodesis may be required to correct genu valgum.

The Ilizarov distraction technique can be attempted for limb lengthening if the knee is relatively stable and the foot is not severely deformed. Some children, however, experience pain and other complications, such as more surgical intervention, with this procedure. Long-term comparison between the function of patients treated with limb lengthening and those with amputation show that both groups function well.[63]

With symmetrical bilateral fibular absence, the young patient can ambulate without assistive devices; surgery is generally not indicated. Eventually, older children can be fitted with prostheses that are gradually increased in height as the child's balance improves and the desire to be as tall as classmates becomes important.

Congenital Absence of the Tibia

Congenital absence of the tibia, formerly *tibial hemimelia*, presents with a shortened limb, pes varus, and deficiencies of the medial rays of the foot. Concurrent instability at the hip, knee, and ankle is not uncommon.

Some patients respond well to foot ablation with provision of a transtibial prosthesis. Others require knee disarticulation, which usually results in good function. Alternatively, with good quadriceps function and an adequate weight-bearing foot, centralization of the fibular head in the intracondylar notch is an option; the procedure includes talectomy and repositioning the lateral malleolus over the calcaneus. The Illizarov fixator is sometimes used to lengthen the fibula, in association with lengthening of the Achilles tendon.

Longitudinal Deficiency, Partial Femoral

This anomaly, formerly designated as *proximal focal femoral deficiency*, is congenital shortening of the femur with varying degrees of hip dysplasia ranging from a normal femoral head to virtually no femur, as well as associated acetabular malformations. Some infants also present unusual facies and anomalies of the kidneys, heart, and vertebrae. The lower limb deformity may also be seen as part of sacral regression syndrome, especially in infants of mothers with gestational diabetes.

When the femur is less than half the length of the contralateral bone, in association with hip and acetabular dysplasia, ankle disarticulation or Syme's amputation with knee fusion and ablation of the foot enables fitting the patient with a transfemoral prosthesis. An alternative is the Van Nes rotationplasty, which entails knee fusion and a 180-degree rotation of the tibia and fibula so that the foot is directed posteriorly and the heel can function as a knee joint.[64] The patient wears a modified transtibial prosthesis and has better gait dynamics than with a transfemoral prosthesis. Most patients achieve better function than with Syme's amputation.[65] Cosmetic considerations must be addressed; however, most boys and girls accept the abnormal appearance. If the knee is stable, the patient can be considered as a candidate for a lengthening procedure with placement of a Taylor spatial frame, in lieu of limb ablation.

Ablative surgery should not be performed when bilateral deformity occurs. Such patients have marked reduction in overall height but are usually able to ambulate without any prostheses in case of an emergency. They can be provided with short rocker-type devices that can be gradually lengthened to maintain socially acceptable height as balance improves.

Children with unilateral deficiency, or their parents, may refuse surgery. An option is a monolithic transfemoral prosthesis with a socket designed to hold the foot in extreme plantar flexion so that it does not markedly protrude anteriorly.

Other Proximal Deficiencies

Patients with hip disarticulations, transpelvic absence, and complete longitudinal absence (phocomelia) have greatly increased energy expenditures when prosthetic ambulation is attempted. Concurrent medical problems may preclude prosthetic use. If a prosthesis is prescribed, a Canadian hip disarticulation prosthesis with a shoulder harness utilized for the younger child is the most common type. This prosthesis has an anteriorly placed broad hip joint that utilizes a spring-loaded extension mechanism at the hip and knee. Those with bilateral high-level lesions may benefit from a standing frame with a swivel base.

Acquired Amputations

Less common than congenital limb absence are traumatic and oncologic amputations among children.

Trauma

Reduction in the number of acquired amputations may result from better medical care of acute illnesses and infections, surgical familiarity with limb salvage procedures, and public safety measures. The Mangled Limb Scoring System (MESS) is widely used to determine whether amputation is necessary. Limb salvage often involves excision of nonviable tissue and installation of an endoprosthesis. Patients may require skin grafts to preserve length of retained portions and osteotomies for correction of angular bony deformities. Advantages include improved psychological and sexual adaptation, lower energy expenditure than with an exoprosthesis, reduced need for an ambulatory aid, and better ability to drive. Most endoprostheses last at least a decade. Complications of limb salvage include length discrepancy, neuropathy, recurrent hospitalizations and surgery, and risk of septicemia and thrombosis.[66]

Tumor

Limb salvage procedures can be utilized in the treatment of osteosarcoma, Ewing's sarcoma, and chondrosarcoma. More effective chemotherapy, ancillary supportive treatments such as anti-emetics and better antibiotics to deal with the complications of chemotherapy, and advanced imaging techniques permit superior tumor-free resection margins. Chemotherapy is initiated to control metastases prior to amputation. Tumors reduce in size and tend to recede from their involvement about the neurovascular bundle. Tumor resection retains the intact neurovascular bundle; the bony defect is replaced with an endoprosthesis with hip and knee articulations as needed. Skeletally immature patients can also be treated with expandable endoprostheses.

Tumor recurrence rate with limb salvage is comparable to the rate with amputation. Complications of limb salvage procedures include loosening of the prosthetic components, infections, neuropathy, compromise of balance, and extracortical bridging. Patients may require knee bracing should instability occur or an AFO to compensate for foot drop. Van Nes rotationplasty is a limb-sparing option when a portion of the femur is resected or after failed placement of an endoprosthesis.

General debility caused by chemotherapy limits functional expectations. Pulmonary metastases, chemotherapy-associated peripheral neuropathy, anemia, and deconditioning due to prolonged bed rest may also complicate care. Immediate postoperative fitting may not be suitable because of the risk of poor wound healing after chemotherapy.

Infection

Sequelae of systemic infection, such as purpura fulminans meningococcemia, are limb loss, damage of the growth plate with growth arrest, shortening of the residual limb, progressive soft tissue contractures, and avascular necrosis, especially of the talus and calcaneus. Patients generally achieve independence in self-care and mobility.[67]

Complications

Regardless of the etiology of amputation, some children are vulnerable to complications. Concerns about spinal and musculoskeletal and other organ system involvements must be addressed to ensure the overall well-being of the patient. For example, a child with sacral agenesis and limb-reduction syndrome may have bowel and bladder incontinence.

Bony Overgrowth

Bony overgrowth is the most common complication among children with acquired amputations, other than local skin irritations. Overgrowth with spur formation is related to appositional (periosteal) growth, rather than bone growth confined to the epiphyses. The distal aspect of the amputation limb may be swollen, warm, and tender. Overgrowth can lead to skin ulceration, skin perforation of the skin by the bone, and refusal to use the prosthetic device. Surgery for bony overgrowth includes resection of the spur with or without capping with cartilage-cancellous bone grafting, silastic or Teflon/felt plugs. Skin traction and skin grafting are usually less effective.

Very Short Amputation Limb

Adolescents with a residual limb so short as to interfere with prosthetic fit may benefit from lengthening, an average increase of 3 inches (9 cm).

Joint Disorders

About one-third of adolescents with transtibial amputation develop genu valgum, patella alta, and patellar dislocation. Painful bursae develop over the fibular head or the tibial tubercle in a few patients.

Hip Disorders

If amputation occurs congenitally or early in life, associated contralateral hip dysplasia with abnormal force application may occur. Surgery, medication, and ambulation aids are options to facilitate functional ambulation.

Phantom Pain and Sensation

Existence of phantom pain in patients with a congenital limb deficiency or who acquire amputation before 3 years of age is controversial. Phantom pain may be latent, occurring in adulthood following minor trauma to the residual limb. Girls are more likely to have psychological triggers for phantom pain.

Phantom sensation occurs in many more patients because cortical representation of the limb persists, associated with a decrease in gray matter of the posterolateral thalamus contralateral to the side of the amputation.

Surgical Requirements

Additional surgery may be required for tumor recurrence, release of contractures, treatment of skin slough, excision or capping of neuromas, and the migration of the posterior heel fat pad after a Syme's amputation.

HABILITATION AND REHABILITATION

To optimize the care of the limb-deficient patient, one needs to train potential and residual abilities, correct dislocations and abnormal postures, provide whatever orthotic/prosthetic and adaptive equipment is functionally indicated, and make a careful and restrained assessment regarding surgery that might improve function. Assuaging any guilt of a parent in regard to the etiology of amputation does much to foster acceptance of his or her child and the youngster's special needs.

Patients should be referred to facilities that are familiar with their deficits so that rational estimation of functional and cognitive abilities occurs. Preprosthetic training can occur when there is advance knowledge that the amputation is going to occur. Early intervention services should be initiated before prosthetic provision to improve sitting balance, developmental transitions, and attempts at weight bearing.

Most children with lower-limb loss should be provided with a prosthesis by about 10 months of age, when infants usually pull to standing and attempt to cruise. A stable base of support is essential for ambulation. Early initiation of prosthetic use decreases the risk of secondary limb atrophy, osteoporosis, and postural asymmetry.

PROSTHETIC COMPONENTS

Components are generally simpler yet can provide the young patient with age-appropriate function. Size

constraints limit options. Infants and toddlers generally do well with solid ankle, cushion heel (SACH; Otto Bock, Minneapolis, Minnesota; Kingsley, Costa Mesa, California) feet. Older children and adolescents make good use of energy-storing foot-ankle assemblies. Gait deviations associated with SACH feet include shortened stance phase and reduced hip and knee flexion. These abnormalities are minimal and often barely detectable among those wearing transtibial prostheses. Energy demand is minimally more than used by an able-bodied child.

For slightly older children, energy-storing feet are excellent choices. Given the rebound effect that such devices provide, patients have better late-stance propulsion, leading to greater sports participation. Such functional gains can result in better quality of life with enhanced cardiovascular fitness.

Transtibial prostheses may not have a patellar tendon bearing-socket if the very young patient has not developed marked bony contours; such people risk lateral subluxation of the patella and angular deformities of the knee. Supracondylar straps and, with a very short amputation limb, a thigh corset or elastic suspension are preferable. Silicone suction sockets are appropriate for those with fragile distal skin. This suspension reduces the need for additional suspension and permits performing higher level motor skills, such as jumping and running. Patients younger than 6 years of age may not be candidates, due to inconsistent reporting of sensory complaints and inattentiveness to skin lesions.

Children with transfemoral loss may start with a monolithic prosthesis lacking a knee joint. Transition to one with articulating knee (and hip) joints should occur at about 36 months of age.[68] Those younger than 4 years often have a manually locking knee, especially if the child has developmental delay or generalized weakness due to systemic illness. A hydraulic or pneumatic knee unit, with or without microprocessor control, is appropriate when the child is large enough to meet the size limitation of the device and can comply with the required training.

The first transfemoral prosthesis may have a quadrilateral or an ischial containment socket. In either case, the lateral socket wall should be adducted to reduce the tendency toward lateral trunk bending. A flexible socket in a thick, rigid frame is desirable because it can be enlarged rapidly, so the child does not miss more than a half day from school when adjustments are made. The prosthetist heats the thermoplastic to accommodate the larger thigh girth and grinds the frame so the larger socket fits properly.

Patients with acquired amputation due to cancer should have a temporary prosthesis with an adjustable socket, a pylon, and a removable foam cover. This prosthesis is extremely lightweight and thus is better tolerated by a young person with medical comorbidities.

The socket can be adjusted to the size of the residual limb as postoperative swelling abates and weight loss or gain occurs with initiation and discontinuance of chemotherapy.

Accommodating Growth

Modifications for growth in height include provision of an intentionally long prosthesis with a lift added to the contralateral (sound) side that can be removed with growth or lengthening the shank. To accommodate increased height, shims can be added to the shank and thigh sections of the prosthesis. The original socket is often delivered extra thick. As girth increases, the socket walls can be ground thinner. Initial use of extra socks is another possibility; socks are subtracted to accommodate the larger amputation limb. A thermoplastic socket can be heated and reshaped to fit the larger amputation limb; the frame portion of the socket is also ground slightly.

On average, a new prosthesis is required every 1 to 2 years until age 12 and then every 3 to 4 years until age 21. This represents an average of 3 prostheses for each 5 years until growth is completed. By age 7, most children don and doff their prostheses independently, assuming normal upper-limb function and average intelligence. A new prosthesis should be prescribed when the current one is uncomfortable after multiple adjustments, height and weight exceed the recommended limit for the components, the child undergoes surgical revision, and/or any angular deformity increases. Funding may be problematic. In New York, for example, Medicaid regulations usually permit provision of a new prosthesis on a triennial basis; specific needs must be documented to exceed this schedule.

Children with multiple upper- and lower-limb anomalies often have systemic medical problems. Covering their reduced body surface area with prostheses can result in thermal instability. As the child develops, often the lower-limb prostheses are abandoned in favor of a powered wheelchair. Most people continue to use upper-limb prostheses to perform daily, recreational, and, eventually, vocational activities.

REFERENCES

1. Lundkvist Josenby A, Jarnlo GB, Gummesson C, Nordmark E. Longitudinal construct validity of the GMFM-88 total score and goal total score and the GMFM-66 score in a 5-year follow-up study. *Phys Ther.* 2009;89:342-350.

2. Bell KJ, Ounpuu S, DeLuca PA, Romness MJ. Natural progression of gait in children with cerebral palsy. *J Pediatr Orthop.* 2002;22:677-682.

3. Rodda JM, Graham HK, Carson L, et al. Sagittal gait patterns in spastic diplegia. *J Bone Joint Surg Br.* 2004;86:251-258.

4. Dziuba A, Szpala A. Foot kinematics in gait of children with cerebral palsy (CP). *Acta Bioeng Biomech.* 2009;10:3-6.

5. Piccinini L, Cimolin V, Galli M, et al. Quantification of energy expenditure during gait in children affected by cerebral palsy. *Eura Medicophys.* 2007;43:7-12.

6. Rose J, Gamble JG, Medeiros J, et al. Energy cost of walking in normal children and in those with cerebral palsy: comparison of heart rate and oxygen uptake. *J Pediatr Orthop.* 1989;9:276-279.

7. Davids JR, Rowan F, Davis RB. Indications for orthoses to improve gait in children with cerebral palsy. *J Am Acad Orthop Surg.* 2007;15:178-188.

8. Brehm MA, Harlaar J, Schwartz M. Effect of ankle-foot orthoses on walking efficiency and gait in children with cerebral palsy. *J Rehabil Med.* 2008;40:529-534.

9. Buckon CE, Thomas SS, Jakobson-Huston S, et al. Comparison of three ankle-foot orthosis configurations for children with spastic diplegia. *Dev Med Child Neurol.* 2004;46:590-598.

10. Smiley SJ, Jacobsen FS, Mielke C, et al. A comparison of the effects of solid, articulated, and posterior leaf spring ankle-foot orthoses and shoes alone on gait and energy expenditure in children with spastic diplegic cerebral palsy. *Orthopedics.* 2002;25:411-415.

11. Van Gestel L, Molenaers G, Huenaerts C, et al. Effect of dynamic orthoses on gait: a retrospective control study in children with hemiplegia. *Dev Med Child Neurol.* 2008;50:63-67.

12. Radtka SA, Skinner SR, Johanson ME. A comparison of gait with solid and hinged ankle-foot orthoses in children with spastic diplegic cerebral palsy. *Gait Posture.* 2005;21:303-310.

13. Balaban B, Yasar E, Dal U, et al. The effect of hinged ankle-foot orthosis on gait and energy expenditure in spastic hemiplegic cerebral palsy. *Disabil Rehabil.* 2007;30(29):139-144.

14. Romkes J, Brunner R. Comparison of a dynamic and a hinged ankle-foot orthosis by gait analysis in patients with hemiplegic cerebral palsy. *Gait Posture.* 2002;15:18-24.

15. Park ES, Park CI, Chang HJ, et al. The effect of hinged ankle-foot orthoses on sit-to-stand transfer in children with spastic cerebral palsy. *Arch Phys Med Rehabil.* 2004;85:2053-2057.

16. Sienko TS, Buckon CE, Jakobson-Huston S, et al. Stair locomotion in children with spastic hemiplegia: the impact of three different ankle foot orthosis (AFOs) configurations. *Gait Posture.* 2002;16:180-187.

17. Flanagan A, Krzak J, Peer M, et al. Evaluation of short-term intensive orthotic garment use in children who have cerebral palsy. *Pediatr Phys Ther.* 2009;21:201-204.

18. Gutierrez EM, Bartonek A, Haglund-Akerlind Y, Saraste H. Kinetics of compensatory gait in persons with myelomeningocele. *Gait Posture.* 2005;21:12-23.

19. Gutierrez EM, Bartonek A, Haglund-Akerlind Y, Saraste H. Characteristic gait kinematics in persons with lumbosacral myelomeningocele. *Gait Posture.* 2003;18:170-177.

20. Bartonek A, Saraste H, Eriksson M, et al. Upper body movement during walking in children with lumbo-sacral myelomeningocele. *Gait Posture*. 2002;15:120-129.

21. Moore CA, Nejad B, Novak RA, Dias LS. Energy cost of walking in low lumbar myelomeningocele. *J Pediatr Orthop*. 2001;21:388-391.

22. Findley TW, Agre JC. Ambulation in the adolescent with spina bifida. II. Oxygen cost of mobility. *Arch Phys Med Rehabil*. 1988;69:855-861.

23. Bare A, Vankoski SJ, Dias L, et al. Independent ambulators with high sacral myelomeningocele: the relation between walking kinematics and energy consumption. *Dev Med Child Neurol*. 2001;43:16-21.

24. Schoenmakers MA, de Groot JF, Gorter JW, et al. Muscle strength, aerobic capacity and physical activity in independent ambulating children with lumbosacral spina bifida. *Disabil Rehabil*. 2009;31:259-266.

25. De Groot JF, Takken T, Schoenmakers MA, et al. Limiting factors in peak oxygen uptake and the relationship with functional ambulation in ambulating children with spina bifida. *Eur J Appl Physiol*. 2008;104:657-665.

26. Schoenmakers MA, Gulmans VA, Gooskens RH, Helders PJ. Spina bifida at the sacral level: more than minor gait disturbances. *Clin Rehabil*. 2004;18:178-185.

27. Thomson JD, Ounpuu S, Davis RB, DeLuca PA. The effects of ankle-foot orthoses on the ankle and knee in persons with myelomeningocele: an evaluation using three-dimensional gait analysis. *J Pediatr Orthop*. 1999;19:27-33.

28. Wolf SI, Alimusaj M, Rettig O, Döderlein L. Dynamic assist by carbon fiber spring AFOs for patients with myelomeningocele. *Gait Posture*. 2008;28:175-177.

29. Bartonek A, Eriksson M, Gutierrez-Farewik EM. Effects of carbon fibre spring orthoses on gait in ambulatory children with motor disorders and plantarflexor weakness. *Dev Med Child Neurol*. 2007;49:615-620.

30. Katz DE. The use of ambulatory knee-ankle-foot orthoses in pediatric patients. *Proc Amer Acad Orthot Prosthet*. 2006;7:P192--P198.

31. Katz-Leurer M, Weber C, Smerling-Kerem J, et al. Prescribing the reciprocal gait orthosis for myelomeningocele children: a different approach and clinical outcome. *Pediatr Rehabil*. 2004;7:105-109.

32. Katz DE, Haideri N, Song K, Wyrick P. Comparative study of conventional hip-knee-ankle-foot orthoses versus reciprocating-gait orthoses for children with high-level paraparesis. *J Pediatr Orthop*. 1997;17:377-386.

33. D'Angelo MG, Berti M, Piccinini L, et al. Gait pattern in Duchenne muscular dystrophy. *Gait Posture*. 2009;29:36-41.

34. Gaudreault N, Gravel D, Nadeau S. Evaluation of plantar flexion contracture contribution during the gait of children with Duchenne muscular dystrophy. *J Electromyogr Kinesiol*. 2009;19:180-186.

35. Bakker JP, de Groot IJ, Beckerman H, et al. The effects of knee-ankle-foot orthoses in the treatment of Duchenne muscular dystrophy: review of the literature. *Clin Rehabil*. 2000;14:343-359.

36. Garralda ME, Muntoni F, Cunniff A, Caneja AD. Knee-ankle-foot orthosis in children with Duchenne muscular dystrophy: user views and adjustment. *Eur J Paediatr Neurol*. 2006;10:186-191.

37. Heckmatt JZ, Dubowitz V, Hyde SA, et al. Prolongation of walking in Duchenne muscular dystrophy with lightweight orthoses: review of 57 cases. *Dev Med Child Neurol*. 1985;27:149-154.

38. Armand S, Mercier M, Watelain E, et al. A comparison of gait in spinal muscular atrophy, type II and Duchenne muscular dystrophy. *Gait Posture*. 2005;21:369-378.

39. Chang CL, Kubo M, Ulrich BD. Emergence of neuromuscular patterns during walking in toddlers with typical development and with Down syndrome. *Hum Mov Sci*. 2009;28:283-296.

40. Galli M, Rigoldi C, Brunner R, et al. Joint stiffness and gait pattern evaluation in children with Down syndrome. *Gait Posture*. 2008;28:502-506.

41. Looper J, Wu J, Angulo Barroso R, et al. Changes in step variability of new walkers with typical development and with Down syndrome. *J Mot Behav*. 2006;38:367-372.

42. Kubo M, Ulrich B. Coordination of pelvis-HAT (head, arms and trunk) in anterior-posterior and medio-lateral directions during treadmill gait in preadolescents with/without Down syndrome. *Gait Posture*. 2006;23:512-518.

43. Smith BA, Ulrich BD. Early onset of stabilizing strategies for gait and obstacles: older adults with Down syndrome. *Gait Posture*. 2008;28:448-455.

44. Selby-Silverstein L, Hillstrom HJ, Palisano RJ. The effect of foot orthoses on standing foot posture and gait of young children with Down syndrome. *NeuroRehabilitation*. 2001;16:183-193.

45. Basel D, Steiner RD. Osteogenesis imperfecta: recent findings shed new light on this once well-understood condition. *Genet Med*. 2009;11:375-385.

46. Graf A, Hassani S, Krzak J, et al. Gait characteristics and functional assessment of children with type I osteogenesis imperfecta. *J Orthop Res*. 2009;27:1182-1190.

47. Losa Iglesias ME, Becerro de Bengoa Vallejo R, Salvadores Fuentes P. In-toeing in children with type I osteogenesis imperfecta: an observational descriptive study. *J Am Podiatr Med Assoc*. 2009;99:326-329.

48. Weintrob JC. Orthotic management for children with osteogenesis imperfecta. *Connect Tissue Res*. 1995;31:S41-S43.

49. Karol LA, Jeans K, El-Hawary R. Gait analysis after initial nonoperative treatment for clubfeet: intermediate term follow up at age 5. *Clin Orthop Relat Res*. 2009;467:1206-1213.

50. Wicart P, Richardson J, Maton B. Adaptation of gait initiation in children with unilateral idiopathic clubfoot following conservative treatment. *J Electromyogr Kinesiol*. 2006;16:650-660.

51. Lincoln TL, Suen PW. Common rotational variations in children. *J Am Acad Orthop Surg*. 2003;11:312-320.

52. Redmond AC. The effectiveness of gait plates in controlling in-toeing symptoms in young children. *J Am Podiatr Med Assoc*. 2000;90:70-76.

53. Vitale MG, Skaggs DL. Developmental dysplasia of the hip from six months to four years of age. *J Am Acad Orthop Surg*. 2001;9:401-411.

54. Hassan FA. Compliance of parents with regard to Pavlik harness treatment in developmental dysplasia of the hip. *J Pediatr Orthop B*. 2009;18:111-115.

55. van der Sluijs JA, De Gier L, Verbeke JI, et al. Prolonged treatment with the Pavlik harness in infants with developmental dysplasia of the hip. *J Bone Joint Surg Br*. 2009;91: 1090-1093.

56. Song KM, Halliday S, Reilly C, Keezel W. Gait abnormalities following slipped capital femoral epiphysis. *J Pediatr Orthop*. 2004;24:148-155.

57. Westhoff B, Petermann A, Hirsch MA, et al. Computerized gait analysis in Legg Calve Perthe's disease: analysis of the frontal plane. *Gait Posture*. 2006;24:196-202.

58. Herring JA, Kim HT, Browne R. Legg-Calve-Perthes disease. Part II: prospective multicenter study of the effect of treatment on outcome. *J Bone Joint Surg Am*. 2004;86A:2121-2134.

59. Ephraim PL, Dillingham TR, Sector M, et al. Epidemiology of limb loss and congenital limb deficiency: a review of the literature. *Arch Phys Med Rehabil*. 2003;84:747-761.

60. Yigiter K, Ulger O, Sener G, et al. Demography and function of children with limb loss. *Prosthet Orthot Int*. 2005;29:131-138.

61. Al-Worikat AF, Dameh W. Children with limb deficiencies: demographic characteristics. *Prosthet Orthot Int*. 2008;32:23-28.

62. Day HJB. The ISO/ISPO classification of congenital limb deficiency. *Prosthet Orthot Int*. 1991;15:67-69.

63. Walker JL, Knapp D, Minter C, et al. Adult outcomes following amputation or lengthening for fibular deficiency. *J Bone Joint Surg Am*. 2009;91:797-804.

64. Westberry DE, Davids JR. Proximal focal femoral deficiency (PFFD): management options and controversies *Hip Int*. 2009;19(suppl 6):S18-S25.

65. Fowler EG, Hester DM, Oppenheim WL, et al. Contrasts in gait mechanics of individuals with proximal femoral focal deficiency: Syme amputation versus Van Nes rotational osteotomy. *J Pediatr Orthop*. 1999;19:720-731.

66. Bryant PR, Pandian G. Acquired limb deficiencies. 1. Acquired limb deficiencies in children and young adults. *Arch Phys Med Rehabil*. 2001;82(suppl 1):S3-S8.

67. Shapiro LT, Huang ME. Inpatient rehabilitation of survivors of purpura fulminans with multiple limb amputations: a case series. *Arch Phys Med Rehabil*. 2009;90:696-700.

68. Boonstra AM, Rijnders LJM, Groothoff JW, Eisma WH. Children with congenital deficiencies or acquired amputations of the lower limb: functional aspects. *Prosthet Orthot Int*. 2000;24:16-27.

Financial Disclosures

Joan E. Edelstein has no financial or proprietary interest in the materials presented herein.

Richard A. Frieden has no financial or proprietary interest in the materials presented herein.

Joan T. Gold has no financial or proprietary interest in the materials presented herein.

Alex Moroz has no financial or proprietary interest in the materials presented herein.

Index

Printed in the United States
by Baker & Taylor Publisher Services